Contemporary Issues in Mental Health Nursing

Edited by

Jonathon E. Lynch

and

Steve Trenoweth
Thames Valley University

Foreword by Professor Peter Nolan

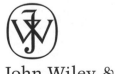

John Wiley & Sons, Ltd

Other Wiley Editorial Offices

John Wiley & Sons Inc., 111 River Street, Hoboken, NJ 07030, USA

Jossey-Bass, 989 Market Street, San Francisco, CA 94103-1741, USA

Wiley-VCH Verlag GmbH, Boschstr. 12, D-69469 Weinheim, Germany

John Wiley & Sons Australia Ltd, 42 McDougall Street, Milton, Queensland 4064, Australia

John Wiley & Sons (Asia) Pte Ltd, 2 Clementi Loop #02-01, Jin Xing Distripark, Singapore 129809

John Wiley & Sons Canada Ltd, 6045 Freemont Blvd, Mississauga, ONT, L5R 4J3

Wiley also publishes its books in a variety of electronic formats. Some content that appears in print may not be
available in electronic books.

Library of Congress Cataloging-in-Publication Data
Contemporary issues in mental health nursing / edited by Jonathon E. Lynch and Steve Trenoweth ; foreword by
Peter Nolan.
     p. ; cm.
   Includes bibliographical references and index.
   ISBN 978-0-470-06055-1 (alk. paper)
1. Psychiatric nursing.   I. Lynch, Jonathon E.   II. Trenoweth, Steven.
   [DNLM: 1. Mental Disorders—nursing.   2. Psychiatric Nursing—methods. WY 160 C7606 2008]
   RC440.C584 2008
   616.89′0231—dc22

                                                                                    2007030204

British Library Cataloguing in Publication Data

A catalogue record for this book is available from the British Library

ISBN 978-0-470-060551

Typeset in 11/13pt Bembo by SNP Best-set Typesetter Ltd., Hong Kong
Printed and bound in Great Britain by Antony Rowe Ltd, Chippenham.
This book is printed on acid-free paper responsibly manufactured from sustainable forestry
in which at least two trees are planted for each one used for paper production.

Contents

Contributors

Dr Joanna Bennett, Senior Research Fellow, Sainsbury Centre for Mental Health.

Gwen Bonner, Senior Lecturer, Thames Valley University.

Lee Bradley, Clinical Nurse Manager, West London Mental Health NHS Trust.

John Cordwell, Trainee Forensic Psychologist, West London Mental Health NHS Trust.

Yvonne Dexter, Senior Lecturer, Thames Valley University.

Dr Peter Harper, Senior Lecturer (Research), Richard Wells Research Centre, Collaborating Centre of The Joanna Briggs Institute (University of Adelaide, Australia), Thames Valley University.

Simon Jones, Senior Lecturer (Research), Richard Wells Research Centre, Collaborating Centre of The Joanna Briggs Institute (University of Adelaide, Australia), Thames Valley University.

Philip Kemp, Principal Lecturer (Mental Health), London South Bank University.

Anna Larter, Service User/Member of the Patient and Public Involvement Forum Organisation (PPIFO).

Carlyle London, Lead Nurse (Education and Training), West London Mental Health NHS Trust.

Jonathon E. Lynch is a Mental Health Nurse in the NHS in London.

Carl Margereson, Senior Lecturer, Thames Valley University.

James Matthews, Mental Health Nurse, West London Mental Health NHS Trust.

Charlie McGrory, Senior Lecturer, Thames Valley University.

Professor Peter Nolan, Professor of Mental Health Nursing, Staffordshire University.

Ian Price, Professional Lead (Mental Health), Thames Valley University.

Helen Robson, Developmental Lecturer, Thames Valley University.

Angela Scriven, Reader in Health Promotion, Brunel University.

Andrew Thornton, Mental Health Nurse, South London and Maudsley NHS Mental Health Trust.

Steve Trenoweth, Senior Lecturer, Thames Valley University.

Foreword
Professor Peter Nolan

Commenting on the myriad mental hospital inquiries of the 1960s and 1970s and why services had reached such a low watermark, Martin (1984) concluded that a network of organizations had turned in on themselves and were aggressively resistant to engaging with outside forces. Much of the apathy, neglect and indifference that prevailed could be attributed to Emil Kraepelin (1856–1926) and his declaration that all psychiatric patients would inevitably deteriorate regardless of what was done for them. We know that badly managed organizations and staff who are ill-informed and poorly motivated are a recipe for disaster, and a thick haze of therapeutic pessimism pervaded much of mental health care for most of the 20th century. Service users were incarcerated within institutions where they were at the mercy of a dysfunctional system, medical and nursing ignorance and general indifference. While criticism of mental health care in the United Kingdom is still warranted, services are nonetheless in far better shape then they were when I entered mental health nursing over 40 years ago. A great deal of credit for this improvement must be attributed to what nurses have done and are now doing.

Highly educated, enthusiastic and inspiring mental health nurses are currently working in a wide range of services across the country. They have been responsible for opening closed minds and letting in the fresh air of intellectual discussion, honest inquiry and innovative practice in the search for better ways to help people who suffer with mental health problems. Contemplating the many mental health colleagues who are such clear thinkers, succinct speakers and elegant writers, I am reminded of Trevor Clay's words when he was President of the RCN, 'The surest way to have a high quality health care system is to have an educated workforce who know what to do and how to do it.'

I consider this book to be a significant contribution to the ongoing development of mental health nursing in the UK. Jonathon Lynch and Steve Trenoweth deserve our appreciation for bringing together a collection of such excellent thinkers and writers; in so doing, they have helped the profession further along the course of maturity. Information, as is frequently stated in the pages of this book, does not stand still. It needs to be reflected upon, synthesized with experience and practice, added to and – when necessary – changed. Our authors are the life-blood of our profession and in the following chapters, you will be informed, challenged and provided with new and illuminating insights that will render your work all the more satisfying.

Copies of this book should be on every reading list of every mental health course, in every mental health care setting and available to all involved in the management and commissioning of mental health services. In the early 1960s, in my first week of training, I was able to read all the books on mental health nursing then available! Now, I am simply amazed when I survey the extent of the literature on nursing. This book is, and will be for some time, top of my reading list and I am proud to be associated with it.

Staffordshire University, June 2007

CHAPTER 1
CONTEMPORARY ISSUES IN MENTAL HEALTH NURSING: AN INTRODUCTION

Jonathon E. Lynch and Steve Trenoweth

This book addresses a number of contemporary issues affecting mental health nurses and the worlds that they and their clients inhabit. We are certain that many, if not all, contributions will also be of interest to users of mental health services and to mental health professionals in other disciplines, and some even to people who have no direct connection to mental health care.

The themes covered could only ever be a sample of those that are of significance today; they could only ever be *some* of the contemporary issues that affect us in the sense that the dynamics of current mental health care bring us all into contact with an ever-increasing number and range of influences, drivers and problems. An analysis of the pace of the changes in the last 10–15 years could be the subject of an entire book on its own! So, too, could the volume of legislation that has touched professional life, whether through direct or indirect influences, and the social ramifications of what Beck (1992) termed the 'risk society'. Although this has perhaps been most visible in the United Kingdom at airports and in city centres in recent years, it has also been evident in the ways in which we carry out and document our clinical care, our interventions and our assessments. So, nurses and other mental health care professionals

Contemporary Issues in Mental Health Nursing, Edited by J. E. Lynch and S. Trenoweth
© 2008 John Wiley & Sons, Ltd

carry out their daily work within societies, and indeed within a world, that has altered profoundly in a couple of decades.

Change is not new to us – it is one of the few things we can be certain will occur! Our nursing predecessors created it, lived with it and coped with it. The contemporary issues presented and considered here may become less significant in the future, and perhaps this will be so even for the authors who deem them important today. Nevertheless, their intention in this volume is to illustrate some of the contemporary complexities, problems, challenges and dilemmas that they feel are faced by service users and mental health nurses alike. In so doing, they provide valid, and we believe useful, insights into the expanding and developing body of critical literature available for practitioners and students of mental health care to draw upon.

If the purpose of this book were to be summed up, it is simply to contribute to the analysis and stimulation of thought about mental health nursing practice and mental health care more widely. As Professor Peter Nolan mentions in his Foreword, several decades ago the available literature on mental health nursing could be read within days. Today, such works are relatively abundant but the critical element in particular has room for improvement and growth, as does that containing other commentaries that fall outside the 'how to' textbook style. While there will always be a need and a market for the latter, the chapters that follow all offer contributions to discussions and dilemmas that touch many spheres of service users' and mental health nurses' lives today.

All of the authors are based in England and their contributions are inevitably focused on matters there as they perceive them today. Overall then, the book's contents are inevitably framed by the health care practices and legislation of England and Wales. However, we believe that most, if not all, of the issues are pertinent to the rest of the United Kingdom. We also consider the text to be pertinent and useful to peers further away. In particular, the literature from Australia and from New Zealand, and from parts of northern Europe and North America, seems to indicate that mental health nurses in these areas encounter, and attempt to respond to, many similar issues. Certainly, there is much for us to learn from how other countries address mental health issues, and we have much to gain from understanding the practices and insights that peers abroad have to offer. Indeed, some form of 'globalization' of mental health nursing care could well enhance understandings, critical thought and evidence bases internationally, and in turn our responsiveness to improving the health care experiences of mentally unwell people around the world.

Each section of this book begins with an overview, which seeks to introduce chapters that are thematically linked. We have attempted to use the overviews to help readers make sense of the whole. Indeed, rather than a collection of unconnected essays, this book attempts to raise and complement awareness of some of the key issues of today and to draw out unifying themes. One such theme is the increasing influence of the political issues that appear to stamp indelible marks on everyday events. Some social scientists would deem all aspects of mental health care 'political' in nature, yet we would argue that any such dialogue is weakened if it fails to take into consideration the entire nature of the subject area. Despite its weaknesses, mental health care in this country *is* striving, sometimes extremely successfully, to assist those who are in need of help with their 'mental health' as we understand the concept today.

However, there are aspects of this book which are quite critical of contemporary mental health nursing practice and of mental health care in general. Some issues that are raised are controversial; some are disturbing. Some are rarely found in mental health nursing books. Readers may not agree with the conclusions that the authors have drawn. Issues are highlighted so as to stimulate discussion and debate, and begin a genuine dialogue as to how we may rectify relevant issues. However, we must also be able to balance such problems with an appreciation, and indeed celebration, of our professional strengths. Indeed, as mental health nurses ourselves, we are optimistic and ever hopeful that our profession can respond meaningfully to the needs of those we seek to care for, and deliver the sort of care and support service users want.

SECTION 1
PROFESSIONAL AND POLITICAL ISSUES

In this first section, a number of contemporary professional and political themes are highlighted and explored by the authors. Certainly, the impact of the recent restructuring and reform of health services in the United Kingdom on mental health nursing care is felt and, indeed, broadly welcomed by the authors. However, the pace and scope of such reforms, and the remarkable growth of the service user movement which may challenge 'orthodox' notions of expertise, have many implications for mental health nursing practice. There is certainly much scope for the enhancement of the profession as one capable of delivering holistic, modern, positive, supportive and evidential care, and responding to the needs of those whom it serves, underpinned by meaningful, interpersonal, professional relationships.

There are, of course, many aspects of mental health care which are unknowable, unpredictable and ambiguous despite our ever-expanding evidence base. Indeed, mental health is a complex phenomenon and as such often requires a multi-dimensional, individualized response by health care practitioners. Furthermore, clinical nursing decisions are often highly contextual and what is an appropriate response for one service user may not be appropriate for, or even acceptable to, another. There are, indeed, many ethical dilemmas and contradictions in relation to service user involvement. Clinical mental health nursing practice may need to base its 'evidence' upon a number of sources, both research and non-research. What is also required perhaps is a broad set of values which assists us to confer our professional identity, allows us a framework within which to operate, and assists us in underpinning and guiding our use of knowledge and clinical decision making.

Here, it is suggested that 'wisdom' is needed to assist in the translation of our professional values, research evidence and personal knowledge into action, particularly when working collaboratively with service users and drawing upon their expertise. This requires self-aware and reflective practitioners as a means to service user involvement, and a shift from the apparently 'objective' to the 'subjective', and 'intersubjective', understandings of experience. This also suggests a recognition that diverse values and perspectives are equally legitimate and emphasises shifts away from the 'right answer' towards seeking negotiated resolutions to complex clinical questions. It is through this process that meaningful outcomes of care can be identified.

In short, there are many contemporary implications arising from the current policy agenda. Mental health nursing needs to develop its definite identity as a profession and with this, illustrate to service users what contribution it can make to delivering the sort of quality-assured and compassionate care they want. There are aspects of clinical practice which may require improvement, but there also needs to be a clear identification and celebration of the significant and positive contributions that mental health nurses make to those whose lives are blighted by mental distress. Attention may also need to be paid to aspects of mental health nursing practice which might, overtly or covertly, be considered discriminatory or contributory to the stigmatization and social injustice faced by many service users. Overall, there is a contemporary recognition that in order for the profession to build upon its successes, and to address its deficits, the service user must be at the heart of mental health nursing care. This necessitates the development of a therapeutic alliance, founded on consensus, negotiation and partnership, in which users' values and perspectives are considered to be of fundamental importance.

CHAPTER 2
REBUILDING LIVES: A CRITICAL LOOK AT THE CONTEMPORARY ROLE OF THE MENTAL HEALTH NURSE

Steve Trenoweth and Anna Larter

INTRODUCTION

Mental health nurses are the largest group of people working with service users and have the potential to make a major contribution to the health and welfare of people with mental health needs (Cowman *et al.*, 2001; Cleary, 2004; Cameron *et al.*, 2005; DH, 2006a). However, the mental health nursing profession, it seems, is in a state of flux and there seems to be uncertainty regarding the profession's primary focus and role (see Chapter 6: Truth, Uncertainty and the Mental Health Nurse). Questions are currently being raised as to what the real nature of mental health nursing activity is, and what it should be (Coleman and Jenkins, 1998; DH, 2005a, 2006a). The authors of this chapter, representing voices from the mental health nursing profession and service users' movement respectively, seek to establish common ground in their exploration of the contemporary role of the mental health nurse. In this chapter, the implications of the contemporary modernization and reform of mental health services for the mental health nursing profession are explored. Consideration is given to that which

Contemporary Issues in Mental Health Nursing, Edited by J. E. Lynch and S. Trenoweth
© 2008 John Wiley & Sons, Ltd

the profession has to offer service users, what challenges might stand in the way of delivering quality nursing care and suggestions offered as to how such challenges may be addressed.

CONTEMPORARY CONTEXTS

The current modernization, restructuring and reform of mental health services in the United Kingdom (DH, 1998a,b, 1999a, 2000a, 2001a) provides the overall contextual backdrop to the delivery of contemporary mental health nursing care (Porter, 1993; DH, 1999b; Dingwall and Allen, 2001; Crowe and Carlyle, 2003; Cleary, 2004). However, arguably the most important policy document for mental health nurses to have arrived in recent years (Arthur, 2007) is the Chief Nursing Officer's (CNO) Review of Mental Health Nursing undertaken throughout 2005 (DH, 2005a), the results of which were published in 'From Values to Action' (DH, 2006a). This document stresses the need to develop a positive modern profession, which addresses the holistic needs of service users, in a positive, evidential and supportive way. Mental health nurses will be required to develop their clinical and research practice in order to respond meaningfully to the complex physical and mental health care needs and wants of the service user group in a modern health care context (Oguisso, 1995; Peck and Norman, 1999; Gournay, 2001; Nolan *et al.*, 2001; Thornicroft *et al.*, 2002; Brimblecombe, 2005; DH, 2006a) (see Chapter 3: User Involvement and the Micro-Politics of Mental Health Care and Chapter 10: The Meaning of Recovery). Another recent important policy framework is that of the 'Ten Essential Shared Capabilities' (DH, 2004a), which seeks to inform educational curricula development at pre- and post-registration levels and interdisciplinary practice in mental health contexts (Figure 2.1). This document details the minimum standards for service and care delivery, and focuses on the development of partnerships with service users in order to promote health and well-being, with the explicit aim of making a real difference to people's lives.

So, in what ways might the profession ensure its responsiveness to service users' needs in a modern and complex health care environment to bring about significant improvement in the health and well-being of those with mental health problems?

WHAT HAS MENTAL HEALTH NURSING TO OFFER SERVICE USERS?

Identifying the specific skills and personal qualities that mental health nursing has to offer service users is a complex task (Towell, 1975; Machin and Stevenson, 1999; Hamblett, 2000; Cleary, 2004), as is identifying the specific contribution that nurses may make to the overall recovery of their clients (Curran and Brooker, 2007). Indeed,

Working in Partnership. Developing and maintaining constructive working relationships with service users, carers, families, colleagues, lay people and wider community networks. Working positively with any tensions created by conflicts of interest or aspiration that may arise between the partners in care.

Respecting Diversity. Working in partnership with service users, carers, families and colleagues to provide care and interventions that not only make a positive difference but also do so in ways that respect and value diversity including age, race, culture, disability, gender, spirituality and sexuality.

Practising Ethically. Recognizing the rights and aspirations of service users and their families, acknowledging power differentials and minimizing them whenever possible. Providing treatment and care that is accountable to service users and carers within the boundaries prescribed by national (professional), legal and local codes of ethical practice.

Challenging Inequality. Addressing the causes and consequences of stigma, discrimination, social inequality and exclusion on service users, carers and mental health services. Creating, developing or maintaining valued social roles for people in the communities they come from.

Promoting Recovery. Working in partnership to provide care and treatment that enables service users and carers to tackle mental health problems with hope and optimism and to work towards a valued lifestyle within and beyond the limits of any mental health problem.

Identifying People's Needs and Strengths. Working in partnership to gather information to agree health and social care needs in the context of the preferred lifestyle and aspirations of service users, their families, carers and friends.

Providing Service User Centred Care. Negotiating achievable and meaningful goals; primarily from the perspective of service users and their families. Influencing and seeking the means to achieve these goals and clarifying the responsibilities of the people who will provide any help that is needed, including systematically evaluating outcomes and achievements.

Making a Difference. Facilitating access to and delivering the best quality, evidence-based, values-based health and social care interventions to meet the needs and aspirations of service users and their families and carers.

Promoting Safety and Positive Risk Taking. Empowering the person to decide the level of risk they are prepared to take with their health and safety. This includes working with the tension between promoting safety and positive risk taking, including assessing and dealing with possible risks for service users, carers, family members and the wider public.

Personal Development and Learning. Keeping up to date with changes in practice and participating in life-long learning, personal and professional development for one's self and colleagues through supervision, appraisal and reflective practice.

© Crown Copyright *Reproduced Under The Terms Of The Click-Use Licence*

Figure 2.1

The Ten Essential Shared Capabilities (DH, 2004a)

studies into mental health nursing are scarce (Gijbels and Burnard, 1995) and 'It seems that not only do we not know what good psychiatric nursing is, we appear to still find it difficult to define what psychiatric nursing per se is' (Gijbels and Burnard, 1995, p. 7). However, as Rungapadiachy *et al.* (2004, p. 723) argue, 'The complexity of the role of the mental health nurse should not be used as an excuse to avoid clarifying the responsibilities of the profession . . .' Indeed, it is essential in a modern health care context for any service providers to be able to transparently explain to its 'users' what it has to offer them (Machin and Stevenson, 1999) and to be clear regarding the values which underpin its practice (see Chapter 5: The Implications of Values–Based Practice in Mental Health Nursing).

Some studies have been conducted amongst mental health nurses in an attempt to establish their perspectives and beliefs regarding the skills and abilities that they perceive underpin their roles. Gijbels and Burnard (1995), for example, sought to identify the skills of mental health nurses in an acute setting. They point to a complex interplay of technical, therapeutic and interpersonal skills related to the provision of care (such as observation: assessing mental and physical states and level of functioning with a view to developing plans and interventions) and further skills related to the structuring, administration, organization and management of the care environment, in order to facilitate the safety and protection. Similar findings were reported by Oguisso (1995), Morrison (1991), Hagerty *et al.* (1995), Beech and Norman (1995) and Tuck (1997). Indeed, the importance of being able to assist service users to meet their mental and physical health needs, holistically, was a central feature of the CNO's Review of Mental Health Nursing (DH, 2006a; Brimblecombe *et al.*, 2007).

In 1999, Barker *et al.* undertook a qualitative study which sought to define the core activities of mental health nurses from their own perspective. Nurses, it seems, perceive a need to be several things at different times depending on context or circumstances. At times, nurses expressed a need to be 'ordinary' and human (characterized by the depth and quality of time spent with clients and the depth of knowledge shared between nurse and client). At other times, the need to be 'professional' was identified, characterized by the exercising of professional judgements for and on behalf of clients. However, a key activity was that of being an intermediary or translator:

Translation emphasised the nurse's need to be multi-lingual: conversing easily with professional colleagues, in the language of psychiatry; yet able to speak with people and their families, in ordinary parlance (Barker *et al.*, 1999, p. 280).

Indeed, service users have often pointed to the need to be treated in a 'human' way (Ricketts, 1996) and with compassion (Cleary and Edwards, 1999) (see Chapter 4: Compassion). They identify the need to be listened to, understood (Shattell *et al.*, 2006) and receive a smile of acknowledgment as well as to be given patient and empathic responses to their questions or requests. As such, mental health nurses are mostly needed to stand alongside sometimes frightened and vulnerable people to provide support and assistance to face, challenge and overcome the devastating effects of the issues which they are facing in their lives (Anonymous, 2006).

CONTEMPORARY CHALLENGES TO MENTAL HEALTH NURSING CARE

There exist, however, a number of issues identified by some authors which may impact on the delivery of the sort of mental health nursing care envisaged by the CNO's Report (DH, 2006a). In this section, we pause to consider some of these challenges.

HISTORICAL LINKS WHICH PERSIST

The origins of mental health nursing can be traced back to the 19th century (Nolan, 1990, 1993; Brimblecombe, 2005), where 'attendants' were charged with looking after and controlling those deemed to be 'mad' (Nolan, 1993). In 1890, a Register of Attendants on the Insane was established (Nolan, 1990), and in the following year formal training was introduced with a clear focus on ensuring that medical orders were carried out. There was a focus on order, tasks and routines and the attendant role was that of rule keeper, servant, spiritual guide and intermediary between doctors and patients (Gijbels and Burnard, 1995). While 'kindness and diversional occupation were keystones' (Brimblecombe, 2005, p. 345), attendants were subject to the absolute power of medical staff who could enforce obedience by instant dismissal.

Mental health nursing has historically been inextricably entwined with activities, interests and aims of psychiatrists (Symonds, 1995). This relationship, it seems, persists today (Barker and Buchanan-Barker, 2005) at both national and international levels (Oguisso, 1995). Indeed, psychiatry still has tremendous influence over nursing in two important ways: influencing the national mental health agenda and more locally, where a direct clinical influence is felt (Brimblecombe, 2005). This may subsequently limit nurses' participation in policy decisions (Oguisso, 1995). However, while there has lately been an increased emphasis on social care and on working in partnership with service users (DH, 1994a), many, including service users (Rydon, 2005), continue to feel that nursing remains under the shadow of medicine and the biomedical approach. Barker and Buchanan-Barker (2005, p. 255), for example, state:

Nursing's traditional subservience to medicine appears to continue to echo this nun–priest relationship. Mental health nurses may have changed from nun-like habits into mufti, but the habitual power relationship between nurses and doctors appears to have changed little (Barker and Buchanan-Barker, 2005, p. 255).

The historical links between the medical and nursing professions played out in many contemporary health care settings often mean that the biomedical model remains alive, well and seemingly unchallenged.

CONTRASTING CONCEPTUAL FRAMEWORKS

The role, function and practice of the mental health nurse has generated much confusion amongst other professionals and service users (Onega, 1991; Machin and Stevenson, 1999) and the general public (Walker *et al.*, 1998). The core activities of the mental health nurse are seemingly complex, difficult to capture and define (Rungapadiachy *et al.*, 2004) and wide-ranging (Cowman *et al.*, 2001). Certainly, a sense of caring concern for the patient as a person is seen to be one of the most important resources nurses bring to patient care (Cleary and Edwards, 1999; Cowman *et al.*, 2001; Barker and Buchanan-Barker, 2005). Caring is, according to Olsen (1997, p. 516), '. . . not part of treatment, it is the reason for treatment. Caring is, then, the very essence of nursing.'

However, there are a number of competing frameworks which currently influence mental health nursing and as such there exist different views as to what 'caring' actually means (Machin and Stevenson, 1999). Mental health nursing, it seems, is a house divided (Forchuk, 2001; Cameron *et al.*, 2005). There are influences from, on the one hand, the medical model (which is seen to perpetuate a scientific view of mental illness and its subsequent treatment) and, on the other hand, the interpersonal approach (which is seen to comprise the art, craft and caring aspects of nursing) (Chan and Rudman, 1998). These views have been summarized by Playle (1995, p. 981):

The art of nursing has been characterised by a humanistic philosophy which values personal meaning, subjectivity and understanding. At the same time, in attempts to become scientific, there has been an acceptance of notions of science which are primarily based in a positivistic, empirico-analytical paradigm (Playle, 1995, p. 98).

The result has been a barrage of claims, counterclaims and challenges to each other's evidence base (Playle, 1995; Barker, 1998; Beech, 1998; Gournay and Ritter, 1998; Parsons, 1998; Rolfe, 1998; Burnard and Hannigan, 2000; Cameron *et al.*, 2005), but above all there seems to be ideological and conceptual confusion about the very nature of the profession itself (Rydon, 2005).

According to Stuart (2001, p. 103), 'The most desirable basis to substantiate clinical practice is the evidence of well-established research findings.' This view typifies the scientific approach to mental health nursing. The scientific paradigm sees mental health problems as illnesses; phenomena which require 'treatment' (Burnard and Hannigan, 2000). Subsequently, the focus of mental health nursing practice should be, within this paradigm, the application of scientifically derived evidence of the effectiveness of particular interventions (for example, cognitive behavioural interventions) with an explicit focus on positive clinical outcomes (Gournay, 1994, 2001). This approach also stresses the importance of mental health nurses developing research skills and becoming research literate (DH, 1994a).

Such an approach has met with official support. The UKCC (forerunner of the NMC) stressed the value of evidence-based practice:

. . . you should use the available evidence to inform and develop your practice. Clients should rightly be able to assume that the type of care they receive is based on sound evidence. However, obtaining evidence through research and/or audit can be complex because of a shortage of published information. Your responsibility is to ensure that you continually update your practice and that you search for the best evidence you can find (UKCC, 1998, p. 12).

Hence, evidence-based practice has been seen by some as a professional, moral and ethical imperative (Cameron *et al.*, 2005). That is, 'psychiatric patients' have the right to receive care which is known to work to help them, and to experience specific goal-directed interventions which maximize clinical outcomes and contribute to an improvement in their experiencing of symptoms.

However, those who believe mental health nursing should focus on the 'art' or 'craft' of caring stress that good nursing cannot simply result from the application of scientific research findings. The 'craft' approach values the individual by listening to what people say, and seeing value in, and exploring meaning arising from, their personal experiences (Barker *et al.*, 1997; Burnard and Hannigan, 2000; Watkins, 2001; Barker and Buchanan-Barker, 2004). As such, 'Understanding the patient's world in this framework is gained through empathic imagination rather than objective, empirical observation' (Playle, 1995, p. 981).

Good nursing, in this sense, is a lifelong apprenticeship '. . . where the tools of the trade are sharpened with every encounter' (Barker and Buchanan-Barker, 2004, p. 18). It is common practice to assert that such an approach is influenced by the humanism of Rogers (1951) and Peplau (1952) (Gijbels and Burnard, 1995). Indeed, this approach often seeks its identity by its opposition to the scientific view. For some who expound the art of mental health nursing, the biomedical approach is seen to over-emphasize the medical origins of mental and emotional distress, which is seen to be stigmatizing and which undermines the therapeutic role of the mental health nurse (Porter, 1993; Barker *et al.*, 1997; Coleman and Jenkins, 1998). There is also a concern that the biomedical approach creates passivity amongst 'patients' who are seen, and may see themselves, as 'ill' and in need of care, and as such:

Working from biomedical models encourages client behaviour related to boredom, lack of choice, disempowerment, fear, confusion, lack of self-esteem and confidence, to be perceived by nurses as symptoms of mental illness (Rydon, 2005, p. 86).

Indeed, there appears to be at least two contrasting frameworks within mental health nursing, with different emphases and assumptions regarding the delivery of care and the needs of service users (Burnard and Hannigan, 2000). The result is that service users may be unclear as to the sort of care they might expect to receive from a mental health nurse, or what 'quality' care might mean, as care offered may differ according to the practitioner's beliefs regarding their needs.

HETEROGENEITY

Another pressing issue is that of attempting to reconcile the apparent fragmentary nature of mental health nursing, not only in terms of its ideological base but also the various unions and nursing associations, which contributes to the heterogeneity of the profession (Barker and Buchanan-Barker, 2005). Whilst some of this may well be '. . . self-indulgent navel gazing . . .' (Lauder *et al.*, 2004, p. 1), it is vital to clarify the practice of mental health nurses, ensuring that it is both transparent and sensitive to the complex needs of service users (Anderson, 1983).

Mental health nursing, then, is not homogenous, but is a remarkably diverse discipline (Barker and Buchanan-Barker, 2005). It seems that 'Each psychiatric nurse develops his/her own style of health care delivery' (Onega, 1991, p. 68), but as Cleary (2004, p. 57) argued '. . . it is the diversity of the nursing role that has been, is, and will continue to be its strength'. Perhaps, there is '. . . no single model [which] is designed to answer all questions; therefore, it is each individual's professional responsibility to search for ways of thinking that allow him/her to best serve the public' (Onega, 1991, pp. 72–73). This point was echoed by Chambers (1998) and indeed Burnard and Hannigan (2000), in their discussion of the benefit of plurality of methods in mental health nursing research. Towell (1975) also noted that many nurses lack commitment to one particular ideology, perhaps because the ideological issues are seen to be irrelevant to their day-to-day work.

Regardless of the specific orientation of mental health nurses, service users rightly expect to receive care which is based on fundamental principles and values that explicitly respect them as human beings. Heterogeneity in values and plurality of approaches is a conceptual issue for the profession, and one that must not stand in the way of the delivery of care which is consistent in terms of its quality and willingness to respond to service user's needs.

INCONSISTENT AND POOR QUALITY OF CARE

Mental health nurses, it seems, have not always been successful in providing good quality or therapeutic care (DH, 1994a; Bray, 1999; Whittington and McLaughlin, 2000; O'Brien and Cole, 2004; Cameron *et al.*, 2005), and current practice does not always seem to meet needs of users (Rydon, 2005). There is also an apparent and marked discrepancy between nursing theory, its stated aims and objectives and the 'reality' of nursing practice (Sullivan, 1998; Machin and Stevenson, 1999; Cameron *et al.*, 2005).

Some studies have indicated a perceived lack of therapeutic skills and self-awareness amongst mental health nurses, although this may not be a new phenomenon (Towell, 1975). Cowman *et al.* (2001), for example, found that some mental health nurses were perceived by nursing students as non-therapeutic. In this study, nursing students perceived that poor quality of care amongst qualified nurses seemed to inhibit the patient's psychological growth and well-being. There seemed to be physical distancing and a 'why bother?' attitude, seen to be a coping strategy to deal with stressful environments where office duties were perceived to be more important than direct patient contact and where talking to patients was only undertaken when the nurse had some free time. Some nurses were perceived to have a self-centred attitude. Indeed, according to Rowe (2006, p. 15), 'Faced with a choice of having a difficult conversation or filling in a boring form, nurses go for the form every time.' Such distancing may assist the nurse to cope with the emotional demands of their job, but this does little to ease the fear many service users experience in some care environments, where nurses are not available to deal with tensions between patients, and where the personal safety of patients is not promoted (see Chapter 16: A Systemic Approach to Violence Risk Assessment and Management).

Inconsistent and poor quality care is perhaps best summarized by those who have had first-hand experience. Faulkner (2004, p. 79), for example, describes a common complaint amongst service users:

In my own experience, long days of watching television and waiting for medication, visiting times or meal times, were underpinned by a total lack of engagement by nursing staff . . . I was far too terrified to approach anyone for help or talk to on the ward: nurses were busy, they stayed in the office or watched television and never offered the space or opportunity to talk. All my fellow patients and I could do in extremity was to express the need for human contact in terms of distress, anger or self-harm.

Care environments often seem to be places of great tension and stress (Rose, 2000; Dale *et al.*, 2006), and often service users feel that they are not listened to (Gadsby, 2006) and that their needs are not being met (SCMH, 2005). For the Standing Nursing and Midwifery Committee (SNMAC), the '. . . experience of admission to in-patient wards has become increasingly custodial, with a greater risk of violence and limited therapeutic activity' (SNMAC, 1999, p. 3). Cleary and Edwards (1999) found that while service users were generally positive towards the care offered to them by nurses, they felt that the busy acute psychiatric wards '. . . may render nurses less sensitive in interpersonal interactions with patients' (Cleary and Edwards, 1999, p. 476). Indeed, in-patient services have been described as an '. . . antithetical therapeutic environment . . . depicted by low staff morale and dissatisfied patients' (Cameron *et al.*, 2005, p. 69). Ford *et al.* (1998) found that nurses working on acute in-patient environments spent much of their time observing clients. Only a minority of patients in such settings seem to feel that they are treated with dignity (SNMAC, 1999; Dale *et al.*, 2006), although there is some evidence that service users receiving community care feel that their care and treatment is respectful (Healthcare Commission, 2006a). Indeed, it is not only service users who appear to be angry, but this is an apparent feature of some nursing teams where there is a lack of cohesion. Working within the mental health nursing profession, it seems, can be challenging, and indeed:

A good deal of nurses' energy is spent in attempting to establish satisfactory relationships with peers, and this is often more difficult than working with users (Glenister, 1997, p. 50).

Some authors have found that some service users seem to be more satisfied with the care offered by unqualified staff, such as health care assistants (HCAs) (Meek, 1998). Indeed, Pashley (1992) argued that health professionals did not use or apply formal theoretical knowledge but relied upon common sense knowledge, a point echoed by Meek (1998, p. 12), who felt that '. . . in reality qualified nurses and health care assistants may apply the same "knowledge base" to practice'. As such, unqualified staff may come to their role ready equipped with this knowledge. Furthermore, as Brown *et al.* (1992) argued, the caring relationship is founded on the carer having developed a number of human qualities (for example, patience, fortitude and compassion) for which training may not be required. However, not all studies have found unequivocally that unqualified staff have benefited their clients. Morrison (1990), for example, found unqualified staff's interaction was minimal and was more concerned with taking a tough approach to control and enforcing ward rules (see Chapter 17: No Euphemisms: The Use of Force in Mental Health Care).

FEAR

Some service users express a real fear of mental health services and the staff who work within them. As many as 50% of service users report not feeling safe in clinical environments, and some, especially female service users, report feeling sexually or physically harassed (Ford *et al.*, 1998; SNMAC, 1999; Dale *et al.*, 2006). According to Beresford (2005, p. 10):

The tabloid press say that people should be frightened of mental health service users. I say many more people are frightened of the mental health system and of ever coming its way.

Service users often express a fear of retribution by mental health workers if they complain about their experiences, which can, in any case, be passed off as an irrational manifestation of some underlying pathology. As Wilson (2006, p. 19) argues:

The fear of repercussions is very real, as is the fear of not being believed. We are disturbed we are told, so we do not have a true perception of reality.

It seems that the very system which exists to support and protect service users from harm may itself be harmful, an example of which Wilson (2006, p. 19) describes:

A woman with a history of physical and sexual abuse was pursued into the shower by male nursing staff, pinned against a wall, her trousers pulled down and injected.

In any human system mistakes can be made, but the fear and anxiety which some service users report regarding the care and treatment they experience within modern mental health services is disturbing. These are not comfortable issues for those who work in mental health practice to confront, but an important way forward for mental health nurses will be to examine their ability to provide protection for those who seek their help, and support to develop a trusting therapeutic relationship (DH, 2006a).

THE WAY FORWARD

RESPONDING TO THE WISHES AND NEEDS OF SERVICE USERS

The role of the mental health nurse must be inextricably linked with meeting the individual needs of their clients. Service users' wishes, it has been argued, should, and must, inform mental health nursing practice wherever possible (DH, 1994a, 2006a; Cameron *et al.*, 2005) (see Chapter 3: User Involvement and the Micro-Politics of Mental Health Care). That is,

To provide structure and direction for psychiatric nursing practice, the patient must remain the focus of attention (Hagerty *et al.*, 1995, p. 431).

Rydon (2005) studied service users' views of the attitudes, skills and knowledge they felt mental health nurses needed. Service users expressed a wish for mental health nurses to convey positive attitudes in the sense of being professional, conveying hope, connecting with, knowing and respecting the person and being interested in people's lives beyond the mental health issues. Similar conclusions have been reached by Jackson and Stevenson (1998), who found the 'gift of time' to be a key element valued by service users.

Rydon (2005) also identified a number of interpersonal and practical skills essential for the role (including exploring problems, using counselling skills, supporting the independence of the person whenever possible, and using organizational and teaching skills). In this study, service users expected mental health nurses to be demonstrably knowledgeable (by sharing their clinical knowledge and ensuring users are better informed about rights), and to possess personal resilience and emotional stability. The study also revealed that service users recognized the power imbalance between themselves and nurses and felt that, at times and under certain circumstances, this power could and should be used judiciously and in a positive way, for example, in protecting the person from themselves.

However, the fundamental needs and wishes of service users are the same for any other sector of society. To have needs is not abnormal (Slade *et al.*, 1999). The way forward in responding to the needs and wishes of service users is to recognize that service users want to be able to trust health care services, to have a decent place to live, money in their pocket, decent employment, friends, support, hope for a future, diversion from boredom, being seen as a complete person rather than as a cluster of psychiatric symptoms, comprehensive physical health care, and assistance to alleviate psychological distress (Cleary and Edwards, 1999; Mortimer, 2006; Cutcliffe and Koehn, 2007).

Furthermore, as mentioned earlier, there is a heterogeneity of ideologies which underpin mental health nursing. Clearly, there is a need to move on from this debate (Burnard and Hannigan, 2000), not least because the tensions and conflicts between these two approaches can be seen to be damaging to the overall care provided due to inconsistencies in perceptions of, and responses to, service user's needs and wishes. While it is true than no-one wants to receive care which is unlikely to work, there is currently much emphasis on care being based on research from within a biomedical paradigm. This may colour perceptions of service user's needs/wants, and may lead to the assumption that the service user's wishes and aspirations are the same as the mental health professional's. As such, we may have a very biased view as to what 'works' or the suitability of an intervention for quantifying 'successful' clinical outcomes (see Chapter 7: Where is your Evidence? Broadening the Scope of Professional Knowledge). Indeed, as Beresford and Beales (2005, p. 7) argue:

Conventional randomised clinical trial-based psychiatric research maintains an artificially narrow focus on personal 'pathology' and individual 'treatment' . . .

Indeed, the best evidence of the 'clinical effectiveness' of an intervention is through the service user's response to, and satisfaction with, treatment and care offered. The service user is, after all, the expert on their mental health problem (DH, 2001b). The fact that under certain clinical scenarios, medication or cognitive behavioural therapy may, statistically speaking, improve the 'mental functioning' of some people within a given population (for example, NICE, 2004) belies the fact that for some people these approaches may not be wanted, acceptable, satisfactory or clinically effective (Gallop and Reynolds, 2004). When considering clinical effectiveness, therefore, it is crucial to consider the sort of bespoke care, delivered sensitively and humanely, which is responsive to the individual needs and wishes of service users and which will help them to improve their lives (CSIP/NIMHE, 2006).

RELATIONSHIP FORMATION

A central role for mental health nursing practice is the development of the nurse–patient relationship (Pollock, 1988; Butterworth, 1994; DH, 1994a; Barker *et al.*, 1999; Trenoweth, 2003; Cameron *et al.*, 2005). Mental health nurses report that clinical contact with service users is the most satisfying aspect of their work (Cleary and Edwards, 1999; Nolan *et al.*, 2007). Indeed, it is argued that the central work of mental health nursing rests on the skilled use of the therapeutic self to promote recovery and to develop relationships with people who have diverse needs and, importantly, to be able to sustain such relationships over time (DH, 1994a, 2004a, 2006a). Here, an emergent theme in the literature is the perceived need to *be* with people (Cleary and Edwards, 1999; Barker and Buchanan-Barker, 2004). That is,

Nurses are 'travelling companions' with patients, not 'travel agents' (Peck and Norman, 1999, p. 235).

Of course, the formation of a trusting and therapeutic relationship and the creation of a positive clinical alliance is often seen to be an essential precursor of effective nursing interventions. Indeed, service users who experience a therapeutic relationship appear to experience a more significant improvement in their mental health and, as such, the potential contribution to recovery is considerable (Hewitt and Coffey, 2005).

Furthermore, people who have significantly improved from the symptoms of 'schizo-phrenia' have frequently reported that they were greatly helped by someone who believed in them, who gave them hope, and who treated them as individuals and not as symptoms of a disease (Kelly and Gamble, 2005; Cutcliffe and Koehn, 2007). Indeed, central to the process of relationship formation is the ability to develop respect for the others (Pollock, 1988) by getting to know, attempting to understand (Trenoweth, 2003) and empathizing with the service user (Gijbels and Burnard, 1995; Cameron *et al.*, 2005). Here, a fundamental requirement for the mental health nursing profession is to be able to base its care on a sound understanding of, and respect for, diversity amongst people in their care (DH, 1994a; Burr and Chapman, 1998; DH, 2004a).

Butterworth (1994), the Mental Health Nursing Review Team (DH, 1994a) and the CNO's Review of Mental Health Nursing (DH, 2006a) have all urged mental health nurses to construct and value partnerships with service users in order to develop realistic individual plans of care with meaningful aims. They point to the importance of the mental health nurse being able to ensure access to appropriate information (including treatment options and rights) and that care plans should be developed with individuals based on their needs and wishes, not the convenience of the service. That is:

People who use [mental health] services should be given real choice in matters of care (Butterworth, 1994, p. 10).

In contemporary practice, the Tidal Model (Barker, 2003) has been cited as offering a theoretical and practical framework by which to structure such practice (Cameron *et al.*, 2005) by '. . . proactively giving voice and bearing witness to the subjective lived experience of [the person's] illness or trauma while simultaneously recognizing as central, the person's need to be understood' (Cameron *et al.*, 2005, p. 69). Within the mental health nursing profession, however, this framework has by no means been universally accepted and has been the subject of criticism and debate (Noak, 2001).

Meek (1998) found that service users appeared most satisfied with the care, contact and support offered by unqualified staff. The suggestion for this study is that the lack of professional power and status of HCAs affords them the opportunity to adopt a 'non-dominant position' with service users that is flexible, humanized and client-centred. Other studies have also stressed the value service users place on the importance of staff being available physically and emotionally and the importance of human contact (Cleary and Edwards, 1999; Olofsson and Norberg, 2001) (see Chapter 4: Compassion). Similarly, Rydon (2005) found that service users felt that community mental health nurses were perceived as friendlier, more able to practice in a way that was congruent with their needs and more sympathetic than in-patient nurses who were perceived to work within the dominant biomedical paradigm which was seen to structure and organize the workplace. Furthermore, Beech and Norman (1995) found service users valued nursing staff availability, and attempts to understand their issues and the creation of a safe clinical environment to promote recovery were seen as important (see Chapter 10: The Meaning of Recovery and Chapter 11: Supporting Recovery: Medication Management in Mental Health Care).

IMPROVING QUALITY OF LIFE

The CNO's Review of Mental Health Nursing (DH, 2006a) points to the need to develop a modern profession, which uses evidence-based therapeutic interventions, including psychological therapies, to underpin a positive approach to care. The review stresses the importance of effective risk management strategies along with an explicit focus on effective health promotion, the improvement of physical care and well-being. Such points have also been underlined by the 'Ten Essential Shared Capabilities' framework (DH, 2004a).

Curran and Brooker (2007) point to evidence which suggests that mental health nurses who use therapeutic approaches (especially cognitive behavioural therapy, and medication management) do so with some success. However, to be truly service user-focused, mental health nurses will need to concentrate on assisting clients to improve their overall quality of *life* rather than the more narrow view on improving the technical quality of care (such as the administration of medication), or the improvement in clinical outcomes seen in terms of an abatement of psychiatric symptoms (NIMHE, 2005) (see Chapter 10: The Meaning of Recovery). As such, a measure of success of an intervention would be incomplete without an evaluation of its effectiveness from the service user perspective. Indeed, this issue has been highlighted in the 'Ten Essential Shared Capabilities' document (DH, 2004a), where 'recovery' is seen in terms of:

. . . *what people experience themselves as they become empowered to achieve a meaningful life and a positive sense of belonging in the community* (DH, 2004a, p. 15).

That is, mental health nursing care will need to be able to assist people, in a committed and compassionate way (McAllister and Walsh, 2004), to meet their mental and physical health and their social care needs (Coleman and Jenkins, 1998). Such interventions must be effective in assisting the service user to overcome their current difficulties but, crucially, must also be acceptable to them (DH, 2004a; NIMHE, 2005). Detailed information regarding treatment must be shared with service users and an explicit involvement in all aspects of care must be the norm (see Chapter 11: Supporting Recovery: Medication Management in Mental Health Care). Individual care will need to be holistic (including an emphasis on responding to physical health care needs), bespoke and flexible, and provided to people from diverse backgrounds (DH, 2004a) (see Chapter 12: Physical Co-Morbidity in Mental Health and Chapter 13: Physical Illness: Promoting Effective Coping in Clients with Co-Morbidity). The mental health nurse must be aware of, and sensitive to, the concept of social justice and how they might tackle social exclusion and promote social inclusion (see Chapter 8: Challenging Stigma and Promoting Social Justice). If the mental health nurse is required to, temporarily, manage the risk a service user poses to themselves or others, then this is undertaken safely, and above all with dignity and respect. Overall, mental health nursing care must be accountable to the people it serves, and undertaken in a climate where the person is protected from harm and where there is no fear of reprisals should a complaint need to be made.

CONCLUSION

Mental health nursing has the potential to make meaningful and significant differences to the lives of people who experience mental distress. There is, of course, much good practice in contemporary health care and mental health nursing practice which needs celebrating (Cleary and Edwards, 1999). The CNO's Review (DH, 2006a) offers a positive framework for responding to service users' needs, even though it is seen to lack operational detail (Brooker, 2007). Similarly, it seems to fail to appreciate the systemic pressures faced by nurses in having to therapeutically respond to the complex needs of service users whilst maintaining a safe and organized clinical environment (Cleary and Edwards, 1999). As such, progress in responding to its various recommendations has to date been rather slow (Vere-Jones, 2007).

However, this will require mental health nurses to adopt a broader perspective regarding the needs and wishes of service users rather than a narrow focus on a bio-medical framework, important though this may be in the delivery of holistic care. Furthermore, for the profession to make its mark it will need to consider the barriers in its contemporary practice which hold it back from being truly responsive to the needs of service users. For example, mental health nurses will need to develop a transparent and unifying framework for practice (Littlejohn, 2003) and to rethink the

'. . . boundaries between our various tribes' (Lauder *et al.*, 2004, p. 1). There is an imperative to ensure a consistency in the quality of care regardless of ideological differences between practitioners, although at a fundamental level there may be little difference between such ideologies, with differences existing merely in emphasis (Burnard and Hannigan, 2000). Perhaps differing perspectives are not incompatible but complementary, and as such we need to capitalize on the benefits of a plurality of approaches. Hence, 'it is expected that nurses have both a professionally objective, scientific stance to and sensitivity to patients and their suffering . . . The ability to quantify must go together with the ability to be present as a fellow human being' (Hem and Heggen, 2003, p. 102). If this is the case, then mental health nurses will still need to demonstrate consistency and quality in terms of practice. They will also need to consider historical links, and whether these ties and allegiances are useful in the context of improving the lives of vulnerable people.

There is indeed much work to be done – and a number of challenges which await the mental health nursing profession, both in the contemporary context and in forthcoming years (Harrison, 2005). At times this may seem overwhelming and the task may seem too great, but as Bertram and Stickley (2005, p. 395) argue:

Individual mental health workers may not be able to change the world, but their attitudes and practices can influence the opportunities of individuals with whom they work.

Perhaps the most important role of the modern mental health nurse, then, is to be able to support service users whose life has been devastated by mental distress (Koivisto *et al.*, 2004), and assist in the rebuilding of a life that is valuable and meaningful to them.

CHAPTER 3
USER INVOLVEMENT AND THE MICRO-POLITICS OF MENTAL HEALTH CARE

Philip Kemp

INTRODUCTION

There is no doubt that over the last two decades there has been something approaching a paradigm shift in the position of service users within the mental health system in the United Kingdom. As Campbell (2005) puts it, 'in 1985 service users were nowhere; in 2005 they are everywhere'. 'User involvement' has become a central policy objective for the National Health Service (NHS) as a whole (Hewitt, 2005). Within the mental health field, service users either individually, or as members of user groups and organizations, are involved in a wide range of activities: national policy formulation; local service planning and development; campaigning; advocacy; service provision; service monitoring; user-led research; and professional training and education. At the level of individual care delivery, policy and professional practice prescribes the involvement of service users (DH, 1999a,b). Indeed, service users themselves now expect to be involved in decisions about their care and treatment (Rose, 2001) and there are increasing requirements for service providers and mental health professionals to develop and offer services that are user-sensitive and based on what users themselves feel are most helpful to them (DH, 1999a, 2000b).

These developments are clearly positive, though it has to be said that mental health service provision has a chequered history. Many have been perceived as disempowering, and some have even been considered abusive at times (Martin, 1984). To some

Contemporary Issues in Mental Health Nursing, Edited by J. E. Lynch and S. Trenoweth
© 2008 John Wiley & Sons, Ltd

extent, mental health service users are an inherently disempowered group and the problem of stigma is well known (Social Exclusion Unit (SEU), 2004a) (see Chapter 8: Challenging Stigma and Promoting Social Justice). Public perceptions and media representations of mental illness can further undermine the status of individuals with mental health problems in society (Philo, 1996).

There is extensive literature on how the development of psychiatry has served to subordinate users of mental health services (for example, Foucault, 1971; Prior, 1993; Scull, 1979 and also see Chapter 9: Homophobia in Mental Health Services) and the institutional context of care is thought to have further reinforced imbalances of power (Goffman, 1963; Barton, 1976). Even recently, concern has been raised about apparent failings in respect of the care and treatment of some individuals with serious mental health problems being cared for in acute in-patient environments (SCMH, 2005) and living in the community (Ritchie et al., 1994; Sheppard, 1996). The pressure to involve service users has arguably had a transforming effect on the way mental health care is delivered in recent years and although this remains unfinished business, there is some evidence that user satisfaction is increasing in relation to the overall service users receive and from mental health nurses specifically (Healthcare Commission, 2005).

Numerous factors have contributed to a change in the position of service users within the mental health system, and these will be explored in this chapter. First will be the 'top-down' policy pressures to involve service users. The second will be discussion of the 'bottom-up' demands from service users for increasing user involvement. Third, the extent to which mental health nurses and other professionals have attempted to adopt user-focused approaches to care will be reviewed. Finally, the chapter will examine the problematic nature of user involvement for nurses. In particular, it will analyse the challenges and contradictions arising from conflicting perspectives of user involvement and how such tensions might be mediated.

'TOP-DOWN' PRESSURE: USER INVOLVEMENT POLICY INITIATIVES

The development of service user involvement in mental health care has taken place in the context of wider societal changes. Recent trends have contributed towards more participatory forms of public decision making, which have been summarized in the term 'collaborative governance' (Newman et al., 2004). One of the effects of globalization is that the power of the state is dispersing (Giddens, 2002). Power has been dispersed in an upward direction, for example, to multi-national corporations and to supra-national political bodies such as the European Union. At the same time, power has been dispersed in a downward direction to sub-national entities, such as the Scottish Parliament and Regional Assemblies. There is an increasing reliance on non-governmental organizations and executive agencies and it is arguable that as societies become more complex, no single agency possesses the necessary information or expertise to tackle contemporary problems. In addition, traditional forms of governance based on hierarchical political institutions and systems are not able to respond effectively to challenges generated by the social diversities that characterize modern societies, such as social exclusion, community regeneration and inequalities in health (Newman *et al.*, 2004). As a result, new forms of governance are evolving in which the state must collaborate with a wide range of stakeholders.

The impetus for increasing public participation in the health and welfare sphere is associated with the marked changes that have taken place over the last 20 years in the way public services are managed. The adoption of a 'New Right' (Mishra, 1990) philosophy by Conservative governments after 1979 introduced market principles into the public sector and with it a stronger consumer focus. The movement towards a more consumer-focused health service was initiated by the introduction of general management in the NHS following the Griffiths Report in 1983 (Griffiths, 1983). This was reinforced by the NHS and Community Care Act 1990, which introduced internal market mechanisms to the NHS and social care. The characterization of these reforms was marked by the notion that health and community care service providers should be responsive to consumer choice. Subsequent changes in NHS structures during the 1990s saw the introduction of a range of consultative mechanisms, including patient satisfaction surveys, consumer audit, Citizens' Juries and Health Panels (Pickard, 1998). These were intended to ensure that health service organizations involved the public and offered them a greater say in health care delivery (NHS Executive, 1996).

With the election of the New Labour Government in 1997, there was a renewed emphasis on public involvement in Britain. The government's strategy for the health service, *The New NHS – Modern, Dependable*, stated:

The Government will take special steps to ensure that the experience of users and carers is central to the work of the NHS (DH, 1997a, p. 66).

New institutional frameworks were put in place following the Health and Social Care Act 2001. These included Patient Advice and Liaison Services (PALS), Patient and Public Involvement Forums (PPIF) and the Commission for Patient and Public Involvement to oversee these structures. At the level of local service planning and delivery, Department of Health guidance expected service users and carers to be integrally involved (DH, 1999b, 2000a). An additional influence that appears to have fuelled the public and patient participation policy agenda might be described as a reduction in faith in health professionals. It would appear that the recent emphases on greater public accountability and tighter professional regulation have been influenced by a series of high-profile cases such as the Bristol Royal Infirmary Inquiry, the Inquiry into Alder Hey Children's Hospital and the case of Harold Shipman.

The concept of citizenship is central to any consideration of an individual's relationship to the state and participation in society. Marshall's classic exposition of citizenship traced the development of the concept through different stages (Marshall, 1950; see also Marshall and Bottomore, 1992). Following the acquisition of *legal* rights (equality before the law) came *political* rights (universal suffrage). Ultimately, the 20th century witnessed the distinct emergence of *social* rights (access to welfare benefits/services) which came of age with the post-war consensus on rights to health care, education and income maintenance—integral components of the Welfare State. More recently, the notion of citizenship has been subject to shifting orthodoxies. The 'New Right' orthodoxy conceptualized the citizen as a consumer articulating individual interests within a free economy. Accompanying this consumerist notion of citizenship was an authoritarian strand that penalized those who did not participate by reducing or withdrawing welfare benefits. A further shift in the way citizenship has been conceptualized was apparent with the election of the New Labour Government in 1997. While the Labour Government continued to espouse the value of private sector input to the delivery of public services, there has been a retreat from an explicit market approach in favour of 'partnerships' (Paton, 1999). Accompanying this change in policy emphasis has been a change in focus of service users from 'consumers' to a new rhetoric of 'active citizens' (Milewa *et al.*, 1998) and the promotion of the idea of a 'stakeholding' society. Under this approach, user involvement is presented as a means of empowerment based on social participation. However, a number of studies (Milewa *et al.*, 1998; Pickard, 1998; Rowe and Shepherd, 2002) have highlighted a disparity between the 'official' discourse of empowerment and the reality of professionalized NHS managers who consider the views of the public and service users as just one source of available data which can contribute to rational decision making.

Rowe and Shepherd (2002) describe two models of public participation in the health service which reflect these conflicting ideological perspectives on service user involvement. Participation within a 'consumerist model' is conceived as a means of eliciting consumer preferences so that services can be developed and shaped to meet needs more effectively. Emphasized are consumer rights, information, access, choice and redress. The second model is a 'democratic model' that values participation itself as an enriching and empowering process for service users. This highlights involving service users in decision making and mobilizing them to participate effectively. Yet while government rhetoric espouses the latter, health service managers appear to favour the former (Rowe and Shepherd, 2002). Hence, there is some uncertainty about policy intentions and the nature of user involvement.

Lister (2001) argues that a further complication stems from two New Labour characteristics: a populist approach that seeks to woo rather than lead the public; and a pragmatism marked by a problem-solving approach rather than by tackling structural inequalities directly. These populist impulses are wedded to the assumption that the general public is essentially conservative in outlook, and leads to a 'moral authoritarianism'. This, in turn, makes it necessary to appear 'tough' in high-profile areas of public policy (e.g. criminal justice or mental health) and to avoid appearing 'weak' (see Lynch and Kemp, 2005).

Discussions about the nature of citizenship are particularly pertinent for people who have experienced mental health problems (Sayce, 2000) (see Chapter 8: Challenging Stigma and Promoting Social Justice). The ambiguities discussed above are reflected in mental health policy and mental health service user involvement. References to user involvement within mental health policy pronouncements, such as the 'National Service Framework for Mental Health' (DH, 1999a) and the 'NHS Plan' (DH, 2000a), similarly adopt the rhetoric of citizen participation. However, the rhetoric on increased participation and empowerment raises a further contradiction within the mental health context – that of government concerns about risk and dangerousness (see Chapter 16: A Systemic Approach to Violence Risk Assessment and Management). Many commentators (for example, Peck and Parker, 1998) have suggested that this is the main driving force behind recent mental health policy initiatives, which have been criticized for leaning towards control and coercion (see Chapter 17: No Euphemisms: The Use of Force in Mental Health Care). This is reflected, for example, in the tense debates concerning proposed reforms to the Mental Health Act 1983 (POST, 2003).

'BOTTOM-UP' DEMANDS: THE RISE OF THE 'USER MOVEMENT'

In contrast to 'top-down' policy pressures, there has been a longer tradition of 'bottom-up' demands from mental health service users seeking greater involvement in their care and treatment. The growth of the 'user movement' has been particularly marked over the last two decades and it is likely that this is a consequence of an interaction between a gradually burgeoning user movement and the societal changes and government policies outlined above.

There had been early initiatives with groups representing and advocating on behalf of service users as well as service users organizing themselves. Three phases of development can be identified (Crossley, 1999). A 'reformist' phase after World War Two up to the early 1960s was characterized by the National Association for Mental Health run on behalf of service users by individuals who were concerned about the way mentally ill people were cared for and treated. Active organizations functioned as pressure groups and helped inform mental health policy. This was followed by a 'radical' phase from the mid-1960s up to the 1980s coinciding with the rise of radical social movements in wider society concerned with the civil liberties of women, people from ethnic minorities, gay and lesbian people and civil rights more generally. It was during this period that the National Association for Mental Health began to transform itself into 'MIND' with a more radical, campaigning agenda. Importantly, it was a user–run organization rather than one run on behalf of service users. New groups also developed, such as the Mental Patients Union and COPE (Community Organization for Psychiatric Emergencies). These tended to be protest groups and often took overtly political stances. To some extent they were influenced by the Anti-Psychiatry Movement, the ideas of which were prominent in the 1970s. Although the impacts made by the early groups are open to debate, it appears that at the very least they had the effect of activating some mental health service users who went on to play important roles in the groups that came to prominence from the mid-1980s onwards (Campbell, 1996a).

A third phase in the rise of the user movement dates from the mid-1980s onwards and can be characterized as 'pluralistic'. The number of service user organizations rapidly grew and they became active in an increasingly wide range of areas. Campbell (1996a) suggests the following characteristics of contemporary user action. First, the flourishing of user activity since the mid-1980s has been characterized by rapid growth. Second, as outlined above, users are involved in a wide variety of activities within the mental health field. Third, service user activity has often developed in response to local needs and demands, such as participation in service developments and alterations. Fourth, user involvement was quickly able to secure 'official' approval – a significant contrast to earlier user movement experiences. Fifth, contemporary user groups prioritize self-advocacy.

So, from its origins within civil liberties movements in the 1970s, the development of the mental health service user movement has followed a democratic model of participation characteristic of other 'New Social Movements' (Crossley, 1999). This could lead to tension or even conflict given the policy ambiguities highlighted above. Nevertheless, the user involvement has become gradually more embedded in many areas, although the quality of 'involvement' has not necessarily been consistent (for example, see Rose, 2001).

PROFESSIONAL ADOPTION OF USER-FOCUSED APPROACHES

Professional developments within mental health practice have gradually incorporated user perspectives into the way care is delivered. The extent to which this is the result of policy pressures, user expectations or progressive advancements within mental health professional practice remains an open question. There have been early attempts in the history of mental health care at more user-sensitive ways of caring for people with serious mental health problems. The reforming approach of William Tuke in the York Retreat towards the end of the 18th century gave rise to the system of 'moral management' in the early asylums involving treating asylum inmates in a more humane and dignified way (Jones, 1993). Unfortunately, such promise dissipated as the asylums became primarily custodial in their function in order to cater for ever-increasing inmate numbers. After World War Two, the therapeutic community movement (Jones, 1968) was influential in spreading ideas about the therapeutic potential of less hierarchical relationships between the mentally ill and mental health workers. There were some attempts by innovative psychiatrists (for example, Martin, 1962) to apply the principles of therapeutic communities to mental hospitals, but with hospital numbers at their peak in the mid-1950s this was likely to have limited success. Nevertheless, there was some liberalization of the culture of mental hospitals, such as the so-called 'open door' policy and the use of 'parole'. The benefits of active rehabilitation (Wing and Brown, 1970) and the significance of social therapies were discovered and with them mental health nurses found new therapeutic roles. With the development of community care policies in the 1980s and 1990s, the momentum towards a more explicitly user-focused approach to care was accelerated. More recently, the increasing incorporation of user perspectives in professional practice has been reflected in areas of nursing and other mental health practitioner activity.

ADOPTION OF USER-FOCUSED PHILOSOPHIES OF CARE

There has been a proliferation of nursing models which have attempted to encapsulate a patient-centred philosophy of care (Walsh, 1998). However, such models have often been found to fit poorly with mental health nursing practice, and the value of theoretical models of nursing has been questioned (Gournay, 1996). However, recent widespread interest in the *Tidal Model* suggests that models per se are not incompatible with practice (and it may be that more attention is required for education on and implementation of these). This paradigm was developed, and its efficacy researched, by Phil Barker and colleagues (Barker *et al.*, 1998; Stevenson *et al.*, 2002; Buchanan-Barker, 2004) and it utilizes the user's unique experience as the central influence on nursing care and the treatment offered. The *Tidal Model*'s user-centredness is highlighted by two critical features: collaboration with the user (and her/his family) and 'empowering the person by putting the narrative experience . . . of illness and health at the heart of the care plan' (Stevenson *et al.*, 2002, p. 272).

Two other notably influential user-focused philosophies have come from outside nursing. The importation of the principles of normalization (Wolfensberger, 1972) from the field of learning disability into mental health services has been one influential ideological theme, informing community care in particular. Wolfensberger analysed not only why and how people with disabilities are devalued by society, but also by the services that are supposed to support them. To reverse this, it was argued, it is imperative that people who are effectively devalued be integrated into wider society and enabled to adopt conventional social roles. The emphasis is thus on providing environments and activities that most 'ordinary' people would want and in promoting socially valued lifestyles.

Normalization was an important influence, particularly in relation to hospital closure programmes and the re-settling of long-stay patients into the community. However, it was not without its critics. Normalization was based on the assumption that there are a set of homogeneous 'valued people' and 'acceptable behaviours' on which to base the lifestyles of people with disabilities. Moreover, nurses have been directly implicated in the practices which devalued people. Yet under normalization, 'the people who are doing the devaluing are the ones whose values we are supposed to help people to aspire towards'

(Smith and Brown, 1992, p. 689). Nevertheless, the ideas of normalization did provide a user-focused principle by which new services could be developed with a critical eye.

A second philosophy that has become increasingly influential is the 'recovery model' (Jacobson and Greenley, 2001; Repper and Perkins, 2003; National Institute for Mental Health (England) [NIMHE], 2005). The centrality of the recovery approach for mental health nurses has been emphasized by the 'Chief Nursing Officer's Review of Mental Health Nursing' (DH, 2006a) (see Chapter 10: The Meaning of Recovery). 'Recovery' is a concept that has been developed largely by service users drawing upon their own personal experiences of overcoming the effects of mental illness and developing personal strategies that contribute to leading meaningful lives; a life that can be defined in ways other than by a diagnosis of a mental illness. The NIMHE (2005, p. 2) defines recovery:

Recovery is what people <u>experience themselves</u> as they become <u>empowered to manage their lives</u> in a manner that allows them to achieve a fulfilling, meaningful life and a contributing sense of belonging in their communities [original emphasis].

So, one aspect emphasized by the recovery model is the personal resources and self-help strategies that service users can draw upon. It is notable that surveys of what service users find most helpful to them frequently illuminate the importance of wider, informal social supports over 'technical' professional interventions (for example, Faulkner and Layzell, 2000). This approach has important implications, then, both for mental heath nurses and for the very nature of service provision. For nurses, emphasis is placed on *enabling* and *facilitating* to support individuals on their journeys to recovery. Most significantly, however, is the need for each nurse to possess positive attitudes towards people with mental health problems and to have and communicate hope and optimism.

Philosophies of care are underpinned by key values which in turn should inform practice. However, if such values and associated attitudes are to have any worth, rather than being merely rhetorical, then it is important that mental health nurses are equipped with the skills to enable them to demonstrate them in practice and in their interactions with service users (Callaghan and Owen, 2005).

APPLICATION OF USER-CENTRED FRAMEWORKS OF CARE

Care and treatment that meets the needs of individuals and is determined collaboratively with service users is a central component of care delivery frameworks that have been developed. A range of 'case management' approaches (Mueser *et al.*, 1998a) have been developed which can be considered a treatment modality in themselves in addition to being a framework for delivering care. The primary framework within which mental health care is delivered in England is the Care Programme Approach (CPA) (DH, 1990, 1999c). The key elements are to ensure that all people receiving support from specialist psychiatric services have a written care plan and that a named care coordinator is identified to oversee and monitor the care plan. An important expectation of CPA is that the service user (and carers) should be integrally involved in the process of formulating their own plan of care.

The introduction of CPA arrangements was far from smooth. It became apparent that in many areas CPA was poorly implemented and a series of mental health inquiry reports lend credence to this, highlighting in such cases systemic shortcomings in communication and care coordination. Revised procedures were introduced in 1999 (DH, 1999c). CPA has become firmly embedded in how mental health nurses and other professionals conduct their practice. Nevertheless, in the years that have passed since its introduction, the extent to which service users have participated in the process has been patchy (Rose, 2001; Social Services Inspectorate, 2002; Healthcare Commission, 2005). Many service users are not clear what CPA is for; many users did not know who their care coordinator was; and fewer feel fully involved in the process. Such findings are important as it is in the care delivery process by which most service users interface and experience mental health services. As such, this can be considered the area where 'involvement' is most crucial and where mental health nurses can potentially make a difference.

Mental health professionals are also required to operate within legal frameworks which aim to protect the interests of service users, notably the Mental Health Act 1983. As suggested above, successive government proposals for reforming the Act since 1998 have been controversial and have provoked much debate because of differing views about the appropriate balance between the protection of the public and the human rights of people with mental health problems (Bertram, 2005). A new legislative framework which aspires to protect the interests of people who lack capacity to make decisions about their own health and welfare is the Mental Capacity Act 2005. This Act became operational in 2007 and as it will impact on certain aspects of professional work, it is important for nurses to appreciate its implications. For example, one particularly interesting feature is the aim to close the so-called 'Bournewood Gap' (Curran et al., 2006), which previously meant that individuals who lacked capacity and had been admitted to mental health units/hospitals voluntarily were less protected under the law than those detained under the Mental Health Act 1983. It also replaces current statutory schemes for enduring powers of attorney and Court of Protection receivers with reformed and updated schemes, and offers a statutory framework to empower and protect vulnerable people. Alterations are also made to lasting powers of attorney. It is too early to estimate the full implications of the Mental Capacity Act for mental health service users, however, it is notable that the protections of the Act do not apply to individuals who are being compulsorily treated under the Mental Health Act.

USER-FOCUSED THERAPEUTIC INTERVENTIONS

A further development in recent years has been the increased use of therapeutic interventions which are predicated on collaborative relationships between mental health professionals and service users (Gournay, 2005) (see Chapter 10: The Meaning of

Recovery). The overarching aim of such psychosocial interventions is to empower service users in aiding their own recovery. Some of the most important are social skills training, family interventions, medication management techniques and cognitive behavioural therapy (CBT) (see, for example, Chapter 11: Supporting Recovery: Medication Management in Mental Health Care). For these interventions to be effective it is essential that professionals develop positive working alliances with service users and vice versa (McGorry *et al.*, 1997; Gamble, 2006). A range of personal qualities are required: being non-judgemental, honesty, warmth, being approachable, being purposeful. These qualities have long been identified as the qualities of effective helping relationships and in counselling (Truax and Mitchell, 1971). What is relatively new is their application to working with people who have experienced serious mental health problems, who have otherwise been marginalized both within society and within the mental health system itself.

Whilst these are encouraging developments, a major challenge is to meet expectations that they should become part of routine clinical practice (NICE, 2002). This is dependent on mental health nurses being able to access the appropriate training and then to be able to transfer new skills to the practice setting, with the necessary organizational support to make this possible, as well as access to clinical supervision. These are challenging requirements for service providers.

THE CHALLENGE OF USER INVOLVEMENT: THE DECENTRALIZATION OF EXPERTISE

It is evident that user involvement has become significantly more wide-ranging and users more influential in recent years. Service user expectations and policy imperatives have combined to cause nurses and other mental health workers to re-think their professional relationships. However, many would argue that there is still some way to go (Campbell, 2005). Many potential barriers to user involvement remain (NIMHE, 2004a), partly, as suggested above, due to ambiguities over policy intentions. Yet barriers can also emerge from differences in perceptions of the values that underpin mental health nursing (see Chapter 5: The Implications of Values-Based Practice in Mental Health Nursing).

The challenge of genuine involvement is brought into sharp focus by considering the activities of front-line practitioners who work directly with service users. This is the location where many policy initiatives take effect and where users' reality of mental health care is experienced. At the centre of all mental health nursing activities is the relationship and the quality of engagement between the mental health nurse and the individual service user. This is as true of the greeting given to a service user newly admitted to an in-patient unit as it is of 'technical' interventions such as CBT. It is often within 'practice relationships' that tensions and contradictions of user involvement can become manifest.

Practice situations usually involve a number of participants: the service user, carers, the mental health nurse and other mental health professionals. Each participant potentially represents a different perspective on a situation and sometimes these perspectives will conflict or contradict each other. Moreover, these relationships are enacted within an ambiguous wider policy context which exerts an influence on day-to-day practice as well as local policies and procedures. The nurse has a role in mediating the different perspectives of each of the participants. This process can be described as the 'micro-politics' of mental health care in contrast to the 'macro-politics' of broad policy debate and formulation.

Sometimes, policies exert pressures in opposite directions. An example of this is that, on the one hand, policy and professional practice aims to promote the involvement and autonomy of service users. On the other hand, policies also emphasize risk management and the protection of the public. It does not mean that these two policy pressures are irreconcilable. However, to overcome this dilemma mental health nurses and other practitioners are required to mediate the systemic pressure (see Chapter 16: A Systemic Approach to Violence Risk Assessment and Management) and tensions between the two policy directions. It is the outcome of such micro-political activity that can make a crucial difference for the mental health service user. Given the current focus on increasing professional accountability the danger is that mental health practitioners will err on the side of caution and favour the latter objective over the former.

Mental health nurses are faced with numerous similar dilemmas in their day-to-day practice. Given the significance of the outcome of such practice dilemmas, mental health nurses are in a potentially powerful position for two contrasting reasons. First, nursing has aspired to professional status. Within this professional perspective practice decisions are based on a body of expertise. Such claims to expertise are seen as a source of professional power. There is an extensive literature on the sociology of professions and debate as to the extent to which nursing matches these characteristics (Abbott and Wallace, 1990). Nevertheless, it is a perspective that the development of 'evidence-based practice' tends to reinforce (Forchuk, 2001).

A second important potential source of power in the micro-politics of care is the role mental health nurses play as front-line practitioners in implementing policy initiatives. Lipsky (1980) conceptualized front-line practitioners as 'street-level bureaucrats'. He examined what happens at the point where policy is translated into practice in various human service bureaucracies such as schools, courts and welfare agencies. According to Lipsky, street-level bureaucrats work in complex situations. Policy aims and organizational goals are rarely prescribed in detail and this means practice situations become socially *negotiated* encounters. This potentially gives practitioners a high degree of discretion in mediating between the different participants within a practice situation and when making practice decisions. One danger is that in exercising their discretion, practitioners can take up partial positions. Such discretion allows practitioners considerable power in relation to service users.

Where different participants within the practice situation have different perspectives, the situation itself is open to different interpretations. This means that mental health nurses cannot always be certain in the professional judgements that they make; their judgements will be open to question (see Chapter 6: Truth, Uncertainty and the Mental Health Nurse). If true account is given to users' perspectives, the relationship between mental health nurses and service users, rather than being hierarchical, as with the conventional understanding of professional expertise, should be collaborative, compassionate, recognizing the validity of service users' interpretations and their lived experiences (see Chapter 2: Rebuilding Lives: A Critical Look at the Contemporary Role of the Mental Health Nurse and Chapter 4: Compassion) (Winter and Maisch, 1996). Professionals, therefore, do not have a monopoly over expertise, and user 'expertise' (for example, expertise in their own experience) should be integrated into the process of reaching 'practice decisions' (DH, 2001b).

Such a process entails a high degree of sensitivity on the part of mental health nurses. Thus, an alternative way of responding to complex practice situations is to adopt the model of the 'reflective practitioner' (Schön, 1991). Schön's well-known exposition of the reflective practitioner points out that 'the technical-rationality' model on which the conventional view of professional expertise is based, has limits. This is because of the very complexity of practice situations confronted by human professions such as mental health nursing. In such circumstances, professional expertise is unable to furnish all the answers as many situations have unique qualities, including different values and interpretations of the situation arising from different participants. Expertise is viewed as situational rather than arising from technical-rationality. Professional expertise and professional judgements are founded on the meanings and interpretations of participants within practice situations.

The reflective practitioner must, therefore, necessarily be a collaborative practitioner. Schön emphasizes that the reflective model of professional work requires a professional–client relationship based on a dialogue with service users. The reflective practitioner:

. . . recognises that his [sic] actions may have different meanings for his client than he intends them to have, and he gives himself the task of discovering what these are. He recognises an obligation to make his own understandings accessible to his clients, which means that he needs often to reflect anew on what he knows . . . The reflective practitioner tries to discover the limits of his expertise through reflective conversation with the client (Schön, 1991, pp. 295–296).

Such an approach has far-reaching implications on the nature of the mental health nurse–service user relationship. The idea of reflective practice is not new and much has been written to guide nurses (for example, Bulman and Schutz, 2004). However, one aspect of this approach which is worth assigning greater emphasis is the potential empowerment of service users through the decentralization of expertise which reflective practice should entail.

CONCLUSION

Service user involvement has become much more of a reality in recent years. However, because of the rapid advances made there is a danger that complacency will stifle developments in this. Policy ambiguities and a failure to translate values into practice are potential barriers to further development. It must also be acknowledged that short-comings in how effective mental health services are at being user-sensitive are unfortunately not confined to history. Current organizational practices that are explicitly intended to be user-focused, such as the Care Programme Approach, have encountered difficulties in meeting this objective (Social Services Inspectorate, 2002; Healthcare Commission, 2006b). Even recent experience of some in-patient settings has led some users to feel unsafe and perceive the environment as custodial and untherapeutic (SCMH, 1998, 2005; DH, 2004b), and some users from minority ethnic groups experience particularly coercive forms of intervention (SCMH, 2002; Bhui *et al.*, 2003; Blofeld, 2004). Recent debates about the reform of the Mental Health Act 1983 (House of Commons, 2005) raise concerns about the perpetuation of power differentials within the mental health system, and many service users continue to experience social exclusion (Healthcare Commission, 2005).

Overall, user involvement still has some way to go then. If it is to develop further, a number of obstacles have to be overcome. These include: achievement of social change through strategies to reduce stigma and promote social inclusion (see Chapter 8: Challenging Stigma and Promoting Social Justice); strengthening service and organizational developments that are predicated on working in partnership with service users (see Chapter 2: Rebuilding Lives: A Critical Look at the Contemporary Role of the Mental Health Nurse); and changes in initial and ongoing education and training of mental health professionals. However, it is arguable that the most important barrier to overcome is the value-bases of individual nurses and other practitioners (see Chapter 5: The Implications of Values-Based Practice in Mental Health Nursing). There is likely to be a need, therefore, to teach nurses the skills for collaborative working and service users' involvement, and as such the role of nurses in day-to-day engagement with service users will be a central issue that requires attention (Callaghan and Owen, 2005). Furthermore, this will require organizational systems which support, facilitate and sustain attempts by mental health nurses to develop user-focused care (Simpson and House, 2003).

CHAPTER 4
COMPASSION

Jonathon E. Lynch and
Steve Trenoweth

How could we understand how someone has become sunk into despair, or a prisoner of their fears, or persecuted by voices, unless we are prepared to be a compassionate presence in their search for meaning in the psychological, social, spiritual or bodily dimensions of their experience? (Watkins, 2001, p. 45)

INTRODUCTION

Despite the widespread belief that compassion is at the very heart of nursing and relationships with clients (Watkins, 2001; Krumberger, 2002; NMC, 2006a; Sabo, 2006), the concept may well prove problematic for some mental health practitioners. This is not to suggest that such individuals are cold and uncaring, rather that they find the concept of 'compassion' unsuitable or inappropriate and, perhaps, out of step with a health care agenda which stresses the importance of sound evidence and transparent clinical decision making. It may imply to them, subjectivity, sentimentality and a subsequent weakness that reduces one's professional capability. However, this is by no means a uniform view. Lakeman (2003), for example, utilizes a less restricted and, arguably, more apposite description, citing compassion as one of several approaches valuable to mental health nursing practice and characterized by values reflective of a capacity to share another person's suffering and appreciate her/his humanity and vulnerability.

'Compassion' is not a common feature of mental health care discourses. While there are some notable exceptions, such as Watkins' (2001) *Mental Health Nursing: The Art of Compassionate Care*, the indices of mental health nursing books, and the keywords cited in articles, rarely list the word. Certainly, there is mention of 'care',

Contemporary Issues in Mental Health Nursing, Edited by J. E. Lynch and S. Trenoweth
© 2008 John Wiley & Sons, Ltd

'empathy' and positive 'attitudes' in many, and these often lead to notions that are relevant to, and supportive of, the point of concern in this chapter. Nevertheless, it will be argued here that there is insufficient attention to 'compassion' in contemporary mental health care provision, despite arguments that a compassionate approach can support ethical dimensions of practice (Lakeman, 2003). Of greatest importance, however, is that approaches which can be described as compassionate mark the type of experiences that remain significant for clients in their recovery and are reflective of high-quality mental health nursing care (Beech and Norman, 1995). In this chapter, we discuss how a lack of compassion might develop within mental health practice, and how the wider socio-political climate can impact on the compassionate delivery of care.

A LACK OF COMPASSION?

Compassion, in its purest sense, represents a sincere, authentic and genuine desire to offer positive help to someone who is suffering or in distress. It denotes concepts of sympathy and kindness, and implies tolerance, acceptance and an empathic understanding and concern for the plight of another. However, being compassionate does not require an overt demonstration of significant emotion in the strictest sense.

There are, of course, many individual examples of day-to-day mental health nursing care which are compassionate and sensitive, given freely by empathic, understanding staff, who feel that care is best facilitated in a positive interpersonal climate within which clients feel understood and supported (Kelly and Gamble, 2005). Such examples of care deserve recognition and celebration. However, anecdotal evidence can also be heard from those who work in mental health nursing and from those who receive care that professionals often seem to lack compassion (Drury, 2006). Furthermore, the health care literature also attests to a lack of empathy and caring concern amongst some professionals (Herdman, 2004), and mental health nurses in particular (Reynolds and Scott, 2000) (see Chapter 2: Rebuilding Lives: A Critical Look at the Contemporary Role of the Mental Health Nurse).

Television documentaries have also sought to highlight the lack of care and compassion offered to some of the most vulnerable members of society. For example, the treatment of the residents of a privately run facility for people with learning disabilities investigated surreptitiously by the BBC's investigative reporter Donal McIntyre and broadcast in 1999 as part of the *McIntyre Undercover* series. Working as an unqualified carer, McIntyre secretly filmed daily life using a hidden camera attached to his clothing. Life for residents and staff, it seemed, was marked not by some mundane though comfortable stability but by a distinct tension between parties who had become polarized. At the root of it all seemed to be an institutionalized lack of compassion for the residents which apparently meant that some members of staff were not sufficiently (if at all) perturbed to challenge others, nor were they moved to complain in the face of overt abuse or neglect. Once such seeds have been sown there is a greater likelihood not only that abuses can occur, but that poor-quality, unprofessional practices can be established and perpetuated. Abuse becomes, in effect, 'custom and practice' – part of the accepted and unchallenged culture of a ward, unit or service into which new recruits are socialized. Though the abuses referred to in the *McIntyre Undercover* programme occurred in a setting for people with learning disabilities, there is no room for complacency in mental health. This is especially so in settings where clients are likely to remain for relatively long periods, as these seem to appear more frequently in reported cases of alleged and substantiated abuse (see Sayce, 1995).

Such practices, once established, can be very difficult to address. People tend to learn from each other and, crucially, as neophytes invariably want to 'fit in' at work they may be particularly inclined to follow what appear to be established ways of working, including unwritten strategies for coping with conflict and shortcuts to getting the 'job' done. Indeed, it is interesting that the acts or behaviour of professionals that can be criticized as lacking compassion are frequently characterized by passivity rather than activity. These failures to act, or, at least, the imposition of limits upon acting, seem more likely to occur when nurses lose sight of a wider picture and fail to recognize or to accept the requirement for basic humanity in the support of vulnerable people. As such, a focus on compassionate care can potentially mitigate abuse and be the driver to deliver proactive and appropriate help to the person in distress.

TOUGH TIMES?

Power is notoriously imbalanced in mental health care. Indeed, Whittington and Balsamo (1998) suggest that some hostility from clients may be rooted in a desire to acquire what Foucalt (1977) famously referred to as a 'temporary inversion' of established power relations. In other words, if clients feel devoid of any power or influence, and this feeling is reinforced by their continuing experiences of care, interpersonal conflict may be one of the few ways in which they can bring about change, albeit briefly.

The tougher the environment appears, the more valuable power becomes. Matters such as toughness and non-compassion may have always existed here and there in mental health care (Morrison, 1990), but could it be that any contemporary concerns are symptomatic of societal shifts and priorities? Garland (2001), for example, has argued that the present era is one of greater 'punitive' ideals from politicians and public alike, who appear to increasingly lack tolerance for those who harm, threaten or abuse others, in any form. Indeed, the first decade of the millennium has already witnessed some startling world events, and modern technology has allowed millions to watch some of these almost as they have occurred, such as the attack on the World Trade Center on September 11, 2001. This 'front row seat' has made tragedies seem even more poignant and more personally relevant. Any personal fear and distress related to such events may reinforce perceptions of the need to effectively and decisively 'deal with' people considered 'problematic' and harmful to society (Lehane, 1996) in order to ensure that such tragedies never occur again. Any such shift in public perceptions, therefore, may not be related to *vindictiveness* but may certainly be more consistent with moral indignation (Young, 2002) and the perceived need for tighter restrictions on freedom to ensure personal and national security. Indeed, some commentators have suggested that, particularly in the Western World, this tough approach may be reflective of a much wider political refocusing on a more fundamentalist and authoritarian structure to control levels of uncertainty and risk in society and a changing geopolitical context (see Chapter 6: Truth, Uncertainty and the Mental Health Nurse). Sorrentino and Roney (2000, p. 2), for example, see such toughness as '. . . a reflection of people's hopes of controlling uncertainty wrought by globalisation, industry downsizing or restructuring, national debt concerns . . . and limited resources for health and education'.

So, are contemporary mainstream social attitudes in England and Wales tough, unforgiving and uncompromising? Certain aspects of social policy may seem to be so. For example, in the criminal justice field the prison population has continued to rise even through times when recorded crime has dropped. The United Kingdom has the highest rate of imprisonment in the European Union (Home Office, 2003) and at the time of writing there are too few prison places to accommodate 'demand'. The imprisonment rate for England and Wales is around twice that of Northern Ireland and higher than Scotland; a contributing factor, no doubt, to the persistent demand for, and pressure on, forensic mental health services. Furthermore, although cautious about drawing conclusions from differing data from differing countries, Goldson and Coles (2005) calculated that children are 130 times more likely to be detained in penal custody here than in Finland. With a similar number of children in the population and some consistencies in social problems, France may be better for 'comparing like with like', yet the custodial rate there is approximately four times lower.

If society has become tougher and less tolerant in recent years, apparently requiring more control over its citizens to combat perceived uncertainty and risk (see Chapter 6: Truth, Uncertainty and the Mental Health Nurse), it should not be assumed that mental health care practitioners and practices are insulated from such pressures. Indeed, it has been argued that pervading societal attitudes and influences are not unfelt at a clinical or organizational level. Indeed, as Playle (1995, p. 982) argued:

Nursing functions within a political climate and the potential influence of this . . . cannot be ignored.

NURSING EDUCATION

Having been short of mental health nurses throughout the decade and with demographic analyses predicting worse to come, the late 1990s saw the start of the recruitment and education of large numbers of people to provide the care that had been available in a patchy fashion in parts of the country. London, in particular, was desperate for registered nurses to work in mental health. As a response, July 2000 saw the publication of the 'NHS Plan' (DH, 2000a), which made formal a drive to expand the numbers and roles of nurses. However, the positive foresight that spurred on the creation of hundreds of places for trainee nurses failed to take into account two significant issues. The first was that they would have to be taught in clinical practice. There were simply too few registered nurses to cope with the large numbers of students and, to make matters worse, too few nurses were able to offer the necessary time required to support students and too little attention was paid to their own developmental needs for the preparation of others. Furthermore, the delivery of the new pre-registration nursing programmes effectively required cultural shifts and different ways of working. Clinical services were required to work in partnership with their Higher Education Institutions (HEI) and to accept more responsibilities for the education and development of student nurses (Watkins, 2000). There were additional requirements for, and pressures on, clinical services within a modernizing health care environment, such as responding to increasing demands for, and expectations of, improved clinical interventions and a more assured responsiveness to improving the health of the community (Scott, 2004). As a consequence, concerns have been raised in recent years regarding the quality of clinical placements for student nurses, both in terms of their ability to offer meaningful learning opportunities and in their commitment to the student's experience (Mullen and Murray, 2002).

The second oversight was the apparent assumption that it would be easy to recruit many times more students than in previous decades. This rested on the notion that large numbers of adequately qualified and suitable people were waiting to apply. In order to meet recruitment targets the net was widened, one 'selling' point being the opportunity for new entrants to acquire both academic and professional qualifications which may have had a subsequent impact on health care education. It is not suggested here, however, that the large cohorts of students recruited over the last 10 years comprise only individuals who would have been rejected in other times and under different circumstances. This is clearly not the case – the majority of students that we come into contact with on a daily basis are thoughtful, committed and caring people. However, the circumstances outlined above were bound to increase the chances of applications from people with more instrumental reasons for becoming mental health nurses. Amid the immense numbers of students recruited and trained, some may have seen mental health nursing as simply an 'insurance policy' – an occupation, at best, but not necessarily a vocation. Such an instrumental, 'means to an end' approach to a mental health nursing career contrasts sharply with a sincere desire to offer compassionate help and care for those experiencing mental distress.

Furthermore, while positive, compassionate mental health care may never have been uniformly present in this country any more than it has been entirely absent, could any perception of a decline in 'compassion' in practice be related to a shift in the focus and context of nursing education? Clarke (1999a) points out that in the 1980s and early

1990s the thinking of mental health nursing students in Britain was influenced (perhaps disproportionately) by the humanistic writings of Carl Rogers, with his emphasis on psychological counselling. Rogers espoused an accessible conceptualization of clinical relations and contexts and the language he used was adopted and used in Schools of Nursing around the country. In the mid-1990s, nurse education left the hospital-based colleges of nursing and moved to HEIs. This was considered necessary to ensure that the professional standing of nursing could improve and then keep up with other disciplines through advances in awareness of research, critical thinking and other fundamental concepts associated with progressive professionalism and ideologies (Thompson and Watson, 2001; Burke, 2003) (see Chapter 6: Truth, Uncertainty and the Mental Health Nurse).

So, with the physical move to HEIs came an apparent ideological shift to more scientific, evidence-based approaches and:

. . . the integration of nursing into higher education has contributed to an emphasis on cognitive skills, which may result in a diminished attention to expressive caring [and] disengagement or lack of empathy, and it is this lack of empathy that is of concern in the nursing profession (Herdman, 2004, p. 97).

If anything, this has thrown the debate regarding the tension between the theoretical and practical nature of nursing (Butterworth *et al.*, 1999; Wilson-Barnett, 2006) into sharp relief and perhaps this debate is of greater importance today than it was before the move to higher education (Fletcher, 1997a). Indeed, nursing, it seems, holds an uneasy position in the academic world (Parish, 2004). Interviewers/recruiters of students to academic programmes may be more focused on the economic survival of the HEI (Fletcher, 1997b) and on an applicant's ability to meet academic demands rather than on their capacity for caring and compassion.

OBJECTIVITY AND INTERPERSONAL DISTANCE

The modern health care policy context seemingly emphasizes the technical aspects of nursing care, reflective of what Herdman (2004) refers to as a 'post-emotional' society. Indeed, emphasis is often placed on the need for a lack of *personal* involvement with the people our work is intended to assist. This allows, it is assumed, a 'clear head' and objective decision making. It is argued that professional carers cannot help their clients if they are too close to their difficulties/problems in an emotional sense. This may lead to an inaccurate assessment of clients' 'real' needs or, at worst, take carers into unprofessional territory characterized by loose boundaries. Such an involvement may render professional judgements subjective and open to accusations of non-professionalism by virtue of having lost a rational perspective.

The 'technical-rationality' model assumed that knowledge precedes practice; 'knowing what' is required before 'knowing how'. Subsequently, a key requirement is the application of one's knowledge of sound evidence to underpin clinical practice and assist decision making in a manner which can be empirically validated (Stuart, 2001). Such 'technical-rationality' is seen to banish subjective probabilities and systematic biases which can lead to 'erroneous' clinical assessments. In this sense, clinical interventions need to be as sterile as the 'aseptic techniques' used for controlling infection. So, just as gloves and apron form a barrier that offers protection against infection, a lack of emotional connectedness, it is assumed, forms a barrier against psychological 'contamination'.

It is little wonder, then, that compassion might be seen to represent the shedding of a professional veneer. We concur that interacting with, and attempting to support, a distressed client would be made very difficult, and perhaps impossible, should the carer be similarly distressed or immobilized by the client's circumstances. Nevertheless, compassion is a realistic and, indeed, a practised feature in mental health care, marking many of the relationships and interventions that clients value highly (Barker, 2004) and feel beneficial to them. Indeed, compassion is unlikely to be perceived on occasions when injustice or punishment is sensed (cf. Kumar *et al.*, 2001; Sequeira and Halstead, 2002). Indeed, those occasions when nurses feel it is necessary to intervene and/or challenge clients may be especially likely to convey messages about how they *really* perceive clients, how confident they feel about their roles and responsibilities, and the durability of relationships at times of difficulty.

While an evidence-based practice 'technical-rationality' model does not necessarily preclude compassionate care (Glazer, 2002), it has been argued that it can discourage it (Herdman, 2004). Slavish adherence to, and unthinking adoption of, such reductionistic, 'psychotechnological' approaches may be out of keeping with the hopes and aspirations of client/service user groups (Barker *et al.*, 1999), for whom trusting and supportive interpersonal relationships are often seen as central to recovery (Kelly and Gamble, 2005). Indeed, for Herdman (2004) the emphasis on 'technical-rationality' has created a 'McDonaldization' of nursing care with a corresponding lack of authenticity characterized by '. . . synthetic, manufactured emotions manipulated and standardized for mass consumption' (Herdman, 2004, p. 95). She continues:

The fast-food restaurant represents a contemporary paradigm of this process of rationalization. It involves increased efficiency, predictability, calculability and control of the labour process. The result is greater productivity, dehumanization and homogenization (Herdman, 2004, p. 96).

Moreover, the increasingly technological context of modern health care (Sabo, 2006) may be 'alienating' for some and create a mechanical form of nursing, reduced to a discrete set of work tasks. In such cases, the client is an 'object' of clinical work or an 'other' who is intrinsically different. And it is here that the seeds of separateness and stigmatization are sown.

For Buber, such 'otherness' found expression in his seminal work *Ich und Du* (Buber, 1923/2004), translated as 'I and Thou'. 'I' and 'Thou' relationships involve meaningful mutual dialogue and authentic engagement, whereas 'Ich und Es' ('I and It') relationships are unidirectional, consisting of egocentric monologues and a distinct separateness. Buber believed these latter, 'Ich–Es' relationships lay at the root of many societal problems including, for example, dehumanization, stigmatization and demonization of the 'other' (see Chapter 8: Challenging Stigma and Promoting Social Justice; Chapter 9: Homophobia in Mental Health Services and Chapter 19: Masculinity as a Risk Variable in Physical and Mental Ill Health). Indeed, separateness was, for Heidegger (1977), a form of 'enframing' – the objectification of nature through technology – which threatens the ability of human beings to understand our world and our 'being' in the Universe.

The objectification of client care potentially leads to a 'production line' mentality (Bevan, 1998), where 'care' is reduced to discrete units of productivity or tasks which are to be achieved. Through such 'conveyor belt' means of production (Herdman, 2004), nursing 'work' may become alienating and disempowering – a means to an end and not something of intrinsic worth, and for Marx, when individuals lose control over their work, they lose control over their lives:

The object produced by labour, its product, now stands opposed to it as an alien being, as a power independent of the producer . . . The more the worker expends himself [sic] in work the more powerful becomes the world of objects which he creates in face of himself, the poorer he becomes in his inner life, and the less he belongs to himself (Marx, 1964, p. 122).

This sort of climate routinizes and dehumanizes work, and facilitates the belief that work can be undertaken by anyone capable of utilizing the appropriate 'technology'. Indeed, routinization of work has been described as a way in which 'staff stay in contact with their patients, but leave them emotionally' (Rees, 2000, p. 44). Without careful thought, mental health nursing may be 'enframed' by reducing it to a set of objectively defined and predetermined targets. When this is complemented by ideologies that see, evaluate and even reward clinical nursing 'competence' through purely behavioural lenses (actions to be completed and recorded), compassion is unlikely to be seen as necessary, and may even be perceived as redundant. As a consequence, the bigger picture (the phenomenology of clients' experiences and its emotional resonance) is neither apparent nor considered relevant to the nursing 'task' being 'performed'.

DEVELOPING COMPASSIONATE CARE

The challenge in developing and supporting compassionate care is the creation of an environment within which it can flourish, and, perhaps, in which it is expected. There are many potential barriers to the development of such environments. Certainly, the working practices and culture of services alluded to previously in this chapter can be a major handicap to the development of compassionate care. Indeed, Morrison (1990) argues that a lack of adequately trained, educated, supervised and supported staff can create 'tough' environments which prioritize physical restraint, enforced rules and the adoption of practices somewhat akin to a police force. Furthermore, an emphasis on a tough approach to controlling others, and on maintaining order, and a general atmosphere of authoritarianism is unlikely to be viewed as compassionate and is more likely to lead to tension and fear (Rees, 2000) or to be a precursor to violent behaviour (Morrison, 1990) (see Chapter 17: No Euphemisms: The Use of Force in Mental Health Care).

It is not possible for every interaction between mental health professionals and clients to be monitored or regulated, and it is not argued here that it would be necessary or desirable even if it was possible. The fostering of suitable and professionally acceptable values and attitudes is crucial, though (see Chapter 5: The Implications of Values-Based Practice in Mental Health Nursing). Self-awareness skills should be (re-)highlighted in clinical and educational contexts to assist the development and maintenance of supportive, professional practices which encourage normative aspects of practice and behaviour. This requires greater emphasis on the socialization of those entering mental health care, at pre-registration education level and also at clinical organization inductions, where explicit attention should be paid to the development of values-based practice imbalances in power relations between providers and recipients of care (see Chapter 5: The Implications of Values-Based Practice in Mental Health Nursing).

Certainly, an awareness of 'self' is often seen as an essential part of relationship development with clients. With ongoing development and reflective analysis, self-awareness can be crucial to the monitoring and maintenance of normative practice standards and a focus upon the clients' experiences of care. One element of this is a public self-awareness, seeing oneself as a *social* being and attempting to identify how one is seen by others (Baron and Richardson, 1994). A second feature of 'self-awareness' is the construction and maintenance of values that encourage matters such as tolerance of clients and acceptable ways of interacting at times of interpersonal conflict. Where they exist, these background conditions reinforce the unacceptability of hostility to clients in a general sense. If hostility occurs, a vicarious lesson may be learned by witnessing repercussions such as expressed peer concern, formal regulation and admonition. Underpinning both foreground and background, solid and resolute, unseen and unmoveable care which is based on genuine and authentic compassion can support and guide nurses. At the most tense of times – for example, when interpersonal conflict peaks and/or potentially serious incidents occur – it assists in ensuring that actions are directed towards the needs of the clients.

Indeed, a marked professionalism is what separates – or should separate – specially trained and educated people from individuals who may be well-intentioned and sincere contributors, but who lack clinical knowledge and professional accountability. Many attitudes towards mentally unwell people stem from wider social contexts and assumptions, including those in which they are portrayed as highly unpredictable (see Chapter 6: Truth, Uncertainty and the Mental Health Nurse), incapable of reason and thereby only manageable through coercion (see Chapter 17: No Euphemisms: The Use of Force in Mental Health Care). Subsequently, some may be treated inconsiderately, harshly perhaps, and without compassion, because of the anxiety they imbue in others (see Chapter 16: A Systemic Approach to Violence Risk Assessment and Management). There is evidence of this in specific occupational cultures (see Green and Ward, 2004), in which force is seen as an acceptable tool in an armoury of pragmatic and symbolic power (Hobbs *et al.*, 2003, p. 150).

Could a lack of compassion also be a form of emotional 'self-defence' – a perceived need to keep people in distress at arm's length for fear of becoming distressed oneself? Sabo (2006) found that caring for people who are suffering and in distress can lead to compassion fatigue, a finding echoed in the works of Menzies (1959) and Mann and Cowburn (2005). Compassionate care is thus a double-edged sword – an essential foundation for nursing practice but a source of distress and 'vicarious traumatisation' which subsequently reduces our capacity to care (Collins and Long, 2003; Sabo, 2006) (see Chapter 18: The Psychological Impact of Restraint: Examining the Aftermath for Staff and Patients). Nurses see and assimilate what goes on in clinical life. Indeed, we are all encouraged to *reflect* upon, and connect with, what takes place in clinical practice and learn from it. For some, however, an emotional distance and lack of engagement may seem to be the best method of self-preservation – a protection against the pain and suffering of others (see Chapter 16: A Systemic Approach to Violence Risk Assessment and Management), particularly when the focus of clinical nursing practice is on the 'doing' rather than the 'being'. As such, '. . . the emotional ingredient in . . . practice has been increasingly devalued, while the instrumental ingredient has been increasingly valued. As a consequence, the cost to the provider of emotional labour has perhaps been overlooked' (Phillips, 1996). Perhaps, one such consequence has been the high levels of stress experienced by mental health nurses in an increasingly outcome-orientated system (Tuck, 1997) and the scant attention paid to how emotional work can be supported and developed in clinical nursing practice (Lützén and Schreiber, 1998; Mann and Cowburn, 2005).

CONCLUSION

Compassion comprises a set of attributes, values, beliefs and behaviours which belies the inevitable simplification and lexicological reductionism found in dictionary definitions. Moreover, as Morrison-Valfre (2005) points out, compassion is a key feature of mental health care, indicative perhaps of the moral health of individuals and services but ultimately an undervalued and poorly recognized attribute. However, from September 2008 'care and compassion' will be a 'visible and identifiable' feature of pre-registration nursing programmes via the introduction of the Essential Skills Clusters

(ESC), which will support and complement existing standards of proficiency (NMC, 2006a). Furthermore, the lost ground in some settings in terms of the development of compassionate care must be regained by nurses and all mental health care professionals, and this can only be achieved through combinations of self-motivation, intolerance of poor practices, and supportive leadership at both clinical and managerial levels.

We do not wish to argue that compassionate care is to be valued over, or should even replace, evidence-based care. That has not been our intention in this chapter. Clearly, compassion is not, in and of itself, enough to assist clients on their journeys to recovery, but then again neither is evidence-based care which is focused solely on improving clinical outcomes. It is our contention that quality mental health nursing care is not only a feature of the skills and knowledge of the nurse, but that a genuine feeling of concern and compassion for another in distress is an important precursor and the foundation for effective care (Watkins, 2001). We further contend that a lack of compassion in contemporary mental health care is a significant obstacle to overall quality care provision.

CHAPTER 5
THE IMPLICATIONS OF VALUES-BASED PRACTICE IN MENTAL HEALTH NURSING

Ian Price

INTRODUCTION

The growth of the mental health service user movement in the United Kingdom over the last 20 years has been dramatic. Whereas there were only six independent user groups available for consultation during the drafting of the Mental Health Act 1983 (Campbell, 1996b), today service users are, in theory and in many instances in practice, an integral part of activity involving mental health services at all levels (see Chapter 3: User Involvement and the Micro-Politics of Mental Health Care). Numerous initiatives are now aimed at embedding such involvement even deeper in all aspects of service planning and delivery. This increase in the influence of the user perspective has challenged many professional practices and, more importantly, the values that underpin these and has resulted in explicit consideration being given to the values necessary for appropriate practice. The concept of 'values-based practice' has emerged from this context and has, in turn, become influential in development of policy and supporting guidance (DH, 2004a). This chapter explores the ethical challenges posed by the growth of user influence on mental health services with specific emphasis on the implications of values-based practice for the ethical basis for the relationship between mental health nurses and users.

Contemporary Issues in Mental Health Nursing, Edited by J. E. Lynch and S. Trenoweth
© 2008 John Wiley & Sons, Ltd

THE POLICY CONTEXT

The development of values-based practice reflects an explicit change in how contemporary care should be delivered. For example, the values of consumerism which characterize the shift from modernism to post-modernism can be seen in the drive towards a patient-led NHS (DH, 2005b) with its increasing emphasis on choice, individualized care and empowerment. In order for services to deliver these goals, preferences, concerns and expectations of patients, their values must not only be identified but also be integrated into decisions about care and treatment. It is this challenge that values-based practice addresses. 'Creating a Patient-Led NHS' (DH, 2005b), while assuming a great deal of progress, sets out intentions to bring about even more profound change. Described as changes to the whole system of providing health care, these ambitions include the introduction of more choice and more personalized care to bring about even more empowerment of the public. This is explicitly identified as requiring a fundamental change in the nature of the relationship between the service and the public from a position where the service does things *for* and *to* patients to a patient-led service which works *with* individuals to help them meet *their* health care needs (see Chapter 10: The Meaning of Recovery). This intention is supported by further best practice guidance (DH, 2005c) designed to help Trust boards respond to the workforce planning and development implications of policy by aligning local workforce strategies with major service goals. One major assumption of the guidance is that the *way* in which practitioners work (as distinct from *what* they do) is key to the success of the government's reform agenda and that for the NHS to become truly patient-led a change of culture is required. The guidance goes on to identify that truly patient-led services will necessitate appropriate behaviour by practitioners in *every* interaction with the public and that 'a step change in working differently' is required.

The values-based practice framework appears to complement the drive towards user and carer involvement seen within mental health services over the last 20 years. Indeed, more specific workforce development initiatives in more recent years have explicitly reinforced the need for such involvement. The Capable Practitioner (SCMH, 2001a) explicitly identifies the necessary values for mental health practice as part of a wider range of knowledge, skills and attitudes necessary to implement the National Service Framework for Mental Health (DH, 1999a). These include the ability to 'encourage self-determination and freedom of choice'. The 'Ten Essential Shared Capabilities' framework (DH, 2004a) identifies the basic building blocks for all mental health staff (whether professionally qualified or not) working in any sector and significantly gives evidence-based and values-based practice equal prominence (see Chapter 2: Rebuilding Lives: A Critical Look at the Contemporary Role of the Mental Health Nurse). The capabilities include ways of working that are clearly compatible with values-based practice, which is not surprising as they are explicitly based on the National Institute for Mental Health England Framework of Values developed by Woodbridge and

Fulford (2004). At the heart of this framework, alongside the need for recognition of the role played by values and for raising awareness of values, is the requirement to practice in a manner 'that makes the principle of service-user centrality a unifying focus for practice'. This means that 'the values of each service user/client and their communities must be the starting point and key determinant for all actions by professionals' (Woodbridge and Fulford, 2004).

The 'recovery approach' is also central to creating a need for change in the nature of the relationship between service users and practitioners (see Chapter 10: The Meaning of Recovery). In many ways, as it has been developed by service users themselves, the increasing influence of the recovery approach is an example of the success of service user involvement (DH, 2001a). The recovery approach attaches importance to the service users' experiences of the process of empowerment that leads to more fulfilling and meaningful lives rather than to what services do *for* people, often in response to crisis (NIMHE, 2005). More specifically in relation to nursing, the Chief Nursing Officer's Review of Mental Health Nursing recommends the adoption of the 'broad principles' of the recovery approach although it stops short of explicitly discussing values-based practice. It also acknowledges that practitioners' values influence their practice (DH, 2006a). This espousal of the recovery approach (and by extension, the underpinning values) challenges the view that the need for greater consideration of values arises more from a lack of awareness rather than from fundamental incompatibility between professional and lay values (Fulford and Williams, 2003) and means that practitioners must be much more aware of the origins of their own professional values.

WHAT ARE VALUES?

To explore the concepts of 'values-based practice' it is necessary to consider what is meant by 'values'. The terms *values* and *values-based practice* are increasingly commonplace, both in government policy and supporting frameworks and guidance and in professional literature. However, as is often the case in health care, defining a term in common usage is less than straightforward and the term is often used to reflect a variety of meanings. This confusion is increased by the tendency to use it interchangeably or in combination with other terms, e.g. 'principles and values' or 'moral values'. A lack of clear meaning is compounded by the fact that a definition or description of values is seldom made clear. The NIMHE Guiding Statement on Recovery, for example, which is based on clearly articulated values, does not explicitly define what is meant by the term 'valuse' (NIMHE, 2005). However, definition is crucial if diverse, taken-for-granted assumptions about the meaning of the term and accompanying uncertainty and confusion are to be avoided. Furthermore, a lack of definition and understanding also creates the risk of a superficial adoption of what is assumed to be values-based practice but which in fact reflects no meaningful change. Indeed, clarification is essential to avoid a 'values myopia' – the inclination to presuppose that our values are the same as others (Fulford and Williams, 2003).

If we are to understand the term in relation to mental health services, it is instructive to look at other possible meanings and contexts in which the word has been used. Values are currently debated in numerous contexts, including political, moral and religious. In such usage, the term is commonly used to describe principles, attitudes or beliefs. The Chambers English Dictionary defines *value* (in the singular) as (among other meanings) 'that which renders anything useful or estimable'. This strongly suggests that when considering actions with which the term is associated (for example, values-based practice) these are assumed to have a *positive* effect. This is supported by other meanings given, which include 'high worth', 'intrinsic worth or goodness' and 'efficacy'. The Chambers English Dictionary also defines *values* (in the plural) as 'moral principles' or 'standards', highlighting a meaning of the term probably closer to that employed when used in a health care context. Pendleton and King (2002) have described 'values' from a professional perspective as 'deeply held views that act as guiding principles for individuals and organisations'. That such views are deeply held suggests that values are ingrained and an integral part of what makes us who we are; in the case of professional mental health nursing practice, a part of what gives nurses their sense of professional identity and shapes their practice.

The term 'values' in health and social care has a more distinct and specific meaning than that used in many lay contexts. Hugman (2005) describes how, in this context, the term is taken specifically to mean a set of fundamental moral or ethical principles, often explicitly and formally set out in codes of conduct or of ethics. It is therefore possible to discuss the values of a particular profession by reference to such codes. This professional interpretation of 'values' is indicative of the belief that the caring professions attach as much importance to the moral or ethical dimension of their practice as to the knowledge or technical skills employed (Hugman, 2005).

WHERE DO OUR PROFESSIONAL VALUES COME FROM?

'Values-based practice' requires that values are explicitly considered when determining professional actions and that appropriate values are developed to enable specific policy imperatives to be achieved (Fulford and Williams, 2003). To understand professional values and the challenges posed by the development of values-based practice, it is helpful to examine the origins of such values. To do so, it is necessary to consider briefly the development of ethics in the modern and post-modern eras and the resultant values and practices (Hugman, 2005).

For the modern era, the principles of objectivity, rationalism, empiricism, universalism and individualism have created the underpinnings of the scientific foundations for health care professions, including nursing. Generally, this is characterized by the objectification of disease in which this is seen as an entity separate from the subjective experience of the sufferer; this was accompanied by a shift in the response to such experiences from private or local level to institutional settings (Bury, 1998). Specifically in the field of mental health, this was inextricably linked to the development of psychiatry as a medical discipline and the power and influence acquired as a result through the development of the asylum system. Consequently, psychiatry became a 'bounded profession', with sole knowledge of and control over the responses to illness and other perspectives becoming marginalized. This involved the lay person becoming a 'patient', passively accepting expert interventions and in the case of the mentally ill subjected to coercive social controls (Bury, 1998). Objectification, therefore, is characterized by an emphasis on the importance of professional knowledge and expertise and a consequent separation of aspects of an individual's experience, in this case mental illness, from everyday life. Porter (1987) felt that one perspective missing from mainstream accounts of the history of mental illness and its treatment is that of the sufferer, which may be seen to render the lay person muisible (Bury 1998). Such invisibility can still be seen in current practice when decisions are made by professionals without consultation with users.

This process, which has been variously described as the development of a 'medical monopoly' and the 'medicalization of everyday life', not only creates professional experts and expertise which stand apart from and above the lay person but also allows for professional views to influence lay society in such a way that it absorbs professional knowledge and adapts behaviour accordingly (Bury, 1998). Ironically, this increase in the acquisition of knowledge by lay individuals eventually creates a shift from compliance in the face of objectification to a more active and increasingly challenging position. As people become more informed about their health and factors that potentially affect this, and about the possible responses or treatments available, their own understanding of and ability to control their destiny increases. This can be characterized as subjectification – a shift from objectivist and rationalist perspectives to that of subjectivity (Bury, 1998) and inter-subjectivity.

Values-based practice can be seen as part of lessening the influence of dominant theories, or meta-narratives, of the modern era. These maintain universal and all-embracing explanations of the social world and provide the basis for practices that establish the primacy of the professional perspective. To examine this issue in more depth, it is necessary to explore what is meant by values-based practice.

VALUES-BASED PRACTICE

Values-based practice starts from the assumption that there exists a plurality of equally legitimate values, in itself a post-modern position. As such, values are the unique preferences, concerns and expectations each individual brings to interactions with professionals and which must explicitly be taken into account by practitioners to ensure that decisions concerning care and treatment serve the interests of the user (Sackett *et al.*, 2000). Values are, therefore, a filter through which individuals view any evidence upon which decisions concerning their care and treatment are made (Lockwood, 2004). It is important to remember that mental health nurses also bring values to the interaction, both as a result of their personal experiences and of professional socialization (with the weight of history behind it). Indeed, the Nursing and Midwifery Council (2004a, p. 27) in the Standards of Proficiency for Pre-registration Nursing Education state that nurses are required to

recognise the effect of one's own values on interactions with patients and clients and their carers, families and friends

However, as we shall see later, a recognition of the effect of one's own values on such interactions is probably not in itself sufficient to be able to deliver values-based practice.

Consequently, in many circumstances there may be no 'right' answer which encompasses the different values of all concerned. In such situations, values-based practice shifts the emphasis away from the 'right' *outcome* (possibly based on available evidence) to consideration of what constitutes good *process* in terms of decision making (Fulford and Williams, 2003).

DESCRIPTION OF VALUES-BASED PRACTICE IN MENTAL HEALTH PRACTICE

Values-based practice can be seen as an attempt to reconcile best research evidence with practitioner expertise (Fulford and Williams, 2003) and patient values through the development of a 'therapeutic alliance' which ensures the best possible 'clinical outcomes' and 'quality of life' (Williams, 2005). Furthermore, the contemporary value attached to greater individualism, the rejection of authority and awareness of diverse points of view, all of which are characteristics of a post-modern world view, have led to a growing dissatisfaction with medical treatments for what are increasingly seen as social or psychological problems. As such, all decisions, it seems, including those of diagnosis and subsequent treatment, are required to be based on values as well as facts (Fulford and Williams, 2003). 'Values-based' and 'evidence-based' practices are therefore potentially complementary rather than antagonistic to each other. For appropriate decisions to be made, both values *and* facts must be considered. This addresses tensions between empirical evidence, constructed from findings and generalizations from samples and populations where the complexities of contexts have been unnaturally reduced, and the individual values of patients.

Contemporary policy, which operates at both government and organizational level, incorporates the need to be 'patient centred', and the ethos of a 'patient-led' NHS

(DH, 2005b) requires that the 'first call' for information is the point of view of the patient (Williams, 2005). This potentially requires a change of locus of control within decision making and addresses the fundamental question 'who decides'? Within values-based practice, answering this question starts from the assumption that there is a diversity of values, that values are increasingly influential and that the values of users are paramount, although not the only perspective that needs to be incorporated into any course of action. Therefore, it is the users (and perhaps carers), and practitioners in clinical practice, who decide (Fulford and Williams, 2003). It is at this point that evidence-based and values-based practices begin to diverge, although the direction of both remains complementary. That is, while evidence-based practice requires objective, perspective-free information, by definition, values-based practice requires exactly the opposite. There is also a need in contemporary practice for multidisciplinary decision making, such that decisions are made in a manner that allows for a balance of *reasonably* different values rather than by reference to a 'rule' prescribing a 'right' outcome (Fulford and Williams, 2003). The shift in emphasis away from outcome towards process allows appropriate decisions to be made when values are not shared or where consensus is not immediately apparent.

Fulford and Williams (2003) identify the need for effective communication skills in values-based practice. Despite the inevitable differences in values between practitioners and users, practitioners have to find practical solutions to challenges, and communication skills are key in combining consideration of evidence with that of values to arrive at acceptable solutions. Again, there is an important difference between the role communication plays in evidence-based practice and values-based practice. In evidence-based practice communication is 'executive' in that it is used to inform about and implement decisions. By contrast, in values-based practice communication skills are substantive in two ways. First, patient perspective skills, listening to and exploring values, are crucial in being able to increase awareness and knowledge of values and improve ethical reasoning. Second, multi-perspective skills are necessary to determine what to do when values conflict. Such skills encompass negotiation and conflict resolution.

THE IMPLICATIONS FOR RELATIONSHIPS BETWEEN PROFESSIONALS AND USERS: MODELS AND ETHICAL FRAMEWORKS

Values-based practice requires awareness and knowledge of the role of values, a different form of ethical reasoning and enhanced communication skills. It also entails a changing of locus of control in the relationship between practitioner and user. This change means that it is necessary to reconsider the ways in which we have understood the nature of this relationship; to reassess the ethical frameworks utilized to govern professional relationships and behaviour in health care. Sabatini (1998) provides a useful framework for considering the relevance of a variety of perspectives on what she terms the 'provider–patient relationship'. This considers the goals of inter-action, the practitioners' obligations, the role of users' values and the conception of users' autonomy (Sabatini, 1998). Sabatini identifies four broad categories of model: the 'informative' (also known as the engineering or scientific model); the 'interpretive'; the 'deliberative'; and the 'paternalistic' (otherwise described as the parental or priestly model).

To address the last of these first, the 'paternalistic' model sees the user's values as being objective and shared by the practitioner, which is suggestive of the 'values myopia' described by Fulford and Williams (2003). This sees the practitioner's role as a guardian and the relationship between the practitioner and the user as analogous to that of a parent and child, with the resultant obligation on the practitioner to do what is seen as being in the user's best interests, regardless of the latter's preferences. In this instance, the user's autonomy is restricted to agreeing to the practitioner's decisions (Sabatini, 1998). On the other hand, the 'informative' model assumes that the user's values are fixed and known to the user. The user will have choice of and control over the care they receive but initially will not have the facts necessary to make this choice. The practitioner's obligation, therefore, is to provide relevant factual information and to implement the user's chosen course of action in their role of a technical expert. Importantly, neither the practitioner nor the user are assumed to be making value judgements as a part of this process (Sabatini, 1998).

The 'interpretive' model involves the practitioner attempting to understand user values and to help the user choose a course of action. This is in many ways similar to the 'deliberative' model; the essential difference lies in the degree to which the practitioner is expected to develop the user's autonomy. In the interpretive model, the practitioner's duty is to reveal and interpret the user's values as they are, whereas the deliberative model requires the practitioner to convince the user of the most advantageous values, to engage in a process of moral development of the user. This takes the relationship beyond that usually thought of as appropriate, counsellor or advisor, into the realms of teacher or friend (Sabatini, 1998). It is arguable, however, that none of these models sufficiently addresses the requirements of values-based prac-tice. The interpretative model probably comes closest, although the requirement for the professional to help choose a course of action does not explicitly take into account the need for the values of the practitioner to be taken into account in terms of the evidence they might bring to bear on the situation.

A critic of traditional ethical approaches, Koehn (1994) also argues that existing models of professional ethics do not provide norms or standards by which professional behaviour might legitimately be understood. Although examining the fields of law, the clergy and medicine from a North American perspective, Koehn's ideas have a reso-nance for health care generally and more specifically mental health services and the role of nursing within these at a time when policy and professional initiatives in the UK require practitioners to consider explicitly the role of values in their practice.

Koehn specifically criticizes two models of professional behaviour typically used to provide professional activities with authority and legitimacy: the 'expert' model and the 'contractual' model. Koehn's critique of these two models is motivated by a question of prime concern to all practitioners within the mental health field: what is it about professional behaviour that warrants the public's trust?

The expert model proposes that professionals' perceived 'superior' knowledge and skills qualifies them to identify problems and to act morally in response. It is because they are experts that the public places such trust in professionals. Many practitioners would agree with this view; given their motivations and desire to use expertise to help, they need autonomy to exercise this as they, and not the public, see fit. Indeed, the very fact that the public seeks out professional help betrays the fact that they cannot help themselves and that they intend to accede to professional advice. Put this way, there is nothing immoral about assisting individuals who cannot help themselves; their need is not created by professionals but is a fact and the public are wise to allow experts to make decisions for them given the time and effort required to acquire the knowledge necessary to help themselves (Koehn, 1994). It is possible to see how such views emerged from the practices that developed within the modern era discussed earlier. However, Koehn argues that expertise destroys authority rather than grants this to professionals by permitting them to establish agendas in their own interests and possibly at odds with the needs of the public. This undermining of authority and therefore of legitimacy is exacerbated by the fragmented organization of professional practice and the consequent deterioration in the distinct and unique nature of professional roles (Koehn, 1994). This last point is particularly pertinent currently in the field of mental health as we see significant challenges to the legitimacy of individual professions and the boundaries between these with the development of new roles.

The contractual model presumes that expertise provides no ground for trusting professionals and is based on three arguments. Professionals should do as the public dictate because (1) professional behaviour needs to be controlled by the public to minimize risk, (2) the public is paying for the professional's service (albeit only indirectly in the case of health care in this country) and (3) if the relationship is to be moral then the autonomy and rationality of the public must be respected (Koehn, 1994). Koehn claims that the contractual model offers no more tenable grounding for professional authority and legitimacy than does the expert model. Difficulties in contracting between unequal partners, a particular challenge in mental health practice in the context of potentially coercive legislation, and the fact that the exercise of professional discretion and expertise is often both desirable and unavoidable, mean that the model undermines professional authority by reducing or removing completely the trust the public must place in professionals in order to obtain assistance (Koehn, 1994).

The failure of existing ethical frameworks to provide an effective guide to practice, combined with criticisms of traditional models of professional practice, have led to the realization that nursing needs to rethink how to make sense of, and more importantly act in, individual instances in practice. These challenges to traditional models of ethical reasoning explicitly raise issues of subjectivity, inter-subjectivity and consideration of context. They also place a great deal of emphasis on, among other issues, communication.

This does not mean that professional knowledge is no longer an important basis for ethical action; rather, that such knowledge is no longer seen exclusively as technical knowledge and skill. Instead, what is required is a practical knowledge, or wisdom (see Chapter 6: Truth, Uncertainty and the Mental Health Nurse), not achieved through formal study but gained by reflection on practical experience. This results in practitioners not only *knowing about* technical aspects of practice but also understanding how to apply these sensitively, taking into consideration the context and the individuals affected (Hugman, 2005).

This has obvious similarities to the processes involved in values-based practice described earlier. However, from a professional, ethical point of view, it would be inappropriate if decision making was based purely on an inter-subjective perspective; that is, if any decision was based solely on consideration of the values of all individuals involved in specific circumstances. This would make it impossible for professional decision making to be consistent and accountable; for example, how could a practitioner provide a rationale for actions with reference to any commonly understood or shared framework (Hugman, 2005). If professionals were to practice in this manner, the public would very quickly lose trust in them. Professionals are also unable to practice in this manner as there are obvious structural limitations on their autonomy in relation to policies and procedures, legislation and existing professional codes of conduct.

TENTATIVE CONCLUSIONS: THE IMPLICATIONS OF VALUES-BASED PRACTICE

Traditional models of professional ethics based on objective approaches to decision making no longer provide a legitimate basis for the relationship between practitioners and the public; however, neither does inter-subjectivity provide an alternative legitimate basis for ethical decision making. A values-based practice approach requires individuals to make and implement decisions giving consideration of *both* objective and inter-subjective approaches. In addition to considering the values of all involved and of autonomy and limitations on this, the knowledge being employed to underpin decisions is also important. Knowledge is potentially even more problematic in a context, such as mental health practice, where this is contested. Indeed, many service users contest the legitimacy and efficacy of numerous supposedly evidence-based treatments. The obvious solution to these challenges would involve professionals helping users reconcile the objective and inter-subjective tensions in making decisions, as is suggested by values-based practice. For example, Hugman (2005) suggests that for knowledge to be valid it must be subjected to open debate involving all potentially affected parties reaching agreement as to its validity. The aim of such a debate would be to achieve consensus, not to exercise professional or other forms of power to 'win' a debate. If this process were not to be undertaken, or consensus as to the validity of knowledge not to be obtained, then the knowledge used to underpin decisions would not be seen as legitimate and any subsequent course of action becomes an exercise in power or coercion (Hugman, 2005).

The criteria that allow professional practice to be judged as 'ethical' include actions that are demonstrably consistent and congruent with stated values and principles, regardless of the ethical framework upon which these are based. However, this assumes that the underpinning values of the framework can be openly explained and justified. This would require a profession's code of ethics to be understandable and acceptable to those potentially affected by the actions of its practitioners; put simply, if service users cannot agree with a profession's code of ethics then this code is not legitimate (Hugman, 2005). Furthermore, at a professional level, codes of ethics or conduct would need to reflect explicitly the values of those with whom the profession works in order to be compatible with the principles of values-based practice. This requires a reconceptualization of the ethical basis for the professional relationship between professional and 'user'.

The implications of values-based practice can be discerned at many levels, but its adoption is not without challenges. The weight of scientific tradition, and the resulting professional values and practice based on this (see Chapter 7: Where is your Evidence? Broadening the Scope of Professional Knowledge) means that professions will not easily relinquish the power this perspective confers. However, there is a very powerful element of current government policy directed towards developing a patient-led NHS which directly challenges the current ethical frameworks used to understand professional practice.

Hugman (2005) asserts that those potentially affected by professional action must consent to the legitimacy of the principles upon which this is based. The capacity for never-ending consultation every time an individual objects to the basis upon which a decision is made would obviously cripple services in terms of meaningful action. Such an approach also runs the risk of replacing one form of professional power and oppression with another (Bury, 1998). That is, the adoption of values-based practice, in this sense, potentially sets professions and services on a route to, at the very least, creating expectations that are unable to be met and in the more extreme cases towards constant paralysing discourse. Whatever the eventual outcomes of any use of values-based practice, it is clear that current government policy requires nurses to develop fundamentally different ways of working with users than has been the case in the past. From an educational perspective this creates a huge staff development issue in terms of values identification and clarification. For the staff of the future, this requires universities to rethink their technical training and their role in the formation of character and qualities necessary for effective and acceptable practice (Watson, 2006) and in stimulating and keeping alive debate and discourse (Rolfe and Gardner, 2006).

Whatever the validity and legitimacy of the policy imperative to implement values-based practice, the congruence of the principles of this with those underpinning the 'Recovery Approach' (NIMHE, 2005) creates fertile ground for public debate concerning the basis of professional practice. It is clear that public desire for such debate exists; the onus now is on professionals to engage meaningfully with such a discourse. This requires clear awareness of the ethical implications to avoid the creation of an unchallenged 'new' orthodoxy that does not essentially change anything and to ensure that practice truly reflects the values of all involved.

CHAPTER 6
TRUTH, UNCERTAINTY AND THE MENTAL HEALTH NURSE

Steve Trenoweth and Ian Price

It may be disturbing to visualize ourselves trying to make progress in a world where there are no firm points of departure immediately accessible to us, no 'givens', nothing that we start out by saying that we know for sure . . . (Neimeyer, 2001, p. 364).

Uncertainty is an inevitable and inescapable feature of decision making in clinical nursing practice (Thompson and Dowding, 2001; West and West, 2002), and one which '. . . prevails in human existence' (Penrod, 2001, p. 238). Indeed, for some, uncertainty '. . . has become the major characteristic of the 20th Century' (Sorrentino and Roney, 2000, p. 1). In everyday life, important decisions often have to be made based on our perceptions concerning the likelihood of uncertain outcomes or probabilities (Tversky and Kahneman, 1974; Thompson and Dowding, 2001). Indeed, this is the very essence of risk assessment and risk management (Vinestock, 1996) (see Chapter 16: A Systemic Approach to Violence Risk Assessment and Management). Furthermore, contemporary mental health nurses are expected to be able to respond to both the complex and ambiguous needs of service users, and the demands of the organization (Machin and Stevenson, 1997). As such, the resultant care can be unpredictable (Gijbels, 1995; Cleary and Edwards, 1999), particularly in in-patient environments. Furthermore, the necessity for action in a multi-professional context (see Chapter 15: Enhancing Effective Multidisciplinary Team-Working: A Psychoeducational Approach), sometimes without 'appropriate' evidence (see Chapter 7: Where is your Evidence?

Contemporary Issues in Mental Health Nursing, Edited by J. E. Lynch and S. Trenoweth
© 2008 John Wiley & Sons, Ltd

Broadening the Scope of Professional Knowledge), changing concepts of 'expertise' (see Chapter 10: The Meaning of Recovery and Chapter 13: Physical Illness: Promoting Effective Coping in Clients with Co-Morbidity) and the possible consequences of a 'wrong' decision can result in considerable personal uncertainty and anxiety.

In this chapter, we explore epistemological issues in the pursuit of truth and certainty and its implications for mental health nursing practice. We consider how wisdom, personal constructivism and quantum physics might help us to understand and appreciate the ambiguity and complexity of the unknown. We examine how mental health nurses are being encouraged to create a climate of certainty regarding their practice, for example, by the use of evidence-based, scientific, external reference points, and consider some potential implications that this might have for their practice and their use of personal knowledge in the care process. We begin from the assumption that uncertainty is unavoidable. Furthermore, we suggest that rather than attempting to pretend that the unknown can be fully eliminated, we should be developing the wisdom and confidence to work in complex and uncertain contexts.

CONTEMPORARY POLICY CONTEXT

Health services in the United Kingdom are currently undergoing a process of modernization and change (DH, 1998a, 1999a, 2000a; Meek, 1998), an agenda which seeks to create a climate of certainty regarding the provision and delivery of health care, thereby ensuring that 'the right thing' is done (Sorrentino and Roney, 2000). For the mental health nurse, there is a requirement to move away from clinical practice based on '. . . untested theories or cherished traditions' (Stuart, 2001, p. 109) or '. . . opinion-based processes and unproven theories' (Stuart, 2001, p. 103). Instead, skills in appraising research evidence and utilizing rigorously assessed research findings in clinical nursing practice (Franks, 2004) are to be developed, to ensure the identification of clear objectives for clinical interventions and with robust measures of outcome (UKCC, 1998; DH, 1999a, 2006a). Evidence-based nursing practice is thus heralded as a means to promote certainty, standardization, sound clinical decision making and the regulation of practice, affording optimum care (Onega, 1991; Stuart, 2001; Franks, 2004). Epistemologically, it seems, 'science' is to be our best and most rational model for dealing with uncertainty in mental health nursing practice (Thompson and Dowding, 2001).

This position, however, requires discussion for it is not clear that the pursuit of certainty can, or will, lead inevitably to 'quality' mental health nursing care. Furthermore, there seems to be an assumption that social and psychological worlds are amenable to quantification or are subject to predictable laws (see Chapter 7: Where is your Evidence? Broadening the Scope of Professional Knowledge). We may argue that the blind pursuit of scientific knowledge may actually undermine the value attached to the personal search for truth and meaning, and, indeed, our ability to respond to complexity and ambiguity. In short, there are epistemological and ontological issues which need to be considered in the delivery of contemporary mental health nursing care.

THE PURSUIT OF KNOWLEDGE AND CERTAINTY

The work and ideas of the British moral philosopher Mary Midgley (1919–) (see, for example, Midgley, 1989, p. 203) are particularly relevant at a time when the drive towards evidence-based practice in mental health care is so powerful. She suggests that, historically, universities which have been the engines that have created the type of knowledge that has become dominant within Western societies, have favoured research over teaching and that this has resulted in a store of knowledge so vast as to be useless by virtue of the fact that nobody has the time to read it all. Perhaps more crucially, one consequence of this emphasis on research has been a lack of attention paid to the *process* of educating people to think critically about the nature and purpose of knowledge. Indeed, Midgley (1989) quotes Einstein as saying that knowledge exists in two forms: lifeless, stored in books; and alive, in the consciousness of individuals. The first, although indispensable, is often seen to occupy a superior position to the second form. If this view of knowledge is accepted, then creating knowledge and storing it as an inert piece of information or property, or indeed presenting it to practitioners in the same format, is far from satisfactory.

Stemming from the work of philosophers such as Aristotle and Plato, who saw knowledge as only one aspect of the broader concept of wisdom, this ability to see a discipline in context involves striving towards an understanding of life as a whole, which makes possible a sense of what is important in life. Aristotle, like Einstein, made explicit the notion of the possession of knowledge as an active process consisting of an interaction between the mind and what it contemplates, which entails much more than mere storage of knowledge. Midgley (1989) also highlights an important aspect of the work of Plato, which suggests that knowledge about what is 'good' (in a moral sense) serves as a reference point for other forms of knowledge. Plato saw knowledge about what is 'good' as controlling, directing and giving value to other forms of knowledge. This stems from the idea that the existence of 'good' and 'bad' as opposites is an essential aspect of the world and as a result, knowledge about what is good and bad is a pre-condition of knowing the world. This notion of the importance of knowledge of what is good cannot be reduced to or equated with the worth of anything else, including other forms of knowledge. One consequence of this is that not all forms of knowledge are equally worth knowing. Both Plato and Aristotle perceived the study of all other topics to be subordinate to contemplation of what is good, and this idea initially formed the basis of much, if not all, of Western scholarship. This means that knowledge is not, as it has come to be seen, an end in itself but merely a means to an end. By contrast, modern science places little or no emphasis on the process of contemplation, although it is unclear historically when and how this shift occurred.

Modern science, therefore, attaches great significance to the discovery or creation of 'facts'. However, are facts in and of themselves 'valuable'? One answer to this appears to be that if these facts have no meaning for anybody then they do not possess any value. Certainly facts have no value if the only utility they can claim is to become part of an abstract entity called 'science'. Midgley (1989) contends that if knowledge is to have any meaning or value then we must possess the ability and the wisdom to interpret it. The role of science is merely to provide the raw material for this interpretation. The dominant position of science as an activity that has come to place value on the accumulation of facts for their own sake and discourages contemplation of these only results in knowledge being further divorced from wisdom.

As far as any academic system or professional practice-based activity is concerned, if scholars or practitioners lose sight of why a particular line of enquiry is worth following then the system becomes distorted and inflexible. As such a system becomes larger and its links with other aspects of society become more numerous and complex, then the mental activities involved in functioning within and understanding this system become increasingly more difficult to sustain; functioning successfully in such a context requires an ability to grasp and own the purpose of actions.

Further criticism of the certainty vested in the scientific approach comes from *within* the scientific perspective and casts a radically different light on the ways in which phenomena might be perceived and understood. Zohar and Marshall (1994) propose that such a different perspective can be found in the form of scientific thinking known as 'quantum physics'. Comprising a number of subdivisions, including relativity theory, quantum mechanics, chaos and complexity theories, these are all based on a common paradigm. This stresses the importance of the indeterminate and the unpredictable. It is holistic in that it sees the whole as being greater than the sum of its parts, emphasizing the multiplicity of possibility. It is also characterized by 'observer participancy' in which individuals help create their own reality.

Many of quantum physics' theories, for example Heisenberg's uncertainty principle, directly contradict the previously held certainties derived from the Newtonian or mechanistic physics of the 16th and 17th centuries – a perspective often seen to be determinist, consisting of cast iron laws that assured certainty and predictability, and reductionist and atomistic in its assumption that a phenomenon is best understood by reducing it to its constituent parts and examining each of these in isolation. In such an approach the observer stood apart from and outside the phenomenon being studied. Zohar and Marshall (1994) describe how this paradigm, based on continuity, hierarchy and a single point of view, not only shapes scientific thinking in such a way as to give rise to a separation between fact and value, but also, and more significantly, influences the structure of social institutions and relationships.

Conversely, quantum physics, although a broad field with many, and at times conflicting theories, is not deterministic in the same way as Newtonian physics, and acknowledges the fundamental impossibility of measuring certain phenomena at the sub-atomic level. Zohar and Marshall (1994), however, are *not* suggesting that the principles of quantum mechanics apply to social and behavioural phenomena. What they do propose is that an understanding of such phenomena from the perspective of quantum physics would allow us to question and ultimately change the way in which we understand ourselves, our actions and the society in which we live.

The Newtonian paradigm has been the inspiration behind nearly all the great social, political and economic thinkers of the 17th, 18th and 19th centuries; Hobbes, Mill, Locke, Adam, Smith, Darwin, Freud and Comte all based their theories on Newtonian principles and these theories have, in turn, helped form the structure of society in which we live today. Zohar and Marshall claim, however, that the institutions that make up today's society are now obsolete because they are so rigid as to be unable to respond to a growing radicalism calling for fundamental change. In practical terms, this translates into a more dynamic view of the world which encompasses the acceptance and valuing of ambiguity, the equal value that can be attached to different perspectives and the acceptance of rapid and unpredictable change. What is needed to improve the quality of life, through actions that are both humane and intelligent, Midgley (1989) argues, is less knowledge and more wisdom.

THE PERSONAL SEARCH FOR TRUTH

What if we hypothesize, then, that there is not a single or universal scientific 'truth' but a plurality of perspectives reflective of a dynamic view of the world (Rowe, 1996; Midgley, 2003)? As such, there may be many and various ways of approaching the same issue or perceiving the same phenomena (Bannister and Fransella, 1986; Winter, 1992; Zohar and Marshall, 1994) and hence '. . . the same event may be construed simultaneously and profitably within various disciplinary systems – physics, physiology, political science or psychology' (Kelly, 1955/1991, p. 10). In contemporary mental health practice, a client's 'problem' or 'need' may be understood and construed differently by the various members of the care team and the client themselves. Indeed, there may exist different disciplinary perspectives regarding what may even constitute a problem. Are, for example, mental health issues symptomatic of an underlying abnormal 'illness' or do they in fact lie on a continuum of normal experiences and behaviours (Bentall, 2003)? Do mental health problems result from defects in a '. . . naturally selected neural computer' (Pinker, 1997, p. 521) or from dysfunctional dynamics within families (Laing and Esterson, 1964)? It seems that 'truth' is rather a matter of personal perspective.

We may further hypothesize that the construal and assumptions made about phenomena we encounter in our world also guide our actions within it. For example, our personal understanding(s) of our world, according to Personal Construct Psychology, is signified by, and reflected, in our behaviour (Kelly, 1977; Bannister and Fransella, 1986; Fransella and Neimeyer, 2005) and our interactions and reactions to and with others. As such, people do not merely react to events to which they are exposed but are active and creative in making sense of their world (Kelly, 1955/1991; Fransella, 1972; Viney, 1987). We interpret, reflect upon our world in our own way (Space *et al.*, 1983; Viney, 1987) or, as Kelly (1955/1991, p. 3) puts it, '. . . each man contemplates in his own personal way the stream of events upon which he finds himself so swiftly borne'. Indeed, it is our own personal experience here which is a crucial source of information in helping us in interpreting our world and to create a sense of predictability in anticipating future events which we may encounter (Kelly, 1955/1991; Bannister, 1983; Space *et al.*, 1983; Villegas *et al.*, 1986; Winter, 1992; Pope and Denicolo, 2001).

Indeed, for personal constructivists, 'truth' is a personal issue – a unique negotiation and interpretation of events within an individual's personal world. Here, personal knowledge may be seen as ephemeral, seemingly subject to change and revision as one's ideas about one's world develop or are altered in the light of personal experience. Thus:

The human quest is not about to be concluded, nor is truth already partly packaged for distribution and consumption. Instead, it seems likely that whatever may now appear to be the most obvious fact will look quite different when regarded from the vantage point of tomorrow's fresh theoretical positions (Kelly, 1969, p. 284).

Of course, the theory of Personal Construct Psychology itself can be seen as another construction – no more right to the construction of 'truth' than any other, and one of many ways in which we seek to '. . . surround our lives with an aura of meaning' (Kelly, 1955/1991, p. 13). However, as Burr and Butt (1992) suggest, its usefulness as a framework comes from helping us describe, understand and construe our own and other's perspectives and the meaning that is attached to the personal and interpersonal world (Winter, 1992).

Science, then, may be seen as one framework by which we seek to gain knowledge of, and seek personal mastery over, our environment, representative of a very distinct way of seeing the world. However, the problem with scientific knowledge is that it is often hard won and there exists a considerable psychological attachment to knowledge empirically derived, and 'a person who spends a great deal of his time hoarding facts is not likely to be happy at the prospect of seeing them converted into rubbish' (Kelly, 1970, pp. 1–2). Hence, there is often an intransigence and a desire to preserve what is known and that anything which challenges the established 'truth' and 'facts' is seen as dangerously subversive (Kuhn, 1970). As Kelly (1969, p. 284) argued:

. . . it is a misfortune that man should be so set on being right at the very outset that he dares not risk stupidities in an effort to devise something better than what he has

As such, knowledge which is personally derived may be seen as invalid, as in a scientific paradigm, '. . . we regard tacit knowledge as useless until it is made explicit . . .' (Jankowicz, 2001, p. 62) and that such knowledge:

. . . does not, in the Western view, have legitimacy. Indeed, it is not considered knowledge at all (Benner and Tanner, 1987, p. 30).

The scientific pursuit of certainty often requires recourse to apparently objective, external reference points and the abandonment and rejection of the subjective, personal construction of knowledge. This has a number of important implications for the mental health nurse.

IMPLICATIONS OF UNCERTAINTY FOR MENTAL HEALTH NURSING

VALUING LIVED EXPERIENCES

Our personal interpretations of events in our world arise from our 'experience' – the term used for the relationship between sentient beings and their world (Jankowicz, 2001). We experience and are experienced. We act and react and are, in turn, acted upon and reacted to. Our experience is an important source of information for us to harvest in our attempts to understand ourselves and our world, both now and in the future. Knowledge derived from experience becomes '. . . the repository of what people have learned, a statement of their intents, the values whereby they live, and the banner under which they fight' (Bannister and Fransella, 1986, p. 14).

Nurses, it seems, do not often use scientific findings in their practice and underpin clinical decisions by utilizing their own personally constructed knowledge derived from their clinical experience (Agan, 1987; Rew and Barow, 1987; Rew, 1988; Burnard, 1989; Easen and Wilcockson, 1996; King and Appleton, 1997; Cutcheon and Pincombe, 2001; Herbig *et al.*, 2001). In this way, our personal understandings of clinical events may not be scientifically precise (West and West, 2002), but they do help to give shape and form to our personal world, without which our '. . . world appears to be such an undifferentiated homogeneity that man is unable to make sense out of it' (Kelly, 1955/1991, p. 9).

However, what might happen if we assume that we can only gain access to 'truth' via the empirical study of phenomena where powerful gate-keepers of such knowledge stand as arbiters of such reality? Some argue that this is the current scenario with the medicalization of mental health problems (Barker and Buchanan-Barker, 2005) – where mental distress is seen as a biological phenomena, and where the psychiatrist decides who is ill and who is sane by the recourse to taxonomic frameworks and by the application of empirical research into mental 'illness'. If we are to assume that the personal constructions of a dominant individual are held to be representative of an 'objective truth', there is likely to be an attempt by the powerful to reinterpret the construing of the less powerful in their own frame of reference. One person's position prevails, one person's views are oppressed and their subjective lived experiences are devalued and undermined. However, if we accept that we are all on a journey to create our own personal meaning, we recognize the inherent value of subjectivity in alternative constructions of reality. By questioning the validity of a universal truth, we can place emphasis upon negotiating shared meanings amongst service users and colleagues, and of understanding and valuing each other's lived experiences.

RESPONDING TO CLINICAL AMBIGUITY

Our clinical nursing world may not fit neatly into scientific boxes derived from empirical knowledge and may not help us respond effectively to clinical complexity and ambiguity (Jordan *et al.*, 2002; West and West, 2002). That is, empirical data facilitate our understanding of a phenomenon under controlled conditions, which will not always help us understand the subjective experiences of another in complex real-life contexts. By narrowing or 'reducing' our clinical field of vision we may fail to see the whole picture. Indeed, as Jolobe (2002, p. 764) points out, there is a danger here of attempting to find '... precise answers to the wrong questions rather than approximate answers to the right questions'. Furthermore, according to Gallop and Reynolds (2004) there is likely to be no single response which is sufficient to address complexities of providing mental health nursing care. While empirical 'facts' can be useful in weighing up clinical evidence for particular interventions, they may fail to capture the reality of clinical situations (Neimeyer, 2001; Thompson and Dowding, 2001) and may be of limited value where rapid decisions have to be made in uncertain, complex and ambiguous clinical situations where an appreciation of contextual factors is vital (Thompson and Dowding, 2001; Trenoweth, 2003). That is:

In contrast to the laboratory setting . . . most problematic situations in the real world are more 'messy', that is, vague and ambiguous, lacking the necessary facts and information, and inadequate in terms of suggesting the appropriate direction or goals for problem solving (D'Zurilla and Goldfried, 1971, p. 113).

Indeed, as West and West (2002, p. 319) suggest:

. . . however much information is gathered, there will always be a degree of uncertainty at the point of making clinical decisions with individual patients

and as such,

. . . evidence, even of the highest quality, is only evidence. There will always be judgements to be made by responsible informed and compassionate people (West and West, 2002, p. 320).

With complexity comes the need to adapt and respond flexibly to the changing needs of service users, requiring us to step beyond narrow paradigmatic frameworks which create an illusion of certainty, potentially restricting clinical decision making (Franks, 2004) and our subsequent ability to offer meaningful support.

UNDERSTANDING OUR 'SELF' AND OTHERS

According to Bannister and Fransella (1986, p. 10) 'each of us live in what is ultimately a unique world, because it is uniquely interpreted and thereby uniquely experienced'. That is, '. . . even if all members of a society told themselves exactly the same stories, the meaning and implications of these stories for different members of the society would not be the same' (Howard, 1991, p. 194). As Kelly argued '. . . individuals can be found living out their existence next door to each other but in altogether different subjective worlds' (Kelly, 1955/1991, p. 56). To remain within our own personally constructed reality is potentially a lonely experience indeed.

However, in clinical mental health care, without the appreciation and understanding of another's internal world, it is difficult to know how care can be conducted at all. Certainly, we would be unable to be compassionate or to develop the ability to empathize with others (Reynolds and Scott, 2000; Gallop and Reynolds, 2004) and this is likely to have consequences for our understanding of our personal and clinical worlds (Rawlinson, 1995). This may also have an implication for the quality of care we provide:

The more skilled the nurse becomes in perceiving and empathising with the lives of others, the more knowledge or understanding will be gained . . . The nurse will thereby have available a larger repertoire of choices in designing and providing nursing care that is effective and satisfying (Carper, 1978, p. 17).

The personal search for meaning clearly needs to involve others – it is thus not only an individual venture but also a social enterprise (Jankowicz, 2001). Indeed, as Walker (1996, p. 13) argued '. . . people are both fashioned within and fashioned of the complex interpersonal worlds they have inhabited and do inhabit'. Social situations are facilitated by an attempt to comprehend the other's unique personal understandings. In interactions with others, we may revise our own personal viewpoint, develop empathy, understanding of another's perceptions or construction of their world. The constructive dynamism within social situations allows us to enter into 'roles' with others and to anticipate other's actions and reactions in social situations – 'If we can predict accurately what others will do, we can adjust ourselves to their behaviour. If others know how to tell what we will do, they can adjust themselves to our behaviour' (Kelly, 1955/1991, p. 96).

Furthermore, by our social interactions we learn more of ourselves as

It is through interactive exploration of others and not through contemplation of our own navels that we come to understand ourselves (Bannister, 1983, p. 385).

To understand ourselves, we must be able to explain our own behaviour and to anticipate how we are likely to act in a given future event (Bannister, 2005). However,
there can be dire psychological consequences of being unable to understand our own
self:

*Central in the stream of unfolding events that we need to anticipate is, of course, self – our own
behaviour. To misread you and fail to anticipate your actions is disturbing: to fail to anticipate
my own actions is grave indeed* (Bannister, 1983, p. 380).

Indeed, an understanding of our 'self' in the world (our roles we assume, our beliefs,
thoughts, feelings and so forth) allows us to harvest our experience, facilitating our
social interaction, which in turn reflexively facilitates us to develop our personal understanding of 'self' in a subjective sense (Jankowicz, 2001).

MANAGING PERSONAL ANXIETY AND STRESS SURROUNDING UNCERTAINTY

In Personal Construct Psychology, 'anxiety' is seen to indicate '. . . an awareness that
our present way of making sense of things is unable to cope with that with which we
are confronted' (Walker, 1996, p. 14). At such times, we become uncertain, unable to
anticipate, or to satisfy our emotional need to cognitively master events within our
world (Viney and Westbrook, 1976; Winter, 1992; Melrose and Shapiro, 1999; Neville,
2003; Franks, 2004). That is, 'anxiety is our awareness that something has gone bump
in the night' (Bannister, 2005, p. 23) but 'it is the *unknown* aspects of those things that
go bump in the night that give them their potency' (Bannister and Fransella, 1986, p.
22, original emphasis).

There seem to be considerable individual differences amongst those who seek out
either certainty or uncertainty in their lives (Sorrentino and Roney, 2000; Neville,
2003; Honkasalo, 2006). Some people, it seems, find meaning in life and comfort from
seeking out clarity from the predictable and familiar (people who are 'certainty oriented'). That is, there are some people who construe the need to be able to anticipate,
to predict, thereby having some notion of control over future events, the absence of
which might lead to their psychological discomfort and anxiety (Kelly, 1955/1991;
Edwards and Weary, 1998).

Indeed, some people it seems prefer to avoid uncertainty – an excess of which can
result in significant levels of personal stress (Sorrentino and Roney, 2000; Sadava, 2001;
Taylor-Piliae and Molassiotis, 2001), and few people seem to tolerate uncertainty well
(Mishel, 1988; Neville, 2003). It seems '. . . we dread the far-reaching implications of
what is about to happen to us' (Kelly, 1969, p. 284) and we feel particularly under
threat in circumstances where deep-seated changes may occur to our deeply held beliefs
or way of life.

However, there are some people who are clearly oriented more towards uncertainty. They seem to find pleasure in ambiguity and in resolving confusion, which they seem to take in their stride, and see such situations as an opportunity to learn from a situation or about themselves. Indeed, there seems to be potentially great value in embracing the unknown representative of an ability, according to Sorrentino and Roney (2000) to be more adaptive to one's environment, more open to new ideas (Kelly, 1955/1991) and less likely to want or need to control others. Indeed, Kelly (1955/1991) acknowledged that facing unfamiliar events may also be exhilarating (Westbrook, 1976), particularly if one's personal frame of reference is sufficiently flexible (or 'permeable') to afford the incorporation of new experiences (Bannister, 1983; Bannister and Fransella, 1986).

The reality of contemporary mental health nursing care delivery, particularly in busy in-patient settings, is one of uncertainty and unpredictability (Gijbels, 1995) as nurses attempt to balance the needs of service users and the demands of the organizations, such as admissions, critical incidents and supporting other wards (Cleary and Edwards, 1999). The tension here lies between such clinical realities and the apparent drive towards certainty and predictability, led by local and national policy frameworks, and an ever-increasing emphasis on accurately predicting the level of risk an individual might pose to themselves or others. Furthermore, there is a perceived lack of clarity regarding the 'primary task' of mental health nursing (see Chapter 16: A Systemic Approach to Violence Risk Assessment and Management) or what the role of mental health nurses should be (see Chapter 2: Rebuilding Lives: A Critical Look at the Contemporary Role of the Mental Health Nurse). Such situations place great demands on nurses' ability to prioritize work, particularly in the face of limited resources. As such, there is perhaps value in assisting people to appreciate and differentiate between clinical situations where certainty is more 'useful' (such as anchoring clinical interventions to 'best' available evidence), and also to appreciate the clinical utility of uncertainty (such as in situations where best available evidence is unsuitable for the client due to apparently complex and ambiguous needs or where it is unclear what the outcomes of a clinical intervention might be).

How clinicians, though, may be best helped and supported to cope with the anxiety surrounding personal and professional uncertainty is unclear (McCormick, 2002). However, a supportive infrastructure is likely to create a climate within which people are facilitated to discuss, explore and resolve such anxieties by increasing knowledge and skills that may assist people to manage uncertainty and increase their personal perceptions of confidence, self-efficacy and control (Penrod, 2001). In this way, nurses may be assisted in being able to transform some situations of uncertainty and ambiguity into opportunity (Buckenham, 1998). Perhaps, however, the best way to manage our own personal uncertainty is to recognize that it cannot be eradicated (West and West, 2002), but only contained. This suggests being able to contain our own personal anxieties surrounding not knowing and recognizing the difficulties with seeking objective and universal truths. Of course, recognizing the transient and ephemeral nature of knowledge can be an uncomfortable realization but '. . . while I do not know the answer to the question, I need not be immobilised' (Kelly, 1977, p. 19). In fact, for Kelly (1955/1991), our uncertainty, and the permeability of our own personal frame of reference and the openness and willingness to other perspectives, can be a useful springboard for our personal change, growth and development as human beings. That is,

The man whose prior convictions encompass a broad perspective, and are cast in terms of principles rather than rules, has a much better chance of discovering those alternatives which eventually lead to his emancipation (Kelly, 1955/1991, p. 16).

CONCLUSION

'Certainty', we may argue, is an illusion (West and West, 2002), the pursuit of which helps us manage and contain our own personal fears of the unknown. As such there is a danger of slavishly applying scientific findings to contain our own personal anxieties. There is, of course, nothing inherently wrong with a scientific/rational way of construing the world – it represents one source of knowledge that we may use to create personal meaning for ourselves. However, such a way of construing, in itself, may be insufficient to grasp complexities of clinical work (Gallop and Reynolds, 2004) (see Chapter 7: Where is your Evidence? Broadening the Scope of Professional Knowledge). The move to an exclusively, and pre-emptively, evidence-based world creates an illusion of certainty, the impact of which can mean that less explicitly scientific forms of knowledge (such as knowledge which forms our own personal understanding and meaning) are devalued because they do not afford empirical 'truth'. This also fails to recognize the richness of the interpersonal world where individuals have different perspectives on 'truth' and are on their own personal search for meaning. Developing the wisdom to embrace uncertainty can help us explore and adapt to our personal world; to develop our personal construal of meaning of the clinical world; and to welcome and value the subjective experiences of others.

CHAPTER 7
WHERE IS YOUR EVIDENCE? BROADENING THE SCOPE OF PROFESSIONAL KNOWLEDGE

Peter Harper and Simon Jones

INTRODUCTION

In this chapter, we will challenge the prevailing notion that the only valid evidence on which to base mental health nursing practice is that derived from research, especially research that focuses on *measuring* phenomena. We will discuss different sources or types of evidence; both research and non-research derived, and reflect on the issue of how the quality of evidence is established. Broadening the scope of what counts as 'appropriate' evidence for practice is not an easy option, and mental health practitioners who follow this route will have to be prepared to justify their actions. Indeed, this becomes more difficult as one leaves the safe confines of convention. The central point in this chapter is that mental health care is a complex phenomenon often involving a multi-dimensional and individualized approach by health care practitioners. Accordingly, we will describe other types of research methods that we consider constitute valuable mechanisms for generating professional knowledge. In what some evidence-based practitioners might consider heresy, we will go even further and propose that non-research evidence can be legitimately used in practice and, furthermore, that there is often no choice but to do so.

Contemporary Issues in Mental Health Nursing, Edited by J. E. Lynch and S. Trenoweth
© 2008 John Wiley & Sons, Ltd

WHAT COUNTS AS EVIDENCE FOR PRACTICE?

For many the simple answer to this question is *knowledge derived from research*, or even more precisely, from doing experimental research, especially a randomized controlled trial (RCT), that is, the testing of a hypothesis in a controlled environment. Such is the potency of this assumption that it permeates the phenomenon generally described as evidence-based practice. Within this conceptualization of *evidence-based practice* the only evidence valued more than that derived from an RCT is that derived from several of them, summarized in the form of a systematic review and/or a statistical meta-analysis. The evidence grading system currently developed by the Scottish Intercollegiate Guidelines Network (SIGN), which is used in England by the National Institute for Health and Clinical Excellence (NICE), illustrates this point (see Figure 7.1) and is typical of other grading systems used internationally.

Using this system, any research that adopts a descriptive approach is automatically consigned to Level 3, regardless of its quality; this category includes all surveys and qualitative research. Why does this model dominate the world of evidence-based practice to the extent that it does? Much of the answer is again fairly straightforward. The origin of evidence-based practice in health care can be traced to the evidence-based medicine movement (Sackett *et al.*, 1996) and the RCT has long been held in high esteem because of its suitability for testing medical interventions such as drug therapy or surgery. Where secondary factors, which potentially influence the intervention being tested, can be adequately controlled, the experimental methods often work well and it would be foolish to deny the benefits that this methodological approach has brought to society historically. Where experimental research does not work so well is in complicated situations with many secondary influencing factors that cannot be controlled adequately, for example in complex interpersonal relationships. This has been recognized by the Medical Research Council (MRC), an organization often perceived as relatively conservative and predominantly reductionist in its approach to research. The MRC have published a framework that is still centred on the use of RCTs as the core component to the generation of evidence, but which places them within a five-stage continuum for the development and evaluation of RCTs for complex interventions (MRC, 2000). This framework incorporates the preliminary examination of theory related to a given complex intervention, modelling of the intervention to aid in-depth understanding, and even the use of qualitative research. Following the 'definitive RCT stage', a final long-term evaluative stage is proposed.

Reaction to the prominence of hierarchies of evidence (such as that shown in Figure 7.1) takes a variety of forms. Some have advocated synthesizing multiple qualitative studies in a way that mimics meta-analysis using what is generically termed meta-synthesis (Weed, 2005). This, on one level, seems quite a good idea but it is problematic in terms of the philosophy of qualitative researchers who rarely aspire to generalization, or the averaging of research findings in the traditional statistical sense, that is, the application of findings from a sample back to the population from which the sample

1++	High quality meta-analyses, systematic reviews of RCTs, or RCTs with a very low risk of bias
1+	Well conducted meta-analyses, systematic reviews of RCTs, or RCTs with a low risk of bias
1 -	Meta-analyses, systematic reviews of RCTs, or RCTs with a high risk of bias
2++	High quality systematic reviews of case-control or cohort studies High quality case-control or cohort studies with a very low risk of confounding, bias or chance and a high probability that the relationship is causal
2+	Well conducted case-control or cohort studies with a low risk of confounding, bias or chance and a moderate probability that the relationship is causal
2 -	Case-control or cohort studies with a high risk of confounding, bias or chance and a significant risk that the relationship is not causal
3	Non-analytic studies, e.g. case reports, case series
4	Expert opinion

Source: SIGN (2001).

Figure 7.1
Levels of Evidence

was drawn. Qualitative researchers instead frequently use concepts like *transferability* or *naturalistic generalization* (Gomm *et al.*, 2002). These are concepts which draw on the assumption that research findings may or may not be widely applicable depending on the context; the emphasis being on the reader to decide the relevance of research outcomes to their own professional situation. Some writers such as Holmes *et al.* (2006) have been more vehement about the concept of evidence-based practice as a whole, likening it to a form of *fascism* or more precisely, a *microfascism* which is considered less brutal but more pernicious than the 'fascism of the masses' practiced by dictators such as Hitler and Mussolini. They describe the objective of their paper as follows:

. . . to demonstrate that the evidence-based movement in the health sciences is outrageously exclusionary and dangerously normative with regards to scientific knowledge. As such we assert that the evidence-based movement in the health sciences constitutes a good example of microfascism at play in the contemporary scientific arena (Holmes et al., 2006, p. 181).

CHALLENGING THE STATUS QUO

We would advocate that a particular clinical question be explored by matching it with the most appropriate research methodology, which may, or indeed may not, be quantitative or 'empirical' in its focus. Sometimes this means researchers may have to abandon attempts to measure the unmeasurable, despite the political, professional and economic consequences of deviating from the so-called 'gold standard approach', namely, the RCT. Starting with a methodology which is deemed professionally respectable or desirable and *subsequently* attempting to shoehorn the clinical question into it is neither appropriate nor desirable. Likewise, many practitioners search in vain for experimental evidence to answer their questions without ever reflecting on the appropriateness of this methodological orientation to their field of interest.

We do not wish to diminish the importance of evidence derived from research in this discussion, but rather to widen the scope of what can be considered as 'appropriate' sources of professional knowledge. By research we mean the process of answering a question through the systematic collection and analysis of data, but we feel it is important to acknowledge the complexity of clinical decision making. It is naïve to assume that every clinical intervention can be supported by experimental research, or any other type of research for that matter. Where the effectiveness of a particular medication has been supported by a thorough RCT, there are still other issues to consider in relation to the use of that drug, such as: the side-effects, the degree to which the patient can or will comply with prescribed therapy, the cost to the health service and alternative therapies (see Chapter 11: Supporting Recovery: Medication Management in Mental Health Care). Even where an experiment is theoretically the most appropriate choice for exploring a particular practice issue, but the research has not yet been undertaken, decisions frequently still have to be made in relation to that issue. It may be that a particular issue is of importance to only a very few individuals and as such resources to conduct research are unlikely to ever be available. Funding may be directed towards issues judged to be more important in terms of the population who might benefit or to research which may lead to significant cost benefits; this is the reality of the world we live in. Many clinical decisions have an ethical dimension and by definition do not have a 'right' answer derived from research (see Chapter 6: Truth, Uncertainty and the Mental Health Nurse). Ethical decisions involve judgements and often practitioners will disagree vehemently on the 'right' course of action (see Chapter 5: The Implications of Values-Based Practice in Mental Health Nursing). Other decisions are highly contextual and what is an appropriate health care response for one patient may not be appropriate, or acceptable, for another (see Chapter 3: User Involvement and the Micro-Politics of Mental Health Care).

It is important then to be realistic about evidence. The bottom line is that mental health nurses should use the best available evidence at any one point in time and if this turns out to be professional consensus, rather than an RCT, then so be it.

WHERE DOES EVIDENCE COME FROM?

SOURCES OF RESEARCH EVIDENCE

The most common source of research evidence is in the form of reports published in professional journals. There are a variety of ways in which practitioners can obtain journals related to their own area of interest, the simplest being to take out a subscription, but whilst many practitioners do just this, it can prove to be an expensive option and even regular diligent reading of the articles in one or two journals is unlikely to result in a comprehensive understanding of the evidence base for a given issue. Most health care practitioners have access to a library with many journals, but again time is a precious commodity and much of it is required, along with considerable dedication and commitment, to gain a comprehensive appreciation of the available evidence (see Chapter 6: Truth, Uncertainty and the Mental Health Nurse). The arrival of the Internet has radically changed the way in which professionals access research studies; large amounts of evidence can now be identified quickly and printed off, frequently without even leaving our homes or office desks. The stumbling block, however, is time to read and absorb the voluminous information retrieved. Filling ring binders full of wonderful, rich, insightful accounts of research can be quite satisfying but is of little use in itself in terms of evidence-based practice. Compounding this issue is the need for practitioners to have the sophisticated research appraisal skills required to be able to evaluate and synthesize what they read. These problems, facing practitioners who want to keep up to date, were identified some years ago and led to an important development which underpins the process of evidence-based practice, namely, the 'systematic review'.

SYSTEMATIC REVIEWS

Literature reviews have always been a means of presenting practitioners with an overview or summary of evidence, but in the past the reader had no way of knowing if the summary presented to them in the review was objective or comprehensive. With regard to research evidence, traditional reviews have a tendency to: include only those studies that support the reviewers' point of view; have no defined inclusion/exclusion criteria for studies; pay little attention to the methodological quality of reviewed studies; ignore a study's sample size, effect size and limitations; rely more on the speciality of the reviewer than on the evidence found; and generally have an element of subjectivity in the way they select and report findings (Mulrow, 1987; Teagarden, 1989; Bourner, 1996; Egger *et al.*, 2001; Rowley and Slack, 2004; Harlen and Schlapp, 2005; University of Melbourne, 2005). Furthermore, it is not uncommon for traditional reviews on the same subject to reach opposite conclusions (Mulrow, 1987) (see Chapter 6: Truth, Uncertainty and the Mental Health Nurse) and '... miss small, but potentially important, differences' (Egger *et al.*, 2001, p. 11). Systematic reviews attempt to address these problems by using systematic and explicit methods to ensure that data from all relevant studies is methodically identified, retrieved and appraised before being rigorously synthesized into a comprehensive review of evidence relating to a clearly formulated question (Egger *et al.*, 2001). Although systematic reviewers will often use a slightly different approach to each review, generally all systematic reviews will follow a similar six-step process:

1. Formulation of a focused review question.

2. A comprehensive literature search.

3. Retrieval of studies that appear relevant.

4. The reviewing of studies against predetermined criteria to identify those which should be included and those which should be excluded.

5. Critical appraisal of included studies.

6. Evidence review, synthesis and summary.

In comparison with a traditional literature review, it is often argued that systematic reviews are generally more objective in their appraisal of the evidence and less prone to bias and error in their analyses (Egger *et al.*, 2001; Harlen and Schlapp, 2005). For these reasons, systematic reviewing has now become a 'worldwide phenomenon' (Andrews and Harlen, 2006), used by policy-makers, health care practitioners and researchers around the globe to produce '... authoritative "state of the art" summaries and syntheses of research in order to inform policy, practice and research' (Andrews and Harlen, 2006, p. 287). As such they have become an essential part of evidence-based practice and a number of highly respected dedicated databases now exist and are freely available to practitioners, e.g. Cochrane, DARE (Database of Abstracts of Reviews and Effects) and the Joanna Briggs Institute. The systematic review process, however, is not without its own problems.

Systematic reviews are based on the idea that by combining the results from multiple studies, either statistically or descriptively, we are able to produce a more powerful result or estimate of treatment effect (Naylor, 1997). The primary means of synthesizing quantitative outcomes is through 'statistical meta-analysis', a process in which studies that explore the same interventions, focus on the same or similar populations, and use the same outcome measurements are statistically aggregated (Egger *et al.*, 2001).

The problem, however, is that in combining these data the reviewer must presume that any differences among studies are primarily due to chance (Naylor, 1997) when in reality the studies that are being combined are often diverse in nature and methodological approach, and there could be any number of reasons for differences among studies (Naylor, 1997; Andrews and Harlen, 2006). For example, studies could have sampled different populations, measured different endpoints, highlighted different confounding factors or even used different statistical methods. If great enough, these differences between combined studies, commonly referred to as *heterogeneity*, can potentially distort a review and lead the reviewer, or reader, to draw the wrong conclusions (Baily, 1987; Thompson, 1995). Furthermore, combining studies may also result in the introduction of *bias*, both through '. . . entrenching the biases in individual studies, and introducing further biases through the process of finding studies and selecting results to be pooled' (Naylor, 1997, p. 617).

The process of systematic review is further complicated by the fact that it is not always that easy for reviewers to find all the studies that are relevant to their question because they may not have even reached publication. For example, a study by Scherer *et al.* (2005) which combines data from 79 studies (29 729 abstracts) reported that, on average, less than half (45%) of all abstracts presented at scientific conferences are later published as full-length journal articles; and it has long been recognized that studies that report statistically significant or 'positive' results are much more likely to be published than studies that report non-significant or 'negative' results (Dickersin, 1990; Easterbrook *et al.*, 1991; Dickersin *et al.*, 1992; Dickersin and Min, 1993; Egger *et al.*, 2001). Subsequently, there is a good chance that systematic reviewers may miss important research (Dickersin *et al.*, 1992; Thornton and Lee, 2000), or that an over-representation of positive studies and an under-representation of negative ones could potentially skew review findings towards a false beneficial treatment effect (Dickersin *et al.*, 1992; Gilbody *et al.*, 2000; Egger *et al.*, 2001), called a 'publication bias'. This, along with other forms of biasing, is a potential problem for reviewers and could have serious consequences for practitioners in the UK since systematic reviews are now widely used to inform decision making in all areas of health care (Muir Gray in Egger *et al.*, 2001). Therefore, basing policy and practice solely on the findings of systematic reviews without first evaluating their potential flaws is ill-advised as it could lead to the construction of a flawed evidence base on the strength of which important clinical decisions may be made.

The impact of systematic reviews and meta-analyses has been such as to generate much discussion about the possibility of applying a similar approach to qualitative research evidence (McCormick *et al.*, 2003; Jones, 2004; Thorne *et al.*, 2004; Walsh and Downe, 2004; Weed, 2005). The debate is wide-ranging, complex, often passionate and surprisingly, not new; Noblit and Hare (1988) made an early contribution with their concept of 'meta-ethnography'.

The processes of searching for and retrieving qualitative research studies are essentially the same as for any type of research. There are distinct differences in the critical appraisal process but the real difficulty, and therefore the controversy, is centred on the process of synthesizing the findings (meta-syntheses). It is a reasonable proposition that findings of several experimental studies that test the same intervention (for example, a particular medication), focus on the same or similar populations, and use the same outcome measures (for example, a physiological phenomenon) might be amalgamated (synthesized). Qualitative research, however, generally does not intervene in the same controlled sense, does not rely on simplistic, clearly categorized outcomes and rarely focuses on population (e.g. people) without considering social context. This illustrates the first problem: how are studies selected as being suitable for synthesis? The second problem is that statistical analysis is predominantly an external process; the same analysis could be performed by a number of individuals on the same data and the statistical outcomes will be the same. In this way analysis is to some extent replicable and verifiable. Qualitative analysis is not external; on the contrary, it always requires some reflexive consideration of the researcher's *self*, and is sometimes deeply personal.

In qualitative research we have come to understand that meta-synthesis must be quite different from simple accumulative logic or averaging across studies. The goal is clearly interpretive, not merely aggregation to achieve unity; it is not a summary portraying the lowest common denominator. Meta-synthesis is not a method designed to produce oversimplification; rather, it is one in which differences are retained and complexity enlightened. The goal is to achieve more not less. The outcome will be something like a common understanding of the nature of a phenomenon, not just a consensual worldview (Thorne *et al.*, 2004, p. 1346).

Synthesis of qualitative data, then, is not just a matter of meta-analysis but rather of 'meta-interpretation' or maybe, most problematically of all, of 'meta-reinterpretation'. It is the degree and nature of reinterpretation which seems to distinguish between the different approaches to meta-synthesis.

SOURCES OF NON-RESEARCH EVIDENCE

There are many ways in which we know about the world other than through research. Hospers (1997) lists the following seven sources of knowledge: perception, introspection, memory, reason, faith, intuition and testimony. Whilst some of these sources of knowledge are implicit in the research process, for example perception and reason, others such as faith and intuition are not. All of us rely heavily on testimony as a source, that is, what we are told by others. What we are told may be derived from systematic inquiry but, on the other hand, it may be rooted in tradition, custom and cultural consensus. We also make sense of what we know in terms of our own experiences, regardless of the objectivity or subjectivity of the knowledge in question. For instance, when we read about some new research findings we ask ourselves: Do I recognize these findings? Do they make sense? Do they relate to my professional practice?

Do these findings fit in with what I know already; or do they conflict? The process of knowing something is a complicated business but something we usually take for granted. Hospers outlines what is described as the '. . . classical analysis of the concept of knowing', which has three requirements: '. . . the statement must be true; you must believe the statement to be true; and there must be good evidence for believing the statement' (Hospers, 1997, pp. 20–21).

Despite being the source of much debate in philosophical circles, this model never-theless provides quite a useful framework for thinking about the complexity of profes-sional knowledge. If I say John has a urinary tract infection then John must, in fact, be infected with a pathogen for the statement to be *true*; it is not enough that I merely *believe* he has an infection. I also need some evidence to support my belief in the form of clinical signs and symptoms. This example illustrates a relatively uncomplicated relationship between evidence, belief and knowledge in terms of how John's infection might be managed, but often the relationship between these three requirements is far from being uncomplicated. Thomas (2006), a general practitioner, illustrates this in terms of his management of a patient suffering from depression:

Although evidence from positivist inquiry helps me recognise the features of depression and consider a range of treatment options, as a generalist, I know that depression is not one entity. It is a feeling that arises from multiple coincidental and interacting factors. Inside depression can be found personal inadequacy, unresolved past hurts, physical abuse, bullying at work, genetic predisposition, dysfunctional families and many other things, all compounding and causing each other . . . When I explore these issues with a patient, I am considering the diagnosis of depression, not as the end of the matter, but the start of an exploration of something more complex. Multiple factors are constantly affecting each other and adapting to changes in each other (Thomas, 2006, p. 451).

Clearly, the business of caring for people effectively in 'real life' contexts is frequently highly individualistic and calls for a more sophisticated approach to the generation of professional knowledge than that embodied in the current realist concept of evidence-based practice (see Chapter 6: Truth, Uncertainty and the Mental Health Nurse). Adopting such a stance, however, involves a willingness to accept uncertainty. Having research evidence for what you do is safe, comfortable and makes action defendable but, in the words of Franks (2004), '. . . the feeling of uncertainty is a reality for most mental health professionals who struggle to understand, make sense of and care for people with multiple, complex behavioural and emotional problems' (Franks, 2004, p. 99). Accepting professional uncertainty involves, in turn, individual and institutional acceptance of risk (see Chapter 6: Truth, Uncertainty and the Mental Health Nurse and Chapter 16: A Systemic Approach to Violence Risk Assessment and Management). Unfortunately, we appear to live in a world where any level of risk is increasingly unacceptable to both the general public and the people who govern them. Again in the words of Franks, the systems within which health care practitioners work are 'based on a fantasy that if everything is performed according to a set of strict guidelines then no accidents or mishaps will occur, disturbed people will not kill themselves or someone else and professional staff will not make mistakes' (Franks, 2004, p. 100). It is perfectly understandable that people want a risk-free existence, but this is perhaps somewhat naïve. It is equally understandable that for politicians to acknowledge the unavoidability of risk in health care would be tantamount to political suicide.

JUDGING THE QUALITY OF EVIDENCE

EVALUATING RESEARCH EVIDENCE

One of the central themes of evidence-based practice is the evaluation of the *quality* of evidence. Just because a research study has been published, even in a prestigious journal, does not automatically mean that the claims made by the researchers are valid and/or reliable. However, learning how to judge the quality of research takes a long time and it is not possible to discuss every aspect of this process in this chapter. We will confine ourselves here to some key points which hopefully will guide further reading.

Appraising research is a sophisticated skill that requires time to acquire and an in-depth understanding of the concept of research in terms of ontology, epistemology and methodology. These are difficult and unfamiliar terms for many but they are important and we make no apology for using them. *Ontology* is the study of, or beliefs about, the true nature of reality. According to Schwandt (2001), ontology is sometimes used synonymously with *metaphysics* and sometimes as a branch of metaphysics. Although there are many different ontological/metaphysical perspectives on reality, there are two distinct ontological orientations to research: *realism* ('. . . the doctrine that there are real objects that exist independently of our knowledge of their existence'; Schwandt, 2001, p. 219) and *relativism* ('. . . the doctrine that denies that there are universal truths'; Schwandt, 2001, p. 225).

Epistemology, on the other hand, is the study of knowledge; this includes how we come to be able to say that we *know* something and different sources of knowledge, for example those described earlier by Hospers (1990). The type of knowledge generated by researchers is closely related to their beliefs about reality, e.g. they may believe that all phenomena are objectively measurable. *Methodology* refers to the collective methods used by a researcher, that is the research design, the data collection/generation methods and the data analysis/interpretation methods. The methodology chosen by a researcher is directly related to the ontological beliefs of a researcher and his or her epistemological orientation. Keeping sight of the relationship between these three concepts is the key to doing valid research as well as to the critical appraisal process.

Crabtree and Miller (1999) highlight this in what they call the 'paradigm question', that is, a failure on the part of researchers to establish explicit congruence between the methods used and the 'operational paradigm' adopted by the researchers. In terms of the critical appraisal process, this results in the application of inappropriate critical criteria.

There are two main requirements to critically appraise research evidence: first, an understanding of the focus of the research, for example, the question being asked, the issue being explored, the problem being investigated and second, a knowledge of the methods being used by the researchers and awareness of alternatives. In our experience, meeting the first of these requirements is not as difficult as meeting the second. Health care practitioners are frequently driven to learn about research because they want to improve what they do. They are familiar with the issues related to their area of practice; they are immersed in them on a daily basis and for most, research is something they only encounter from time to time. This is as it should be; even though research findings influence practice, it is professional practice that drives research in that all research starts with a focus, a question, a problem or an issue. The first stage in judging the quality of a piece of research, then, is an examination of both the rationale for and purpose of the study. Understanding the precise purpose of the research is crucial to being able to judge the appropriateness of the chosen research methods. You should ask yourself, has the researcher chosen the best way of generating the knowledge required? To answer this question you need your professional knowledge but you also need the second requirement outlined at the beginning of this section. You will not be able to judge whether the 'best' method has been chosen unless you have some familiarity with what methods are available.

Meeting the second requirement involves knowing the research 'rule book'. The better you know the rules of research the more able you are to apply them in your appraisal of a research study. The problem is that, unlike the rules of golf or football, there is no single recognized international rule book that applies to all professional spheres. The rules are to be found spread across a wide range of sources and whilst the rules relating to some areas of research are subject to high levels of agreement, for example statistical analysis of quantitative data, others are open to personal interpretation and historical change, for example, the analysis of qualitative data. It is possibly better to think in terms of not just *rules* but also of *conventions*. Probably the single most common error people make when attempting to appraise a research study is to use the wrong set of rules and/or conventions. This is particularly evident when moving from a study based on quantitative data to one based on qualitative data. Sample size is one of the best examples; having a representative sample is crucial to the use of inferential statistics. If you want to 'infer' or *generalize* your research findings from a sample, back to the population from which the sample was drawn, then your sample must be large enough to be representative of the population. If we are talking about a population of human beings, the degree of variability frequently means that samples must be fairly large. This process of generalizing from the sample to the population in this way is mathematical in nature. Qualitative research, however, often explores small samples in great depth and the sort of generalization described above is neither appropriate nor intended by the researchers.

Qualitative researchers sometimes talk about *transferability* instead; this means that what is discovered may be transferable to other situations or similar contexts. In other words, we can learn from our own experience and that of others and we can recognize that people have similar experiences, interpretations, needs, interests, problems and so on without losing the uniqueness of individual experience. It follows that to judge a qualitative study primarily on the basis of the small size of its sample is incorrect. The person who does this has not understood the rules and/or conventions associated with qualitative research.

There are a number of appraisal tools used to systematically evaluate research studies and many, such as those used by the Scottish Intercollegiate Guideline Network (SIGN, 2001) and the Critical Appraisal Skills Programme (CASP) (CASP, 2006), are publicly available. The latter is unusual in that it offers an appraisal tool designed specifically for evaluating qualitative research. This move away from the traditional epistemological orientation to evidence-based practice is also reflected in recent work by the Joanna Briggs Institute, which has developed computerized instruments for the appraisal and synthesis of both qualitative and quantitative research (Pearson *et al.*, 2006), a development to be welcomed in that it represents a broadening of the scope of what counts as valid professional knowledge within the evidence-based practice world, but is not without problems as it requires the kind of shift in ontological and epistemological orientation outlined earlier. Some approaches to the meta-synthesis of qualitative research data are plainly reductionist in nature; the result of the crude transference of the meta-analytical ontology and, as such, we would suggest, incongruent with the essentially relativist and holistic nature of qualitative inquiry.

EVALUATING NON-RESEARCH EVIDENCE

Evaluating non-research evidence varies according to the specific type of evidence. Clearly, evaluating or verifying a personal belief is conceptually problematic. If, however, the evidence takes the form of consensus then evaluation is easier, if not totally free of problems. If the evidence constitutes the consensus of a highly respected professional organization and represents practice as agreed by the majority of the leading practitioners within that organization, then this evidence can be considered a fairly sound basis for professional practice. The problem with consensus is that simply equating agreement with reality is dangerous. The consensus of the fans at a home football match might be that the referee was biased against their team. But just because they hugely outnumber the away team fans does not make their appraisal of the referee accurate. There are consensus approaches that potentially could be used as a bridge between formal and informal knowledge. These include the Delphi and Nominal

Group techniques (Plunkett *et al.*, 2005) that attempt to systematically summarize and sometimes quantify opinion, but as far as we are aware have not been incorporated into the concept of evidence-based practice.

Interestingly, and innovatively, in addition to the tools outlined previously, the Joanna Briggs Institute have developed a tool called NOTARI (The Narrative, Opinion and Text Assessment and Review Instrument) within their portfolio that aims to appraise, extract and pool evidence arising from text, expert opinion and discourse. This makes the Joanna Briggs model of evidence-based health care unique in terms of attempting to include not only qualitative research but some types of non–research evidence in what counts as valid evidence for practice (Pearson *et al.*, 2005).

CONCLUSIONS

What does all this mean in terms of professional nursing practice? Consider the following question: even if you had infinite resources would you be able to research every single aspect of your work? Or perhaps this question could be phrased in another way: could you function at work if you only undertook activities that you could provide written, explicit research evidence for? An interesting exercise is to record a day's activity in detail and try to match each action with some research evidence. You will probably find that much of what you do in a working day is not research based; some of it will be, some of it perhaps should be or could be, but some of it will be guided by informal knowledge, sometimes consensual but at times very personal. As illustrated earlier, often formally and informally acquired knowledge intertwine; the contention in this chapter is that an understanding of this complexity is crucial to meeting the needs of patients and clients in a comprehensive way.

Our position in this chapter, however, does not represent licence to ignore or denigrate the concept of evidence-based practice. Neither does it support a reversal of the hierarchy of professions in which personal knowledge takes precedent. Our aim is to promote the idea that there are many sources of valid professional knowledge; no one source takes precedent over another in the form of a universal external hierarchy. Precedent should be given to a particular type of knowledge, and/or to the process by which it is generated, only in terms of the context of the phenomena under scrutiny.

There are times when experimental testing of a theory is entirely appropriate; there are, however, times when it is not. There is a place for consensus and times when taking individual or collective perceptions of morality or beliefs into account is unavoidable. There are instances when the exploration of the experience of one individual gives more valuable insight into a phenomenon than the aggregated, collective experience of the many. It may even be appropriate at times to accept the potentially adverse consequences of acting intuitively.

The beginnings of a shift to a more sophisticated orientation to professional 'evidence' can be seen within the Joanna Briggs model:

The term evidence is used in the model to mean the basis for belief; the substantiation or confirmation that is needed in order to believe something is true. Health professionals seek evidence to substantiate the worth of a very wide range of activities and interventions and thus the type of evidence needed depends on the nature of the activity and its purpose (Pearson *et al.*, 2005, p. 210).

But the place of personal knowledge remains problematic and it may be that it is contradictory and conceptually unrealistic to attempt to formalize it within a model of professional behaviour. By its very nature, much of personal knowing may have to remain recognized, acknowledged and expressed but essentially internalized; playing its fundamental and cohesive part in the epistemological background.

CHAPTER 8
CHALLENGING STIGMA AND PROMOTING SOCIAL JUSTICE

Carlyle London and Angela Scriven

INTRODUCTION

The relatively recent emphasis placed on care in the community and social inclusion (DH, 1999a; Social Exclusion Unit (SEU), 2004a; DH, 2006b) has brought into sharp and contemporary focus the stigma that has long been associated with mental ill health (London *et al.*, 2006). This chapter explores this theme, beginning with an examination of the meaning of stigma and how it manifests itself from the perspective of the mental health service user and that of the mental health nursing profession. Media representations of stigma and how these continue to affect attitudes towards mental ill health will also be considered. The ramifications of stigma are profound and particular attention will be devoted to an analysis of the implications for social justice and social inclusion. This will lead to an identification of the challenges that confront mental health nurses when dealing with stigma and recommendations will be made for change and development to mental health nursing practice in relation to reducing stigma and promoting social justice.

WHAT IS STIGMA?

The word stigma is derived from the ancient Greek word *Stizein*, which referred to a distinguishing mark burned or cut into human flesh (Goffman, 1963). These

Contemporary Issues in Mental Health Nursing, Edited by J. E. Lynch and S. Trenoweth
© 2008 John Wiley & Sons, Ltd

distinguishing marks were employed to identify slaves or criminals so that others would know their status as less-valued or excluded members of society. The contemporary use of the term, however, does not refer to a visible mark, but still denotes societal attitudes towards those in the population who are deemed to be less valued or are excluded in some way (Porter, 2004). Stigmatization occurs through interactive social processes and in a manner that can be deeply discrediting to those who are stigmatized (Link and Phelan, 2001). When one applies this notion to people with mental health problems, it can refer to the reactions of the public and can include the attitude and behaviour of both the victims and the perpetrators of stigma (Sayce, 2000).

Oliver (1992) argues that existing explanations of stigma are unhelpful because they are too individualistic in approach. In Goffman's (1963) seminal work, for example, stigma is defined as an attitude of discredit or disgrace and it is argued that the focus on individual self-perception and micro-level interpersonal interactions detracts from what is widespread and patterned exclusion of stigmatized people from economic and social life. Link and Phelan (1999) agree with this and assert that stigmatization is both caused by, and results in, a lack of access to social, economic and political power. They contend that stigma results in discrimination through the identification of differences; the construction of stereotypes; the separation of labelled people into distinct categories, with the subsequent disapproval, rejection, separation and status loss (Sayce, 2000). Indeed, an emerging consensus view is that a greater concentration on the discrimination that is a direct outcome of stigma would shift the focus to the individuals and groups that perpetrate stigma, rather than on those that are being stigmatized (Chamberlin, 2001; Hitchon et al., 2006; Thornicroft, 2006).

HOW DOES STIGMA MANIFEST ITSELF?

Stigmatization of and discrimination against people with mental health problems appear to be common throughout society (Crisp et al., 2000; Byrne, 2001; DH, 2003). Indeed, it has been suggested that these negative attitudes are a direct result of the growth of psychiatry and the medicalization of mental illness in the 19th century, and attempts to describe mental distress in terms of diagnostic categories and syndromes (Hitchon et al., 2006; Lyons and McLoughlin, 2001). Furthermore, in addition to the media influences outlined above, general ignorance and fear of the unknown can be significant contributory factors to stigmatization and social exclusion (Royal College of Psychiatrists (RCP), 2000) (see Chapter 6: Truth, Uncertainty and the Mental Health Nurse) as service users are perceived to be uniformly unpredictable and dangerous. This simple perception is far from accurate, though, as they are far more likely to be victims of violent crime (Walsh et al., 2003; Lalani et al., 2006). A review of homicides committed by people with a mental illness over a 38-year period showed them to be extremely rare, with minor fluctuations and a 3% annual decline (Taylor and Gunn, 1999; DH, 2001c). There may also be an assumption that the situations of service users are hopeless in that their problems are untreatable or that their prognosis is poor. However, Harding and Zahniser (1994) found that between a half and two-thirds of users, including those with chronic mental health problems, significantly improved or recovered (see Chapter 10: The Meaning of Recovery).

Stigma impacts on mental health service users in a number of ways. It can result in distress, poor prospects of training for employment and associated socio-economic restrictions, loneliness and feelings of self-worth, and hopelessness, or in extreme cases deliberate self-harm (SEU, 2004). The discriminating effect of stigma is ultimately marginalization from society with obstacles to engaging as a full citizen, and being free of discrimination, exclusion and oppression (Bracken and Thomas, 2005). People with mental health problems can be amongst the most excluded in society, and one consequence of this is that despite higher rates of physical illness, service users often have poorer access to medical care services than other groups in society (DRC, 2006) (see Chapter 12: Physical Co-Morbidity in Mental Health).

Evidence suggests that stigma may have a negative impact at the outset of mental health problems (Penn and Wykes, 2003). Perceived alienation, for example, is a stress factor in the onset of psychosis with an increased rate of reported delusional ideation in individuals who experience more discrimination at the onset of the disorder (Janssen et al., 2003). The experience of stigma is such that many mental health service users may internalize the problem and suffer further loss of self-esteem and personal confidence (Guimon et al., 1999; Corrigan and Lundin, 2001). Families and friends can also feel stigmatized by association (London et al., 2006) and self-stigma can negatively affect family relationships and reduce social interactions (Link et al., 2001). Indeed, the fear of being stigmatized may lead to an increase in the time to initial treatment, which may have an effect on the long-term recovery rates in psychosis (Norman and Malla, 2001) (see Chapter 10: The Meaning of Recovery).

Indeed, both the experiencing of mental health difficulties and receiving a diagnosis of 'mental illness' can be potentially disempowering. The processes inherent in psychiatric care and treatment may actually add to an individual's sense of this, such as creating a climate of dependence based on an unchallenged assumption that mental 'illness' stems from a physical or biological cause, thereby requiring medical treatment to effect a 'cure'. As such, one of the commonest forms of disempowerment is the failure to attribute proper value to service users' personal narratives, especially their experiences of living and coping with mental health problems (Barker and Stevenson, 2000). Chamberlin (1998) argues that psychiatric diagnosis is an invalidation of the personal experience of mental distress, which has meaning and value in the context of the service user's life.

The use of words to describe mental health and illness is also an important factor in stigmatization (Finzen and Hoffmann-Richter, 1999). These terms can violate the identity of sufferers. A similar source of stigmatization is the use of diagnostic labels. Such 'iatrogenic stigmatization' does not stop at labelling through application of a diagnosis. The concomitant assumption and justification of the need for chemotherapeutic interventions via a medical diagnosis may produce side-effects, which will further mark an individual and make her/him 'stand out', in some cases more so than any original symptoms (Sartorius, 2002).

Mental health nurses may also inadvertently promote social exclusion and stigma by applying disempowering practices and attitudes that have emanated from particularly institutionalized forms of care (Campbell, 1999) (see Chapter 3: User Involvement and the Micro-Politics of Mental Health Care and Chapter 5: The Implications of Values-Based Practice in Mental Health Nursing). Bertram and Stickley (2005), for example, found that in a residential rehabilitation unit, staff attitudes impeded clients' opportunities to become socially included by defensive practice, paternalistic attitudes and the stagnant views that are embedded in the cultures of many mental health services (see Chapter 16: A Systemic Approach to Violence Risk Assessment and Management). Frequently, mental health professionals fail to see that users have the same needs as the people who use other types of health service (Fox, 1999). Some may view users as 'childlike' and dependent upon others, and may seek to make all decisions on their behalf (Corrigan, 2000) (see Chapter 20: Some Considerations for Mental Health Practitioners Working with those who Self-Neglect). Service users also report that inadequacies in services are ignored and they are held solely responsible by mental health professionals for failures in improvement (Granat-Goldstein, 2001). Bassman (2000) supports this position and argues that what is interpreted as behaviour resulting from poor functioning can be reframed as a response to contexts and environments which deprive service users of opportunities and resources to maintain their competencies and skills. There is also evidence of stigma-laden information being disseminated during treatment (Corrigan, 2005).

One outcome of relatively long and frequent admissions might be diminished social networks and increased contact with health care professionals and other service users (Holmes-Eber and Riger, 1990). People from minority ethnic groups may experience greater levels of stigmatization when in contact with services. Indeed, there is evidence to suggest that young black men are more likely to have a negative experience of mental health services and more likely to be detained formally under mental health legislation (SCMH, 2002; Healthcare Commission, 2005b). Gender can also influence the experience of stigma (DH, 2003) (see Chapter 19: Masculinity as a Risk Variable in Physical and Mental Ill Health) as can sexuality (King and McKeown, 2003) (see Chapter 9: Homophobia in Mental Health Services), sensory or physical disability (DH, 2005d) and learning disability (DH, 2005e).

MEDIA REPRESENTATIONS AND THE REINFORCEMENT OF STIGMA

The news media possess the power to confirm opinions and influence attitudes and beliefs (Lalani and London, 2006) (see Chapter 19: Masculinity as a Risk Variable in

Physical and Mental Ill Health). As such, they constitute important sources of information and have a continued impact on knowledge and contemporary understandings of 'mental illness' (Taylor and Sorenson, 2002; Stark *et al.*, 2004). There is evidence to suggest that negative, stereotyping media representations of mental illness reinforce prejudice and correlate with negative public attitudes towards people with mental health problems (Cutcliffe and Hannigan, 2001; Olstead, 2002; Edney, 2004). Moreover, continued television and newspaper sensationalization of homicides committed by mentally unwell people may reinforce misconceptions and serve to strengthen the perceived but largely erroneous link between violence and all mental health problems (Guimon, 2001; SEU, 2004). Thus, the media may compound and reflect stigma, and whilst media coverage of people with common mental health problems is slowly becoming more balanced and sympathetic, positively inclined coverage of serious mental illness appears to be evolving at a slower pace (Cutcliffe and Hannigan, 2001; Rethink, 2006).

SOCIAL JUSTICE

A sense of belonging and access to social networks can bring significant benefits to both individual citizens and to society as whole. However, Bracken and Thomas (2005) argue that loss of citizenship and downward social mobility are the ultimate outcomes of stigma. These outcomes result from social exclusion and a lack of access to employment opportunities and ultimately, rejection and discrimination are the more serious ramifications. One's mental health status, both real and imagined, is based on a capacity to manage, to communicate and to form and sustain relationships – this is often determined by how people think and feel about themselves and about others and how the world is interpreted (Health Education Authority, 1997). As such, one's designation as 'mentally ill' can in itself be a precursor to social isolation, which is a compounding factor in deterioration of mental health, and the diminished likelihood of participation as an 'included' citizen, which has implications for the creation of a just and fair society.

The implications for society are far-reaching. Indeed, the concept of 'social justice' is founded on the principles of equal worth of all; entitlement to basic necessities; opportunities and life chances for all; and the reduction of unjust inequalities. It refers to the notion of equality of distribution of resources within society and can also describe the movement towards human rights and equality. Manifestations of social injustice for mental health service users can be seen via many of the issues discussed in this chapter, namely restricted access to employment (SEU, 2004), marginalization, segregation and loss of status (Link and Phelan, 1999) and discrimination, stigmatization and labelling (Link and Phelan, 2001). Health inequality is a further social injustice for people with mental illness who experience barriers and discrimination in seeking and accessing primary health care, have higher rates of obesity, smoking, coronary heart disease, hypertension, diabetes, stroke and respiratory disease and are more likely to die at a younger age than the rest of the population (Herman, 2001; DRC, 2005, 2006). It is not just the increased risk of disease but also that a significantly high proportion of their physical illness lies undetected (Phelan *et al.*, 2001). Furthermore, the excess morbidity and mortality for people who experience mental health problems is preventable through supportive health education/promotion advice, proactive and comprehensive health screening, lifestyle changes and the treatment of common diseases (Connolly and Kelly, 2005) (see Chapter 12: Physical Co-Morbidity in Mental Health).

Indeed, it could be argued then that many of those who encounter recurring mental health problems experience some violation of Article 14 of the European Convention on Human Rights, which calls for no discrimination of persons on any ground, regardless of any status, including mental health (World Health Organization Project on Human Rights, 1991). Mental health nurses have, therefore, a crucial role to play in addressing this infringement of the fundamental human rights of those in their care.

CHALLENGES FOR MENTAL HEALTH NURSES

Recent research by Campbell *et al.* (2006) indicates that being socially excluded can lead to poor decision making and a diminished learning ability. This will clearly impact on citizenship, which Bracken and Thomas (2005) argue involves being regarded as a full human being, free from discrimination, exclusion and oppression. It is, therefore, crucial that mental health nurses do not ignore the social injustice created by stigma and the associated loss of citizenship.

Corrigan (2005) suggests that the stigma that stems from mental ill health is a form of social injustice, and places the responsibility for its removal on professionals and institutions, which should recognize the harm caused by stigma and embrace their duties to find means for its eradication. To this end, a specific recommendation in the Chief Nursing Officer's Review of Mental Health Nursing (DH, 2006a) is that nurses strive to remove stigma and promote social justice. As such, nurses face a serious challenge to de-stigmatize mental ill health and facilitate social justice and inclusion for mental health service users. This issue may require a coordinated effort that asserts itself on two fronts simultaneously. One aspect must ensure that the processes inherent in contemporary care and treatment do not add to users' disempowerment, both real and imagined (Barker and Stevenson, 2000) (see Chapter 3: User Involvement and the Micro-Politics of Mental Health Care). The second aspect is similarly enduring but one might hope that its existence is time-limited – it is the elimination of the disempowering practices and attitudes that have emanated from mental health care over a long period of time (Campbell, 1999), such as institutionalization – the embedding and constraining of an individual's actions to normative requirements of an organization (Goffman, 1963; Barton, 1976).

To enable and actively promote social inclusion, mental health nurses should priori-tize developing positive and collaborative working relationships with service users and carers (DH, 2006a; Hitchon *et al.*, 2006) (see Chapter 2: Rebuilding Lives: A Critical Look at the Contemporary Role of the Mental Health Nurse). To this extent, Repper and Perkins (2003) postulate three core, interrelated components that would enable health care professionals to address the social justice issue:

1. Developing hope-inspiring relationships as a foundation for growth and develop-ment, and recovery.

2. Facilitating personal adaptation, understanding and empowerment inspiring the confidence necessary to mobilize internal resources.

3. Promoting inclusion, by helping people to access the roles, relationships and activi-ties that are important to them.

In doing this, the robust values that underpin nursing practice should be translated into practices that can ameliorate stigma (see Table 8.1 for examples).

A clear example as to how this may be translated into contemporary mental health nursing practice may be in the area of medication management. Objective, non-judgemental information about mental health problems, medication and its manage-ment and sound evidence regarding interventions and the various treatment modalities

TABLE 8.1

Values and practices in mental health nursing which ameliorate stigma

Values	Practices
Respect	• Respecting service users as partners in care
	• Respecting service users' autonomy
Honesty *Tolerance*	• Adhering to the laws of the land
	• Undertaking non-discriminatory practice
	• Endorsing social justice
Equality *Trust*	• Promoting and protecting the interests and dignity of service users
	• Giving truthful, accurate information to service users
	• Acting to identify and minimize risk to service users
	• Upholding the duty of care owed to service users
	• Maintaining knowledge and competence

and outcomes should be provided (see Chapter 11: Supporting Recovery: Medication Management in Mental Health Care). Mental health nurses can then use their knowledge to facilitate the empowerment of service users and carers in making meaningful choices about treatment. There also needs to be a shift from some inherited practices, namely the focus on symptom management and containing disturbed behaviour which reinforce medical ideologies of sickness or illness (see Chapter 16: A Systemic Approach to Violence Risk Assessment and Management and Chapter 18: The Psychological Impact of Restraint: Examining the Aftermath for Staff and Patients).

In attempting to respond to stigma, the move should be towards taking a positive approach to risk, and supporting service users in developing and maintaining social links and roles, education and opportunities for employment and challenging stigma and discrimination (DH, 2006b).

Service users can be helped to overcome stigma when nurses display sincere human qualities, build valuable relationships and reach out to them as unique individuals (Connor and Wilson, 2006). Humanity, empathy, common sense, sensitivity and understanding, respect, trust and compassion are important qualities for nurses (see Chapter 4: Compassion) who strive to challenge stigma and promote social inclusion (see Table 8.2).

Overall, mental health nurses also need to adopt a holistic view of a service user's life, including not only their clinical mental health needs but also the physical, emotional, spiritual and social aspects of their experience (NIMHE/Care Services Improvement Partnership (CSIP), 2006).

CONCLUSIONS

The stigmatization and exclusion of people with mental health problems remains a contemporary and a prevalent issue. Despite various strategies to address social exclusion and justice, many remain stigmatized and isolated from 'mainstream' society. It is crucial that mental health nurses play full and active parts in promoting inclusion and social justice and take active steps to acknowledge and appreciate the personhood of each individual. These actions can help service users to perceive themselves not as 'mentally ill' or 'schizophrenic', for example, but as valued human beings (Lyons and McLoughlin, 2001).

Service users benefit from feeling supported by professional (and other) carers (see Chapter 10: The Meaning of Recovery). Support is essential for them to be able to work through and beyond experiences of mental distress and to acquire from life as much as anyone else, and meet their own (current and future) needs (Watkins, 2001; Repper, 2006). Nurses will need to empower and support service users to manage their lives in a manner that is fulfilling, meaningful and capable of offering a positive sense of belonging to, and being able to contribute to, their communities (NIHME/CSIP, 2006). In other words, nurses should consider service users as citizens of the

TABLE 8.2

Challenging stigma and promoting social justice

Summary of points necessary for challenging stigma and promoting social justice

- Treat all clients as individuals

- Respect personal values of each person

- Develop therapeutic relationships which inspire hope and confidence

- Increase frequency and amount of time spent in direct clinical contact with service users

- Provide opportunities for service users to maintain and/or to enhance their competencies and skills

- Ensure that minority groups receive an equitable service

- Support users in accessing and sustaining roles and relationships which they deem to be important

- Be aware of own attitudes and values and how these may influence practice

- Empower service users so that they are able to make choices about treatment and care

- Demonstrate understanding and empathy

- Adopt holism and apply principles of the Recovery Approach to practice

- Challenge public and professional stereotypes of mental ill health

- Engage in participatory approaches with users, families and carers

- Provide objective, non-judgemental information

Factors that may oppose those above and facilitate social exclusion

- Adoption of paternalistic attitudes and defensive practices

- Use of diagnostic terminology carelessly, e.g. John is a schizophrenic

- Viewing service users solely as 'patients', i.e. ignoring important social roles

- Assuming that service users do not know what is best for them

- Labelling service users and using labels as barriers to working in partnership

wider community, with full social roles (Sayce, 2000). Finally, mental health nurses also need to reflect on and examine their own attitudes and beliefs towards mental ill health and the needs of service users, so that they do not inadvertently become agents of social exclusion. It is only when the rights and abilities of service users are valued that social justice and social inclusion can be promoted and stigma and its effects mitigated.

CHAPTER 9
HOMOPHOBIA IN MENTAL HEALTH SERVICES
Andrew Thornton

INTRODUCTION

Gay men and lesbians often, it seems, have very negative views of health services, which have been described by such groups as homophobic and discriminatory (McFarlane, 1998). This chapter is concerned with the effects of such homophobia and related prejudices on the experiences that gay and lesbian people have of mental health services. It considers the implications of negative attitudes that health care professionals may hold towards service users' sexuality and the subsequent implications for their overall health and well-being. Overt evidence of homophobia in mental health services will be considered, and highlighted will be the fact that such hostility may invariably leave the gay or lesbian service user (and indeed homosexual staff member) marginalized and vulnerable – exactly the opposite of what is considered compatible with contemporary health care and is effectively outlawed by the Equality Act (2006) (Women and Equality Unit, 2006). It may be four decades since homosexuality was decriminalized in this country, and much anti-discriminatory progress has been made since then, but it seems much remains to be done if services really are to provide equal, non-discriminatory and quality care for all who use them.

BACKGROUND

Historically, psychiatry has had an ambivalent attitude to 'sexual deviancy' and only in recent years has it ceased to view homosexuality as a pathological condition (Smith

Contemporary Issues in Mental Health Nursing, Edited by J. E. Lynch and S. Trenoweth
© 2008 John Wiley & Sons, Ltd

et al., 2004). In the past, treatments to 'cure' homosexuality were mainly administered in NHS hospitals (Smith *et al.*, 2004) and ranged from the most common behavioural aversion therapy, with electric shocks or nausea-inducing 'apomorphine', to oestrogen treatment, electroconvulsive therapy (ECT), psychoanalysis and religious counselling (Smith *et al.*, 2004).

A range of studies have demonstrated consistently that gay men and lesbians continue to receive unequal and unfair treatment when accessing health care services. For example, a large UK study of the standard of mental health services experienced by gay men and lesbians reported that 33% of gay men and 40% of lesbians recounted negative or mixed positive and negative reactions from mental health professionals when being open about their sexuality (King and McKeown, 2003). These ranged from overt 'homophobia' (the irrational fear or even hatred of homosexuals with often concomitant discriminatory or abusive behaviours; Stonewall Scotland, 2003) to a lack of acceptance of diverse sexual orientations (see Chapter 19: Masculinity as a Risk Variable in Physical and Mental Ill Health). King and McKeown (2003) also identified poorer experiences of mental health, mental health services and general quality of life for gay men and lesbians when compared with heterosexuals. The study used over 2300 general and standardized questionnaires and a further smaller-scale study explored the experiences of gay and lesbian mental health service users and concluded that:

- Gay men and lesbians reported more psychological distress than heterosexuals.

- Their levels of substance abuse were higher than those of heterosexuals.

- Lesbians were more likely than heterosexual women to drink alcohol excessively.

- Violence and bullying in adult life were more commonly reported by lesbians than heterosexuals.

- Self-harm was also more common, affecting 30% of gay men and 12% of lesbians.

An earlier study by McFarlane (1998), for the Project for Advice, Counselling and Education (PACE), of 35 gay and lesbian mental health users and 35 mental health workers reported that a majority of respondents experienced or identified homophobia and 'heterosexism' (the belief that heterosexuality is the 'normal' or 'natural' form of sexual expression; Stonewall Scotland, 2003) as having an impact on their mental health care (McFarlane, 1998). Amid McFarlane's (1998) findings, anecdotal evidence indicated reluctance amongst gay men and lesbians to contact mainstream mental health services. This was largely due to perceived and reported fears about expressed homophobia and ignorance within the mental health services, and a perception that their sexuality would be pathologized. Declining to seek help for these reasons could, of course, leave individuals more vulnerable to mental ill health, prevent the early intervention for health problems which may subsequently lead to an individual's mental state deteriorating, and increase their feelings of social isolation and marginalization. In the study by McFarlane (1998), participants expressed the view that good health care practice depended on the awareness and commitment of individual staff members, a point that may be unsurprising to some readers but is fundamentally important feedback from those who receive care. Worryingly, the study (McFarlane, 1998) also pointed out that the very physical safety of gay men and lesbians cannot be guaranteed within mental health services – women especially feared or experienced intimidation, sexual harassment and sexual assault.

A further, qualitative study of 37 gay men sheds light on the mental health care experiences and needs of gay men (Robertson, 1998). In this case, findings provide further evidence of a reluctance amongst gay men to disclose their sexuality in health care settings. Whilst it could be argued that few service users 'disclose' their sexuality routinely when coming into contact with health care professionals (and this is a personal choice that an individual is entitled to make), it is important to note that the reluctance identified here is due to concern about subsequent hostility or other poor treatment based on a declared sexual orientation, a feature that is bound to compromise relationships between professionals and service users. In the mental health context in particular, circumspect, self-protective attitudes of service users essentially mean that they may not feel able to trust those whose job it is to care for them. This is serious enough yet it is exacerbated by the corollary that mental health needs may then remain unrecognized and unaddressed. There can be no room for complacency when studies such as that by Dorais (2004) in North America have led to the conclusion that there is a link between the social stigmatization of homosexuality and higher levels of suicide attempts. Overall, the importance of the Nursing and Midwifery Council's (NMC) *Code of Professional Conduct* (NMC, 2004b) is worth emphasizing and re-emphasizing as some service users appear to be receiving care that falls below the standards of professionalism that are required in nursing.

REVIEW OF RISKS FOR GAY MEN AND LESBIAN SERVICE USERS

It is, however, not only an increased risk of suicide and being the victim of violent attacks from others that gay men and lesbian service users may experience. There is considerable evidence that gay men and lesbians have significantly poorer overall physical and mental health (Stonewall Scotland, 2003), which compromises their overall quality of life. Service users may also be exposed to risks associated with emotional harm and a significant loss of personal dignity. Indeed, the risks of emotional harm may increase if a gay man or lesbian's sexuality is not accepted or acknowledged within the assessment process and understood as an important aspect of his or her personal identity and psychological well-being.

The risks that can jeopardize gay men and lesbians' mental health are complex and are by no means the same for each person. There are many variables that can influence the resistance of a person from a 'minority' group to withstand discrimination from a predominantly heterosexual society. This is reflected in the 'stress vulnerability' model (Zubin and Spring, 1977; Brennan, 2006), which links different components of stress vulnerability with the personal abilities of someone to cope with environmental stress. Support structures such, as the interrelatedness of the family, social networks including the influence of peers and the progressive approaches within schools or colleges, can all contribute to the strengthening of one's personal ability to cope.

Homophobia may accentuate the feelings of rejection and stigma gay men or lesbians experience in a mainstream, predominantly heterosexual society. Isolation and its effects may be especially potent when their sexuality results in some individuals losing the support of their families and friends (Mind, 2007) (see Chapter 8: Challenging Stigma and Promoting Social Justice). This negative view may affect an individual's sense of self-worth and ability to integrate socially – this can lead to withdrawal and further isolation (McFarlane, 1998; Mind, 2007). As well as generalized anxiety and sleep disturbance, homophobia can trigger, in vulnerable people, panic attacks, depressive moods or thoughts, poor memory and concentration, compulsive behaviour and obsessive thoughts (BBC, 2004). There may be an increased risk of self-harm or a suicide attempt, although this can depend on how much support an individual has (BBC, 2004; Mind, 2007).

Furthermore, with unchecked homophobia and heterosexism within mental health services, there is a danger that the legal status of an individual's civil partner (under the introduction of the Civil Partnerships Act 2004) may not be recognized or acknowledged. As such, the civil partner of a gay or lesbian service user may not be accorded the same rights or respect as their heterosexual counterpart. This has clear implications for next of kin considerations under the Mental Health Act 1983 and the Care Programme Approach arrangements (DH, 1990, 1999c).

POLICY CONTEXT

So what can mental health services do to enable gay men and lesbians to feel more welcomed and able to access mental health services earlier? The answer to this question is important as it can make a difference to whether or not individuals proactively seek support. Indeed, Platzer (2005), for PACE, identified and suggested a number of practical guidelines in working with the families of gay men and lesbians in mental health services and as such is recommended as a useful guide to local health authorities and practitioners alike in accommodating the needs and wishes of gay men and lesbians. Furthermore, Stonewall Scotland (2003) offers recommendations for improving the overall health and well-being for gay men and lesbians, focusing on the need for such views to be challenged within services and society in general, and also for the development of polices which reach out to and actively seek to engage gay communities, whilst ensuring that health care practice is explicitly, and demonstrably, anti-discriminatory.

Encouraging service users to engage and express themselves fully is currently being encouraged on professional and political fronts. In *From Values to Action: the Chief Nursing Officer's Review of Mental Health Nursing* (DH, 2006a), service users and their carers stated clearly that they want skilled and knowledgeable nurses who possess positive human qualities. The report indicates that users want their personal values to be acknowledged and that recovery can be assisted by recognition of individual worth. Showing acceptance and working towards meaningful goals collaboratively set out with gay and lesbian clients will be a positive step towards fulfilling some of the recommendations set out in this timely review.

Recent initiatives by the Department of Health have sought to promote anti-discriminatory care and practice. The *Ten Essential Shared Capabilities* (DH, 2004a), as well as the National Institute for Mental Health in England's (NIMHE) *Guiding Statement on Recovery* (NIMHE, 2005), will help to focus the drive for changes and prevent behaviours that are subjective, negative and discriminatory. This, it is hoped, can encourage the development of user-focused resources and help speed up the changes required to meet the needs of gay men and lesbians. By providing resources and up-to-date information for service users and their carers, rights to evidence-based and individualized care can be promoted.

THE WAY FORWARD

It is clear that individual mental health workers and services more generally have progress to make to provide care which is sensitive to the needs of gay and lesbian clients and to counteract the prevailing heterosexist orientation of care delivery. This may be difficult to achieve and to maximize chances of success, it is clear that a multi-faceted strategy will be needed.

Perhaps the greatest challenge will be to enable mental health nurses to become aware of possible heterosexism (intentional or unconscious) and homophobia (overt or covert). Setting up a reflective group that meets regularly to discuss issues in an open and frank forum could help all professionals think about values, beliefs and attitudes that are incompatible with anti-discriminatory practice. Such a group might help individuals develop an empathic understanding of the needs of gay and lesbian service users. A better and more visible representation of gay and lesbian nurses will facilitate this, and may support the creation of a mutually respectful environment where all nurses can learn from each other. Indeed, such groups may be supported by ongoing individual clinical supervision which can help nurses reflect and adapt themselves to the needs of comprehensive, modern mental health care.

Such an approach could also help remind staff of the need to implement changes collectively, underlining the positive impact that they can generate by thinking about sexuality in creative ways and with unbiased perspectives. This may offer a collective sense of pride and will be a positive step within team building efforts and initiatives.

Nurses with different beliefs can then see the benefits from valuing each other's life experience and what this can bring to team identity. Indeed, R.D. Laing and his anti-psychiatry perspective on mental health suggested the creation of 'therapeutic communities' (Clay, 1996). This approach welcomes and values people with different perspectives, united by their common respect for humanity. A clear, visible and widely consulted philosophy of care could include stressing the need for respect for all types of sexuality, as the expression of this is a basic human need and right. This could be evaluated regularly to see whether changes had been made and allow good practice examples from other services or agencies to influence further development.

Education can play an important part here – there are many learning packages and teaching events available from organizations that offer support to gay men and lesbians, such as PACE or 'Gay Men Fighting Aids'. These may help nurses challenge their own values and assumptions. It means that the nurse can respect the client's separateness and accept their unique differences (Nelson-Jones, 2003; McMillan, 2004). Furthermore, it is incumbent upon Higher Education Institutes (HEIs) to ensure that their pre-registration nursing programmes highlight issues of homophobia and heterosexism in health care services and the subsequent potential impact on physical and mental well-being. However, this is unlikely to have any major impact if students are socialized into clinical environments within which discriminatory behaviour is normalized and unchallenged.

Indeed, achieving a better representation of gay and lesbian nurses in clinical practice, reflecting the local population, poses challenges for workforce planning. One way to enhance such recruitment will be to advertise mental health nursing jobs within the local gay and lesbian media. Furthermore, interviewers could include questions and exercises that focus on issues regarding 'values-based practice', as recommended within the Chief Nursing Officer's review (DH, 2006a) (see Chapter 5: The Implications of Values-Based Practice in Mental Health Nursing). This could, in turn, help interview panels ascertain each candidate's values towards notions such as social inclusiveness and respect for diverse sexuality. Trusts need to ensure that their equal opportunity policies are updated and well publicized and that steps are taken if such policies are transgressed.

Challenging homophobia and heterosexism in clinical services will require effective clinical leadership and support. To instigate effective changes in attitudes towards gay and lesbian sexuality, the role of the clinical leader or other change agent will be to assist colleagues who possess homophobic attitudes to begin to question their under-standings of homosexuality. Indeed, Thyer (2003) states that, by its very nature, nursing is suited to transforming health care environments. This is because it is creative, visionary, empowering, communication focused and involves decision making which has a practical impact. Thyer (2003) goes on to say that 'transformational leadership' will have positive effects on team development and collaboration. The most effective and respected leaders are often those who keep a regular presence in clinical areas and offer colleagues a chance to contribute their views. This way of working ensures that consensual change can be brought about. Conflict within a team can hinder change and Almost (2006) argues that positive outcomes for nurses and health care organizations can be achieved when conflict is properly managed and understood. Therefore, conflict resolution requires nurses to view problems as a means of enabling their teams to move through a variety of differing standpoints and towards a collectively resolved and managed conclusion that allows team development and genuine learning from each other. This can only benefit the quality of care that gay and lesbian service users receive as staff will have already confronted conflicts regarding sexuality. This experience can not only foster stronger team approaches to finding collaborative solutions to difficulties; it also helps teams acknowledge that they can deal with conflicts and that they are able to move forwards by not being afraid of open and honest discussion.

IMPLEMENTATION OF CHANGES

To implement changes successfully, consideration will need to be given to the nature and extent of anti-discriminatory views that may be held. One way in which this could be done is through anonymous questionnaires, whether Trust-wide or at ward level. However, the wording and format would need to be carefully thought through as this may have an influence on how honest respondents are to relevant issues. Ensuring anonymity will help prevent respondents providing answers they think they *should* provide as opposed to honest ones which, if reflected upon, can assist in identifying beliefs and attitudes that can lead to negative experiences for some service users. Baker *et al.* (2000) state that for genuine and meaningful cultural transformation to succeed there should be a process and an environment that is comfortable and non-threatening in language and actions, as well as participatory and engaging.

Those organizations in which management works closely with clinical staff are usually more adaptive and flexible (NHS Service Delivery and Organisation, 2006). Therefore, the process that this chapter suggests to set up would be first to launch a Trust-wide consultation process before any changes are made. This will be more likely to bring about effective changes as employees will be more likely to feel equipped to deal with the dynamics of change. In large organizations it is of course unlikely that the ideas concerning change will be perceived and approved in the same ways by all members of staff.

Effective clinical governance will be established if service managers are seen to be supporting and facilitating change processes that aim to benefit service users. This sort of use of clinical governance is merely one example of its potential to influence and steer change at local level. Ford (2004) suggests that organizations with successful clinical governance frameworks have staff with a range of attitudes and a greater openness and willingness to tackle quality issues in a collaborative way. Thus, managerial governance which is committed to a team approach can foster the responsible clinical leadership that is essential for implementation of changes in the care that gay men and lesbians receive from mental health services.

CONCLUSION

In this chapter it has been argued that many gay men and lesbians receive mental health care that falls far below the standard of that received by others as a consequence of their sexual orientation. This has the potential to leave them at greater risk of further deterioration in mental health and marginalization from mainstream service and society. In the present climate of exploring what mental health nursing stands for, especially its values, it is important to acknowledge that prejudices of any description form one of the main barriers to quality care. Through a combination of education, professionalism, team work and management support this can be addressed, but a long-term and indeed perennial commitment from health care staff at all levels is required. This will ensure that mental health care is open to all sections of the community. Every patient's sexuality should be acknowledged and respected when care is provided by mental health services. Mental health nurses can, and must, take a lead role in improving the health-related experiences of gay men and lesbians in their care.

SECTION 2
CLINICAL ISSUES

- **The Meaning of Recovery (James Matthews)**

- **Supporting Recovery: Medication Management in Mental Health Care (Joanna Bennett)**

- **Co-Morbidity in Physical and Mental Ill Health (Helen Robson, Carl Margereson and Steve Trenoweth)**

- **Physical Illness: Promoting Effective Coping in Clients with Co-Morbidity (Carl Margereson)**

- **Responding to the Needs of Younger People: The Bereaved Adolescent (Yvonne Dexter)**

- **Enhancing Effective Multidisciplinary Team-Working: A Psychoeducational Approach (John Cordwell and Lee Bradley)**

In this section, the authors draw our attention to a number of prominent and contemporary clinical themes, such as the issues of 'holistic' care delivery and a focus on 'recovery'. Indeed, the concept of recovery has become a recurring theme within the contemporary field of mental health care, and as such is of particular relevance to the practice of mental health nurses. The perception of recovery in purely medical terms (that is, an absence or abatement of symptoms) has been challenged in recent years. There is an increasing emphasis, from within the profession and at governmental level, on a much wider view of recovery and a more explicit focus on assisting service users to improve their quality of life and well-being. This requires a redefinition of the 'end goals' of mental health nursing care, and a requirement that the subjectivity of the service user's views, their wishes, experience and expertise are at the centre of attempts to support their recovery. With changes to nurse prescribing and a continued need for mental health nurses to be proactive in medication management, the need for service user partnership and on-going collaboration is vital. As such, the need to listen to, acknowledge and understand the personal experiences of service users in relation to their health and problems is an important undercurrent throughout this section. Clearly, there are many benefits that working within a cohesive and well-led multi-professional team can have on improving the health and well-being of clients. Indeed, complex problems, such as bereavement in adolescence, or those resulting from a 'personality disorder' are most likely to be effectively managed within a multi-professional and multi-agency context.

Physical health care has quite rightly become an important issue in recent years. Mental health services' readiness to deliver 'holistic care' is, of course, an important policy issue for the UK government and a central feature of the Chief Nursing Officer's Review. This aside, it is becoming all too obvious that people with mental health problems have some of the poorest physical health in society and unequal access to medical care. Mental health nurses have a professional duty and moral obligation to support service users in their attempts to improve, cope with and recover from physical illnesses. This may have implications for the education and training of mental health nurses, now and in the future.

Much of the research referred to in this section comes from fields other than mental health nursing. It is crucial that we are able to increase our efforts to research clinical nursing interventions, using a variety of different methods and approaches, which will allow us to assist service users in their attempts at recovery. This is especially true in the area of adolescent bereavement, within which myths abound.

CHAPTER 10
THE MEANING OF RECOVERY

James Matthews

INTRODUCTION

The concept of recovery is a recurring theme within the field of mental health, and of particular contemporary relevance to the practice of mental health nurses (Repper, 2000a; Took, 2002; NIMHE, 2005; DH, 2006a). It is, however, a multifaceted and complex issue (Badger and Nolan, 2007). As such, it can be difficult to fully appreciate what is meant by the term 'recovery', and what it means to those affected by mental health problems. In this chapter, the concept of recovery is explored along with an appreciation of why the client's personal and internal frame of reference is so valuable within modern mental health nursing practice. Factors which are held to be important in assisting and supporting recovery are also considered.

RECOVERY MODELS

Warner (1985) proposed that a distinct difference exists between what he termed 'complete recovery' and 'social recovery'. In the former, he described the experience of recovery from schizophrenia in which the affected individual returns to his or her level of functioning as before the onset of symptoms – recovery is seen to be 'complete'. Social recovery, on the other hand, focuses on beliefs and aspirations *towards* recovery, and involves an emphasis on social support, realistic planning, significant working relationships, encouragement, appropriate treatment, choice and self-management. Indeed, some have suggested that contemporary emphasis should be placed not on

Contemporary Issues in Mental Health Nursing, Edited by J. E. Lynch and S. Trenoweth
© 2008 John Wiley & Sons, Ltd

complete recovery, but on the on-going process of *recovering* from mental health problems (Corrigan and Phelan, 2004). Here, an emphasis is placed on enabling a person to move on, in a climate of optimism, acceptance, hope and positive determination by all those involved in the process (Took, 2002; Kelly and Gamble, 2005). This, it is felt, can lead to real and significant improvements in an individual's quality of life (Mitchell, 2001; Fisher, 2003; Ochocka *et al.*, 2005; NIMHE, 2005) whilst assisting in the achievement of personal goals despite experiencing 'symptoms'. Hence, recovery in this sense:

. . . is not about regaining a problem-free life – whose life is? It is about living life more resourcefully, living a satisfying and contributing life, in spite of limitations caused by a continuing vulnerability to disabling distress (Watkins, 2001, p. 45).

Indeed, many aspects of the social recovery model described by Warner (1985) more than two decades ago have gained a wider acceptance in the United Kingdom and have been integrated into broader governmental health policy frameworks such as the National Service Framework for Mental Health (DH, 1999a) and the guiding principles set out by the National Institute for Mental Health in England (NIMHE, 2005). Indeed, NIMHE sees 'recovery' as a multifaceted concept which they describe as:

A return to a state of wellness (e.g., following an episode of depression); Achievement of a personally acceptable quality of life (e.g., following an episode of psychosis); A process or period of recovering (e.g., following trauma); A process of gaining or restoring something (e.g., one's sobriety); An act of obtaining usable resources from apparently unusable sources (e.g., in prolonged psychosis where the experience itself has intrinsic personal value); To recover optimum quality of life and have satisfaction with life in disconnected circumstances (e.g., dementia) (NIMHE, 2005, p. 2).

It is also worth noting that many of these aspects of the social recovery model were highlighted in the recent review of mental health nursing (DH, 2006a). As such, the future development of mental health nursing will necessitate:

. . . working in partnership with service users (and/or carers) to identify realistic life goals and enabling them to achieve them; stressing the value of social inclusion (clear evidence exists which demonstrates that inclusion has a strong link with positive mental health outcomes); stressing the need for professionals to be optimistic about the possibility of positive individual change (DH, 2006a, p. 17).

If we accept a social model of recovery as an important approach for mental health nursing practice, then we must also accept that there are individual meanings that people attach to their experience of health and illness (Watkins, 2001). As such, perceptions of recovery itself can be subjective, particularly in respect to the definitions of 'end goals' for each individual involved in the process. An appreciation of the service user's personal perception of recovery, identification of goals desired and the meaning attached to experiences, hopes, aspirations and fears is, therefore, vital (Rethink, 2005a). Indeed, it might be that the individual may need support to clarify realistic personal goals, as whether or not these 'end goals' are explicit and achievable can have a profound effect on an individual's motivation in the recovery process. This may require nurses to help people develop a realistic understanding of their mental health problems and their coping abilities. For example, a medical approach may perceive recovery from mental health problems to be as an abatement of clinical symptoms or a 'cure' (Cohen, 2005). Indeed, if one aligns a personal recovery to being 'symptom free' then one may see oneself as ill until 'cured' (Corrigan and Phelan, 2004), with a concomitant perceived need for on-going treatment. At such times, the individual may react passively to his or her illness, feeling at the mercy of the symptoms which may be perceived as being out of his/her personal control. However, helping people to regain control over their lives and, moreover, active engagement by the service user are seen as important aspects of the process of recovery (Coodin-Schiff, 2004; Rethink, 2005a). Indeed, it has become apparent that those individuals who have a clearer and more comprehensive understanding and acceptance of their health problems, and engage more positively with support mechanisms around them, have a greater chance to improve their quality of life, and as such seem to be less limited by their condition (Cunningham *et al.*, 2005) (see Chapter 15: Enhancing Effective Multidisciplinary Team-Working: A Psychoeducational Approach).

PERSONAL EXPERIENCES OF RECOVERY

Inevitably the path of recovery from some form of health problem or illness will be experienced by most of us in some way at some point in our lives. A serious health problem can be a personal and unique experience (Rethink, 2005a), and to some extent can affect the very core of someone's individuality and their relationship with their immediate and perceived reality (Anthony, 1993; Roe *et al.*, 2004). Similar to the process of recovery from physical illness, recovering from a mental health problem is said to represent a determination to move forward and is linked to the basic human motivation for survival and growth (Ochocka *et al.*, 2005).

Indeed, there exists considerable subjectivity and uncertainty regarding the recovery process both in theory and in practice (Repper and Perkins, 2003; Skärsäter *et al.*, 2005) (see Chapter 6: Truth, Uncertainty and the Mental Health Nurse). In the sort of recovery envisaged by NIMHE (2005) and Rethink (2005a), individuals affected by mental ill health should be actively (as opposed to passively) involved in the overall process (Roe *et al.*, 2004). However, Dorrer (2006) reviewed the topic of recovery extensively and suggested that there is a significant gap between how clinicians and researchers measure recovery and users' definition of their own progress. Indeed, Dorrer (2006) highlights the risks of endeavouring to quantify the recovery process in purely medical terms, and stresses that mental health practitioners need to listen to, and hear, what those who have experienced mental health problems have to say.

For Coodin-Schiff (2004, p. 215), recovery from mental health problems was associated with feelings of '. . . being at peace, being happy, feeling comfortable with the world and others, and feeling hope for the future'. Others report that one of the core concepts in recovery from mental health problems is an endeavour to be honest with oneself, and to this extent the person affected will have to accept, reconsider or reject some of his or her values and search for meaning and personal truth in the face of mental distress (Mitchell, 2001; Watkins, 2001). That is, mental health problems can be life changing and life damaging, but recovery from such difficulties can also be life affirming. In this sense, the concept of recovery incorporates purpose, hope, inclusion and draws on the personal resilience, strengths and efforts of those affected to tackle the barriers that impede progress towards health and well-being (Anthony, 1993; Lunt, 2001; Kelly and Gamble, 2005). An important area for mental health nursing care, therefore, will be to understand how an individual perceives his or her problems. Indeed, one factor which can affect an individual's personal experience of, and may act as a barrier to, recovery is that of social stigma – the individual's feeling of being spurned or avoided as a result of having a mental health problem (Wahl, 1999) (see Chapter 8: Challenging Stigma and Promoting Social Justice). As such, mental health nurses will need to carefully consider how stigma may affect an individual's feelings of self-efficacy and self-esteem (Link and Phelan, 2001; Link *et al.*, 2001) and how such views may undermine the recovery process (Sirey *et al.*, 2001; Watkins, 2001).

SUPPORTING RECOVERY

According to NIMHE (2005), contemporary emphasis in mental health care should be placed on the personal *process* of recovery rather than focusing purely upon the achievement of positive clinical *outcomes*. This has considerable implications when considering the many and diverse factors which may affect recovery. For example, consideration needs to be given to the psychological climate within which mental health care takes place, as the collaboration and involvement of service users in their care is likely to be a significant factor in their recovery (Rethink, 2005a). This is an issue which is of particular importance to service users who have indicated the importance they attach to involvement in their own care and having their own contribution to their recovery acknowledged (Badger and Nolan, 2007). Indeed, it is felt that the recovery process is facilitated when:

Hope is encouraged, enhanced and/or maintained; Life roles with respect to work and meaningful activities are defined; Spirituality is considered; Culture is understood; Educational needs as well as those of families/significant others are identified; Socialisation needs are identified; They are supported to achieve their goals (NIMHE, 2005, p. 4).

That is, to support the recovery of clients with mental health problems, services and practitioners will need to ensure their willingness and ability to listen to their service users' hopes and fears, and to collaborate with them, delivering care which is explicitly service-user focused (Rethink, 2005a) (see Chapter 2: Rebuilding Lives: A Critical Look at the Contemporary Role of the Mental Health Nurse).

We are reminded here by Reisner (2005) that the personality and style characteristics of the carer can be a significant factor in the recovery process (Luborsky *et al.*, 1999). Thus, the emotional responses, the ability to solve problems, the willingness to engage and the overall performance and functioning of mental health nurses and other carers can significantly influence the service user's experience and perception of the recovery process (Dixon, 2000; Kelly and Gamble, 2005). Indeed, 'people who have significantly recovered from schizophrenia have frequently reported that they were greatly helped by someone who believed in them' (Kelly and Gamble, 2005, p. 249) and here, the support from family and friends, as well as a wider social network, is likely to be a major factor in supporting recovery (Rethink, 2005a; Badger and Nolan, 2007).

In recent years, a number of approaches have been developed which, ideologically and practically, seem to facilitate recovery. Barker (2000), for example, proposed the use of the Tidal Model to address issues of situational and individual crises experienced by users at various times in their lives. That is, according to Barker (2003, p. 99), 'by emphasizing the centrality of the lived experience, of the person and her/his significant others, the need for mutual understanding between nurse and the person in care is also acknowledged and the need for a personally appropriate, contextually bound form of care, established.' Barker also suggests that the Tidal Model may assist practitioners to understand their own responses whilst assisting in the service user's recovery (Barker, 2001).

Motivational interviewing (MI) is another technique which may assist in supporting and facilitating user-focused recovery. MI is a client-centred, directive approach which enhances an individual's perceived intrinsic motivation to change by exploring and resolving ambivalence (Miller and Rollnick, 2002). As such, MI may assist clients to identify and clarify their personal goals whilst affirming their inherent right to make informed choices about their treatment and care. Indeed, Miller (1994) argues that it is inappropriate to think of MI as a technique but as an interpersonal style, not necessarily restricted to formal counselling settings (see Figure 10.1).

For some, 'self-help' organizations may be significant to support an individual's recovery (NICE, 2004; Richards, 2004), especially amongst those with limited social

- *Expression of empathy* – seeing the world through clients' eyes and sharing their experiences

- *Supporting self-efficacy* – belief that change is possible (an important motivator)

- *Rolling with resistance* – not fighting the client's resistance but using the client's 'momentum' to explore his or her views further

- *Developing discrepancy* – enabling client to perceive a discrepancy between where he is and where he wants to be

Source: Miller and Rollnick (2002).

Figure 10.1

General principles behind motivational interviewing

support networks (Badger and Nolan, 2007). Self-help groups '. . . draw upon the experience of members to provide support, information, coping skills, problem solving and advocacy. Group members are empowered to take control over their lives, support others, and develop positive attitudes about themselves and their condition' (Peterkin, 1993, p. 817). As such, self-help groups may assist in the development of self-efficacy and assist people to marshal their own internal resources to support their own recovery (Richards, 2004). Furthermore, an important and embryonic area here is that of 'self-management' approaches, where the individual is acknowledged as an expert in recognizing and responding to his/her own mental health needs and 'symptoms', and which assists people to explore and understand their personal experiences (DH, 2001b; Rethink, 2003) (see Chapter 13: Physical Illness: Promoting Effective Coping in Clients with Co-Morbidity). For some service users, the use of medication may have been an important aspect of their recovery (Badger and Nolan, 2007) and as such, involvement of the service user in prescribing decisions, and their subsequent satisfaction with the medication, will be crucial (see Chapter 11: Supporting Recovery: Medication Management in Mental Health Care). However, recovery is likely to be inhibited by dosages of medication which impact on the person's ability to engage in the process of recovery or where side-effects are experienced (Took, 2002).

FACTORS AFFECTING RECOVERY

While variations remain in the way each person will experience recovery, a number of factors have been identified as having possible effects on the overall process. Recovery can be significantly affected by social and spiritual issues relating to the individual, such as culture, employment, faith and views of the 'self'. Indeed, there can be important differences in relation to how one's culture may affect the recovery process. Snowden and Wu (1997) found that compared with White Americans, some Latino, African-American and Asian-American clients were more likely to utilize out-patient and community services than in-patient services, although the same study also found the reverse was true in some other parts of the United States. In another study, Guarnaccia and Parra (1996) found significant variations in the readiness by some peoples to accept a professionally applied label of an illness over others (European-Americans more so than others), and a greater expectancy of complete recovery for family members (Hispanic-and African-Americans had stronger beliefs that their relatives would be 'cured' than European-Americans). Strong religious beliefs amongst ethnic minority groups in the latter study were believed to be a significantly prevailing factor resulting in this optimism. However, while it is worth considering that although belief systems may play a role in how some ethnic minorities experience the process of re-covery, it is also clear that issues such as discrimination, language, low socio-economic status, unemployment and education may skew findings in relation to how some ethnic minorities perceive or access health services (Lambo, 1970; Holzer *et al.*, 1986; Robins *et al.*, 1991; Guarnaccia and Parra, 1996).

Employment is widely accepted as an important variable in the recovery process for those who have experienced mental health problems (Rethink, 2003; Rinaldi *et al.*, 2004). However, 'the transition from benefits to work can be difficult, given that people tend to progress in stages, e.g. through voluntary work, part-time work before full-time work. Some may never be capable of full-time paid work yet may engage in meaningful activity that keeps them well and out of expensive hospital care' (Took, 2002, p. 636). Helping people to realize their aspirations, or reframe their expectations, of careers and employment in the light of their difficulties is, therefore, an important aspect of mental health care (Rethink, 2003). Indeed, the concept of employment may equally apply to job or career opportunities but also to employment of time. For example, the playing of sport, undertaking voluntary work and study have also been described as facilitating recovery (Badger and Nolan, 2007). This finding has been reiterated by others who have noted important associations between self-esteem, hope and employment (Marwaha and Johnson, 2005).

Faith or religious beliefs have also been found to have a significant effect on the rate of recovery in some people with mental health problems (Basky, 2000; Rethink, 2003, 2005a). Other findings that have supported this theme have also noted a strong association between hope, spirituality, comfort and reassurance in the recovery process (Deegan, 1993; Lunt, 2001). Initiatives that include peer and family support have also been identified as helpful in the process of adaptation and functioning for those recovering from mental health problems, as have well-structured psychoeducational training programmes (Stromwall and Hurdle, 2003) (see Chapter 15: Enhancing Effective Multidisciplinary Team-Working: A Psychoeducational Approach). There is some evidence to suggest that self-management programmes can be an effective way in helping some people with phobias, panic disorders and obsessive–compulsive disorders (Barlow et al., 2005). That is, the recovery process may depend not only on the severity of their symptoms, but also on an individual's personal perception of self-efficacy in terms of being able to control and manage symptoms (Markowitz, 2001) (see Chapter 13: Physical Illness: Promoting Effective Coping in Clients with Co-Morbidity).

Contemporary emphasis, therefore, has rightly been placed on the importance of psychological working to create a climate to support recovery, such as goals clarification, hope, optimism and so forth (Kelly and Gamble, 2005). However, in order to assist people in the recovery process in a holistic sense, attention also needs to be paid to issues which affect people's physical and biological functioning. For example, good nutrition is said to play a role in the prevention of, and recovery from, some mental health problems (Mental Health Foundation, 2006). In a study that looked at the relationship between dietary supplements and depression, researchers in Finland found that after adjusting for variables such as smoking, alcohol consumption, body mass index, socio-economic status, marital status, appetite, education and total fat intake, they could not exclude the possibility that a relation exists between depression and dietary folate – the water-soluble B vitamin that occurs naturally in food and is synthesized as Folic acid in supplements and fortified foods (Tolmunen et al., 2003) (see Chapter 12: Physical Co-Morbidity in Mental Health).

Another study that looked at the effects of food on age-related cognitive functioning and decline found that the consumption of antioxidant-rich foods such as fruit and vegetables (especially apple juice) can help in the prevention of oxidative damage and cognitive decline that can occur through the aging process and dietary and genetic deficiencies (Chan et al., 2006). In their laboratory-based study of animals, Weaver and colleagues (Weaver et al., 2004) found a relationship between specific amino acids and genes that affect the way some species mediate stress. This suggests that diet can have a significant effect on how stress is managed and how confidence is affected in relation to exploring new environments. Drawing from these findings, Motluk (2005) suggests that in the future, some aspects of diet may be able to manipulate, alter or reverse certain illnesses, including Huntington's disease, schizophrenia and cancer.

Indeed, the NICE (2006a) guideline on the management of bipolar disorder recommends that, to support recovery, dietary advice along with exercise should be integrated into any proposed treatment plan. However, this advice appears to be specifically directed at those who have had significant problems with weight gain as a result of medication. From a clinical standpoint, decisions in relation to choice of diet, dietary supplement and how both may affect a client's recovery will most likely be an agreed decision between the client and the appropriate key worker. However, this remains a controversial area as other findings from trials and reviews in the area of diet, dietary supplements and mental well-being have suggested that there is no conclusive evidence to imply that dietary supplements or herbal remedies can improve mental well-being (Walter and Rey, 1999; Jorm *et al.*, 2002; Ellinson *et al.*, 2004; Vaughan and McConaghy, 2004; Petersen *et al.*, 2005). However, we should not underestimate the relationship between diet, our subjective experiences of well-being and the effects food is likely to have on human physiology (Benton and Donohoe, 1999).

Finally, the importance of the relationship between, and impact of, substance misuse and mental health cannot be underestimated in the recovery process (DH, 2006c). While the debate as to how prognosis and recovery are affected by those with a 'dual-diagnosis' (for example, concurrent substance misuse issues and mental health problems) remains open to significant discussion and reviews (O'Sullivan, 1984; Black *et al.*, 1991; Bartels *et al.*, 1995; Drake *et al.*, 1996), it is clear that there are increased rates of substance misuse amongst those with serious mental health problems (SNMAC, 1999; DH, 2002a). For example, there is likely to be a reduced concordance with treatment plans, increased physical needs, higher incidence of re-hospitalization, a propensity towards violence and increased incidents of self-harm in clients with a 'dual diagnosis', which can seriously undermine their recovery attempts (Gournay *et al.*, 1997; Graham *et al.*, 2001; DH, 2002a, 2006b). However, while this is an issue which affects both primary and secondary health services in terms of the overall treatment and care of this client group (DH, 1999a), many health care professionals may overlook the complexity of the associated needs of those who misuse substances (Gafoor and Hussein-Rassool, 1998). Furthermore, as there can be significant variations in support services for those with a dual diagnosis, with a recognition that many services have a primary or specific function (for example, specialized alcohol, drug or mental health teams rather than a combined service), there is a concern that the needs of large numbers of such clients will be ignored, not identified or will go unmet (Weaver *et al.*, 2003; Galletly and Watson, 2006).

CONCLUSION

Recovery, then, is a journey rather than a destination. The concept is not new by any means to many professionals working in this field. However, the contemporary focus on social recovery (Warner, 2005) requires mental health nurses to possibly reconsider their practice. A holistic approach needs to be taken, and nurses need to develop a broader understanding of what they may be able to do to improve their care for clients in the process of the recovery. Listening to, and taking account of, the experiences of those involved in the recovery process is certainly crucial.

Obviously, change is one of the most important and meaningful issues to consider in the recovery process. For some, this change may prove to be a difficult process (Davidson, 2005), characterized by anxiety, changes in perception, an awareness of loss (what they may have lost during their illness) and issues of self-control (Forchuk *et al.*, 2003). Indeed, it is likely that the experience of recovery is likely to be intensely personal with associated individual meanings and resonances. As such, we as mental health nurses may have to define recovery beyond the realms of biology and psychiatry if we are to fully appreciate the subjectivity of this experience.

Reviewing the ways in which we work with our clients, and our ability to listen to, and instil hope and optimism, may invigorate our existing methods of practice. It is also likely to assist our clients in relation to the way they cope and live with the difficulties they may encounter on their own journey towards and through recovery. Embracing the concept of recovery may also offer mental health nurses a fresher and possibly more innovative way in which they can approach the delivery of care (Andresen *et al.*, 2003; Lakeman, 2004; Leung and Arthur, 2004; Oades *et al.*, 2005).

CHAPTER 11
SUPPORTING RECOVERY: MEDICATION MANAGEMENT IN MENTAL HEALTH CARE

Joanna Bennett

INTRODUCTION

A recent report by the Healthcare Commission (2007) suggests that the management of medication must be a top priority in mental health services. The report highlighted a high level of medication use, with 92% of mental health service users having taken medicines for their conditions in the previous 12 months. However, it was also suggested that in mental health services the issue of medication management receives less support than is found within medical services, although mental health service users are more likely to have problems with their medicines.

Utilizing a description from an earlier document published by the Audit Commission (2001), the Healthcare Commission's report (2007, p. 3) describes medicines management as '. . . the entire way that medicines are selected, procured, delivered, prescribed, administered and reviewed, to optimise the contribution that medicines make to producing desired outcomes of patient care'. This chapter, however, is primarily concerned with the clinical use of medication as a care and treatment option in mental health care. Emphasis is thus given to the prescription and administration of medications within psychiatric contexts and the processes involved in the care and

Contemporary Issues in Mental Health Nursing, Edited by J. E. Lynch and S. Trenoweth
© 2008 John Wiley & Sons, Ltd

management of service users. This chapter also outlines the key elements of a proposed framework for the clinical management of medication by mental health practitioners. This includes:

- Developing a therapeutic alliance with service users and their carers.

- Rational prescribing based on the best available evidence and focused on facilitating recovery.

- Monitoring the adverse reactions and side-effects of medication.

- Promoting concordance.

CONTEMPORARY CONTEXT

The Commission's report confirms that medication continues to be the main treatment approach in mental health, traditionally seen as the domain of the medical practitioner. The main focus in many contemporary health care settings seems to be on the reduction of symptoms and the assumed, potential risk resulting from mental ill health. Indeed, there continues to be the view that the mental health and subsequent status of those prescribed medication renders their views 'unreliable'. Furthermore, the 'patient' may be generally viewed as a passive recipient of medication and expected to tolerate whatever is prescribed, including any unpleasant side-effects (Healthcare Commission, 2007).

However, it is becoming increasingly clear that medication alone is insufficient to prevent relapse and chronicity of mental health problems. Though still developing, evidence has highlighted several key features that can assist these goals: providing wider psychosocial supports; working in partnership with service users, carers and families; offering greater treatment choices; and enhancing concordance so service users can be enabled to utilize prescribed medication to best effect. As such, the goals of treatment have developed from merely objective improvements in symptomatology to incorporate factors such as users' subjective responses, perceived well-being and quality of life (DH, 2004a).

With the introduction of non-medical prescribing, mental health nurses and pharmacists specializing in mental health are now receiving training as supplementary or independent prescribers. These developments require a framework for the clinical management of medication that goes beyond an understanding of the assumed biological matrix of mental disorders and the types and actions of medication. A suitable framework should emphasize how the use of medication is managed in a broader sense. Indeed, the evidence that emerges from the views of service users indicates that many desire greater partnership and respect from professionals, and would prefer to see the use of medication as one means of facilitating recovery.

DEVELOPING A THERAPEUTIC ALLIANCE

One of the core skills that all contemporary mental health practitioners are expected to develop is the ability to work in partnership with service users and their families and carers. At times this requires that practitioners possess and feel able to use assertive engagement techniques so that relationships can be built and/or maintained. In its guidelines on the use of antipsychotic medication, the National Institute for Health and Clinical Excellence (NICE) (NICE, 2002b) recommends that the choice of medication should be made jointly by the individual and the clinician responsible for treatment, and based on an informed discussion of the relative psychopharmacological benefits and side-effect profiles. It is also recommended that the individual's advocate or carer should be consulted where appropriate. Hence, the development of a partnership between the practitioner and the service user is the first step towards deep-rooted and meaningful user involvement.

Achieving a true partnership will require significant changes to some relationships and practices. Indeed, factors that can facilitate such partnership working include: the attitudes and personalities of professionals; effective communication and information sharing; the ability to sustain interpersonal relationships; a willingness to share power and decision making; and skills in understanding and resolving conflict (Jordan *et al.*, 2002). It may mean a transformation of the professional's perception of their role from 'expert' to 'partner', and the subsequent transformation of the service user's role from passive recipient to partner (see Chapter 10: The Meaning of Recovery). Indeed, this is a fundamental assumption behind the 'expert' patient initiative (DH, 2001b) where it is envisaged that health professionals will provide evidence-based information and share their own clinical expertise with service users who are subsequently encouraged and enabled to contribute to discussions about medication treatment. During this process, compromises will inevitably need to be made on both sides in order to reach a decision which is mutually acceptable – in terms of clinical effectiveness, as well as in terms of suitability for the particular client (see Figure 11.1).

Some critics have argued that many service users do not want to participate in decisions; that revealing the uncertainties inherent in medical care could be harmful; and that increasing involvement in decision making will lead to greater demand for unnecessary, costly or harmful treatments (Coulter, 1997). However, there is considerable evidence that 'patients' do not feel as involved as they would like to be in decisions about medication and want more information and greater involvement in their treatment (Scottish Association for Mental Health (SAMH), 2004). Furthermore, it has been shown that the quality and amount of contact with health professionals positively influences service users' willingness to take medication (e.g. Oehl *et al.*, 2000; Nose *et al.*, 2003).

Despite the available evidence, it is arguable that many doctors have not recognized the need to alter practices. Some have not yet made the transition from prescribing

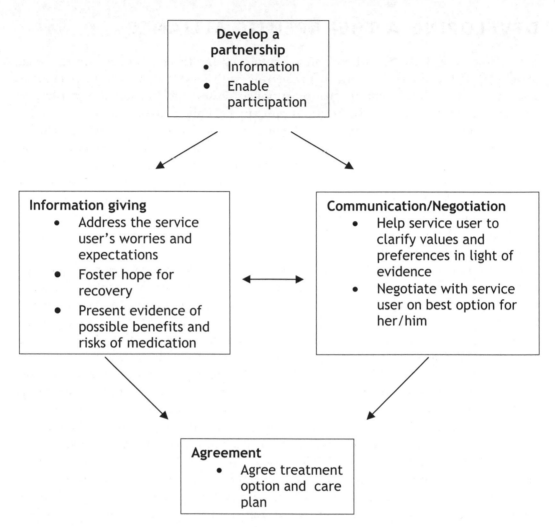

Source: Adapted from Jordan *et al.* (2002).

Figure 11.1

Stages to achieve partnership and shared decision making

'to' and prescribing 'for' patients to prescribing *with* service users (White, 2003). A therapeutic alliance based on partnership will enable mental health practitioners to give appropriate information to enable choices about medication to be made, and to discuss the possible implications of not taking medication. Where appropriate, partnership also enables practitioners to provide support to those who choose a non-medication treatment option.

PRESCRIBING MEDICATION

A number of sources provide guidance on prescribing for medical and non-medical prescribers, such as the British National Formulary, and various NICE guidelines (e.g. NICE, 2002b). Of course, there are many other resources (e.g. Healy, 2005), various reports (e.g. Healthcare Commission, 2007), professional bodies (e.g. NMC, 2006b) or local organizations that may also make recommendations or offer guidelines to influence prescribing practice. Some of the general principles which are suggested to underline contemporary prescribing include the following:

- Medication should only be prescribed when appropriate and necessary.

- Service users should be fully informed about their medication, including both positive and negative outcomes.

- Prescribers should maintain up-to-date knowledge of the medication they prescribe and ensure evidence-based prescribing.

- Dosing should be individualized, starting at a low dose and building up gradually to the dose that achieves optimal effect for the individual.

- Medication interactions should be anticipated and prevented.

- Prescribers should establish a working partnership with pharmacists, nurses and other relevant individuals to monitor therapy and ensure effective support for service users.

Although medical staff undertake the majority of prescribing, Ferner (2003) suggests that many medical schools no longer teach the skills, knowledge and attitudes needed to make good prescribing decisions. Ferner suggests that the key skills for a rational prescriber include:

- Deciding the aim of prescribing.

- Reconciling the prescriber's view with that of the service user.

- Deciding whether the treatment is likely to achieve the aim.

- Learning how to use the British National Formulary, the Cochrane Database of Systematic Reviews and other guidelines.

- Deciding whether the risk of harm might outweigh the possible benefits.

- Turning the general information on efficacy and safety into specific action for an individual sevice user.

Furthermore, the Healthcare Commission (2007) has also raised concerns about the continued competence of non-medical prescribers. The Commission's audit found that of the 187 nurse prescribers reported by mental health Trusts, only 81 (43%) reported prescribing at least once a week and none of the nine pharmacist supplementary prescribers were prescribing. The Commission suggested that to maintain competence, non-medical prescribers need to use their skills regularly once they are trained. Indeed, the Healthcare Commission report places great emphasis on the need to include a pharmacist in the multidisciplinary team to provide specialist knowledge on medication. However, to ensure rational prescribing, it is essential that prescribers and other mental health practitioners have knowledge of the effectiveness of medication and at least a working knowledge of psychopharmacology. This will enable discussion amongst the multidisciplinary team members and the service user on the most effective use of medication and the integration of different treatment approaches.

The following sections will consider evidence concerning our current understanding about the effectiveness of antipsychotic and antidepressant medications and associated issues. Space restrictions forbid any attempt to include psychopharmacology in this chapter, thus the reader is referred to other relevant texts (e.g. Healy, 2005; Taylor *et al.*, 2005).

ANTIPSYCHOTIC MEDICATION: EFFICACY AND SERVICE USERS' EXPERIENCES

TYPICAL ANTIPSYCHOTIC MEDICATION

The first-generation antipsychotic medication, referred to as 'typical' or 'conventional', includes the phenothiazines, butyrophenones, thioxanthenes, dibenzoxazepines and dihydroindolones. Although these medicines are not generally considered first-line treatment today, there is evidence of their continuing prescription. For example, a recent audit found that 31% of people were prescribed both first- and second-generation antipsychotics (Healthcare Commission, 2007).

There is some evidence of the overall effectiveness of 'typical' antipsychotic medication. Many clinical studies have shown this group of medications is more effective than placebo in reducing positive symptoms of schizophrenia, such as auditory hallucinations. However, these medications have little effect on negative symptoms, such as withdrawal, apathy and a lack of motivation (Davis *et al.*, 1989; Baldessarini *et al.*, 1990; Kane and Marder, 1993). Additionally, maintenance therapy with 'typical' antipsychotics results in an improvement in relapse rates compared with no antipsychotic medication treatment. However, effectiveness in practice is substantially less than efficacy in clinical trials. All 'typical' antipsychotic medications can produce a range of unwanted side-effects, including extrapyramidal side effects (EPSE) such as dystonic reactions, parkinsonism, akathisia and tardive dyskinesia. These symptoms are often distressing and lead some service users to discontinue their medication.

ATYPICAL ANTIPSYCHOTIC MEDICATION

The 1990s saw the introduction of the majority of 'atypical' antipsychotic medication – also referred to as second-generation antipsychotics. Those currently in use in the UK include amisulpride, aripiprazole, clozapine, olanzapine, quetiapine, risperidone, sertindole and zotepine. NICE (2002b) has evaluated the effectiveness of atypical medications in the UK and published guidelines on their use. The evaluation of clinical effectiveness was based on a review of 172 randomized controlled trials (RCTs) and other relevant studies. The evidence considered showed that the 'atypical' antipsychotics are at least as efficacious as the 'typical' agents in terms of overall response rates, though they may vary in their relative effects on positive and negative symptoms and relapse rates. In the short to medium term, all these 'atypical' medications are associated with a reduced incidence of EPSE compared with those in the 'typical' category. In the long term, however, there are limited data to support a reduced incidence of EPSE with some in the 'atypical' category. Additionally, there is little evidence on comparative rates of tardive dyskinesia – a serious neurological condition associated with long-term use of antipsychotic medication, marked by involuntary and repetitive tics and movements – between the various atypicals, or, indeed, between the typical and atypicals, due to the paucity of long-term trial data.

The Clinical Antipsychotic Trials of Intervention Effectiveness (CATIE) study provides the most comprehensive set of data on the effectiveness of antipsychotic medications in the treatment of schizophrenia in routine clinical practice (Lieberman et al., 2005). The study compared the relative effectiveness of 'atypical' antipsychotic medications with that of a conventional one (perphenazine) in a double-blind study. The results showed that overall, all of the medications exhibited comparable efficacy but they were also associated with high rates of discontinuation. As many as 74% of users discontinued medication for any reason within 6–8 months, olanzapine having the lowest overall discontinuation rate. The efficacy of the conventional antipsychotic agent perphenazine appeared similar to that of quetiapine, risperidone and ziprasidone. Similar among the groups were the amounts of time until discontinuation associated with intolerable side-effects. Olanzapine was associated with the highest level of discontinuation for intolerable side-effects, in particular weight gain or metabolic effects, and perphenazine was associated with more discontinuation for extrapyramidal effects.

One 'atypical' antipsychotic, clozapine, is restricted to individuals with schizophrenia who are unresponsive to or intolerant of 'conventional' antipsychotic therapy. Although rates of movement disorders are lower, clozapine is associated with increased drowsiness, seizures and excess salivation. The committee for the NICE guidelines concluded that more widespread use of the 'atypical' antipsychotics would benefit individuals with schizophrenia because of the likelihood of a reduced incidence of EPSE and that these medications should be considered in the choice of first-line treatments for individuals with newly diagnosed schizophrenia (NICE, 2002b).

SERVICE USERS' EXPERIENCES OF ANTIPSYCHOTIC MEDICATION

It should be noted here that changes in symptoms and the incidence and severity of side-effects are generally the criteria used to evaluate the efficacy of psychotropic medication. However, the ultimate criterion of effectiveness is how the person receiving medication feels and functions in everyday life (Awad, 1992). Indeed, a survey of the use of antipsychotic medications (SAMH, 2004) found that while 62% of users rated antipsychotics as helpful, overall nearly 70% reported unwanted effects, and 40% reported unwanted effects even when they stopped taking the medication. Interestingly, more unwanted effects were reported on stopping with newer atypical medications than older (typical) medications. Overall, the 'atypical' medications were viewed as marginally better than the older group. The best 'performing' antipsychotic overall was sulpiride, an older 'typical' medication, while depot antipsychotics consistently received poor ratings with under 40% of respondents considering them to be helpful overall.

PRESCRIBING ANTIPSYCHOTICS

Despite extensive guidelines regarding the prescription of antipsychotic medication, there is evidence of 'polypharmacy' (the concurrent use of more than one medicine) and excessive dosing in everyday practice. A one-day census of 44 psychiatric in-patients services in England found that high-dose prescribing and polypharmacy were common, with 50.5% of patients receiving more than one type of antipsychotic medication (Lelliott *et al.*, 2002). A key point here is that available evidence does not support high-dose prescribing and polypharmacy. In fact, the evidence suggests adverse consequences of this approach to prescribing. According to Taylor (2002), there is very little evidence to suggest that two medications are effective in cases where one alone is ineffective. The only exception is that of augmenting response to clozapine, which has the backing of some clinical trials. Additionally, polypharmacy has been associated with early death (Waddington *et al.*, 1998; see also Ito *et al.*, 2005).

NICE (2002b) has recommended that 'atypical' and 'typical' antipsychotics should not be prescribed concurrently. The co-prescription of such medications has been shown to increase the frequency of acute EPSE. In terms of the safety of 'high-dose' treatment, Taylor (2002) also highlights dangers such as prolongation of the cardiac QT interval that may cause *torsades de pointes* (atypical, rapid ventricular tachycardia) and sudden death.

There is a growing body of research to suggest that an individual's response to psychotropic medication may be related to her/his ethnic background. Frackiewicz *et al.* (1997) reviewed data generated by studies that examined different responses to antipsychotic medication according to ethnic/racial background. They stated that reported differences in response may be due to genetics, kinetic variations, dietary or environmental factors, or variations in the prescribing practices of clinicians. Studies suggest that satisfactory responses of certain groups to lower doses of antipsychotic medication may be due to differences that are pharmacokinetic and pharmacodynamic (i.e. related to the disposition of medications in the body, and to medication action respectively). Research relevant to the experiences of service users of African descent in the USA and UK is limited, but some studies suggest that apparently different responses and experiences of some in this group may be due to clinician biases and prescribing practices, rather than to pharmacokinetic or pharmacodynamic variability. (For thorough discussions see: Littlewood and Lipsedge, 1997; Fernando, 2003.)

ANTIDEPRESSANT MEDICATION: EFFICACY AND SERVICE USERS' EXPERIENCES

The two original types of medication used for the treatment of depression were the monoamine oxidase inhibitor (MAOI) Iproniazid, and the tricyclic antidepressant (TCA) Imipramine. Unfortunately, these produced a range of intolerable and potentially fatal adverse reactions and side-effects, and other medications from both groups were subsequently developed and used. 'New-generation' antidepressants have been developed over the last 20 years. When compared with the older type, new antidepressants, such as selective serotonin reuptake inhibitors (SSRI), have not demonstrated any clinically or statistically significant difference with respect to efficacy (Anderson, 2000; Williams *et al.*, 2000). Generally, newer antidepressants are considered to have a more tolerable adverse effect profile than older agents. However, the side-effects of SSRIs include nervousness, nausea, agitation, insomnia, diminished sexual libido and anorgasmia. Recent concerns have been associated with evidence that SSRIs increase suicidal thinking and behaviour, particularly in children. Other side-effects include increased agitation and aggression, and severe withdrawal effects (NICE, 2005b).

In the study by SAMH (2004), while antidepressants were found to be helpful for 56% of users, 60% reported side-effects and 45% had problems when stopping medication. To this extent, the newer medications were not found to have less adverse side-effects than older medications. Overall, SSRIs were not rated better than older tricyclics.

PRESCRIBING ANTIDEPRESSANTS

Since the introduction of the SSRIs and other new antidepressants in the 1990s, there has been a major increase in prescribing this class of medication in many countries including the UK (McManus *et al.*, 2000). NICE (2004) has issued guidelines for the British National Health Service on the treatment and care of people with depression (NICE, 2004, 2007). The guidelines recommend that for mild and moderate depression, psychological treatments specifically focused on depression such as problem-solving therapy, cognitive behaviour therapy and counselling can be as effective as medication treatments and should be offered as treatment options. The guideline further recommends that:

- Antidepressants should not be used for the initial treatment of mild depression, because the risk–benefit ratio is poor.

- Where antidepressants are prescribed for moderate or severe depression a SSRI should be chosen because these are as effective as tricyclic antidepressants and their use is less likely to be discontinued because of side-effects.

- All patients prescribed antidepressants should be informed that, although the medications are not associated with tolerance and craving, discontinuation/withdrawal symptoms may occur on stopping or missing doses or, occasionally, on reducing the dose of the medication.

- For severe depression, psychological treatment (specifically cognitive behaviour therapy) should be used in combination with antidepressant medication.

Additional analysis of existing data indicates that besides Prozac the SSRIs offer more risks than benefits in children. Suicidal thoughts or attempts increased by 14 times compared with placebo. In terms of effectiveness in mild and moderate depression, SSRIs are no better than placebo (Whittington *et al.*, 2004). In the wake of this evidence, NICE (2005a) has published new guidelines which recommend that antidepressants should not be prescribed for under-18s because of the serious risks. The guidance recommends that children or young people with moderate to severe depression should not be prescribed antidepressants other than when this is in conjunction with psychological therapy. Additionally, advice on nutrition, exercise and sleep should be more readily available to help combat depression. A recent study by Aursnes *et al.* (2005) found that the increased suicidal activity observed in children and adolescents who were taking certain antidepressant medications may also be present in adults. These authors suggested that the recommended restrictions on the use of SSRIs in children and adolescents should be extended to adults.

DETECTION AND MANAGEMENT OF ADVERSE REACTIONS AND SIDE-EFFECTS

Like virtually all medications, psychotropic medications can produce both unwanted and beneficial effects. As has been mentioned, a large proportion of individuals report side-effects from both antipsychotic and antidepressant medications – 70% and 60%

respectively (SAMH, 2004). Side-effects can be distressing and socially disabling and are a major factor in decisions not to take medication (Liebermann *et al.*, 2005).

Typical antipsychotic medications often produce a range of common side-effects, including the extrapyramidal symptoms of akathisia, dystonia, parkinsonism in the early stages of treatment and tardive dyskinesia (TD) after longer term treatment. In most cases, the symptoms of TD are subtle, and are often unrecognized by the individual (see Table 11.1). Atypical antipsychotics have a much lower risk of producing extrapyramidal symptoms than the older antipsychotics, but are not entirely free of this risk except in the case of clozapine. However, atypical antipsychotics have been associated with metabolic side-effects, which are of considerable concern in clinical practice. These include obesity, diabetes and dyslipidemia (a disorder of lipoprotein metabolism). Overall, metabolic disturbance significantly increases the risk for premature heart disease. Research suggests that between 2% and 36% of individuals treated with atypical antipsychotics develop metabolic complications (American Diabetes Association *et al.*, 2004), so it is clear that further research is required and improvements have yet to be attempted in this field. Available guidelines (e.g. American Diabetes Association *et al.*, 2004) recommend a protocol for baseline screening and ongoing monitoring and the need for referral to specialist services is emphasized. It is suggested that the best approach to prevent a cardiac event is to address obesity, inactivity and insulin resistance.

The general approach to the treatment of side-effects is to reduce the dosage of medication. If this is ineffective, another medication with a reduced propensity for the relevant side-effect may be chosen (Taylor *et al.*, 2005). In the case of dystonia, the response is treatment with anticholinergic medications. The treatment for akathisia is often propranolol or benzodiazepines, as anticholinergics are generally ineffective.

Balanced decisions about medication require reliable evidence on the positive as well as negative effects. Bennett *et al.* (1995a) suggested that a standardized approach to monitoring side-effects in mental health practice was essential to effective medication management. Subsequently, they developed a measuring tool to assist in monitoring side-effects including both the objective assessment of clinicians and the subjective reports of service users (Bennett *et al.*, 1995b). The Side Effects Scale/Checklist for Antipsychotic Medication (SESCAM) showed good reliability and benefits in clinical practice and it continues to be used by a number of clinicians. There are a number of other standard scales that have been developed to assess medication side-effects (see, for example, Guy, 1976; Day *et al.*, 1995). Several small-scale evaluations suggest a standardized approach improves the detection and management of side-effects (see, for example, Jordan *et al.*, 2004; Walker and MacAulay, 2005).

MEDICATION CONCORDANCE

Around 50% of people who are prescribed antipsychotic medications do not actually take them in accordance with the prescription (Nose *et al.*, 2003). Furthermore, the

TABLE 11.1

Common side-effects and adverse reactions of antipsychotic medications

Systems	Side-effects	Signs/symptoms
Cardiovascular	Hypotension Cardiotoxicity	Low blood pressure, dizziness
Nervous system	Functional	Drowsiness, over-sedation, psychomotor retardation
	Dystonia	Muscle spasm in any part of the body – torticollis (twisted neck), oculogyric crisis. Inability to speak or swallow. Back may arch or jaw dislocate
	Akathisia	Restlessness, inability to sit/stand still, crossing/uncrossing of legs. Linked to suicide, and violence and aggression
	Parkinsonism	Rigidity, slowness in movement and thinking, tremor, 'masked' face, excessive salivation, shuffling gait
	Tardive dyskinesia	Abnormal mouth/tongue movements (chewing, tongue flicking in and out of the mouth or worm-like movements in the mouth), other jerky or writhing movements. Difficulty speaking, eating or breathing
	Neuroleptic malignant syndrome	Muscle rigidity, hyperthermia, fluctuating consciousness
Autonomic	Gastrointestinal	Dry mouth, constipation
	Urinary	Retention or incontinence
	Blurred vision	
Endocrine	Weight gain Diabetes Sexual problems	Decreased libido, erectile and ejaculatory difficulties, amenorrhoea, galactorrhoea (persistent secretion of breast milk), gynaecomastia (excessive development of male mammary glands)
Haematological	Agranulocytosis	Hyperthermia, sore throat
Other	Skin problems	Photosensitivity, rashes, urticaria

discontinuation rates for antidepressants have been reported to be between 29% and 42% at 4 weeks, and between 63% and 76% at 6 months (Hunot *et al.*, 2007). Not taking and discontinuing prescribed medications are termed 'non-compliance' or 'non-adherence'. These words imply that the individual concerned has failed to follow the instructions they were given by the prescriber. The commonly held view in mental health care is that non-compliance/non-adherence with psychotropic medication is an irrational decision by the service user, due to a range of illness factors such as 'lacking insight' into her/his circumstances. From the individual's perspective, though, there are often rational reasons why the decision is taken to stop medication. A service user's decision to discontinue medication is generally related to perceptions of treatment, and social/environmental factors. For example, Hunot *et al.* (2007) suggest that matters such as concerns about antidepressants and incompatibility between preferred and pre-scribed treatments act as significant barriers to sustained adherence. This study high-lighted the central roles played by: the relationship between each doctor and service user; working with identified treatment preferences; and providing supportive and continued management of medication.

Much effort has been devoted to developing methods to improve 'compliance' and 'adherence'. This has included compliance therapy for antipsychotic medication (Kemp *et al.*, 1998; Gray, 2000). However, a recent multi-centre randomized controlled study of adherence therapy found that such an approach had no effect in improving confor-mity to antipsychotic medication regimes amongst individuals with schizophrenia (Gray *et al.*, 2006). Increasingly, 'concordance' is being recommended as a more appropriate approach to prescribing and managing medication (Royal Pharmaceutical Society of Great Britain, 1997). It is argued that the term 'compliance' embodies a traditional model of prescriptive care, whereas 'concordance' encompasses elements that can enable full therapeutic partnership. The main features of the concordance approach are:

- Respect for the person's beliefs and wishes in determining whether, when and how medicines are to be taken.

- Agreement is reached after negotiation between the individual and health care professional.

- Respect for the aims of both parties.

- Non-concordance describes an inability of both parties to come to an understanding, not merely a failure of the individual service user to follow the health professional's instructions

Indeed, concordance is an approach to the use of medication that treats each person as an individual who makes meaningful personal choices. Use of this model encourages mental health professionals and service users to work together to reach a shared under-standing of the best way to help the service user. Differences of opinion need to be openly acknowledged and respected, as is the desire to work towards negotiating a compromise which meets the challenges of clinical efficacy whilst being commensurate with the service user's wishes. Medication concordance is achieved when the professional has: developed a rapport with the service user; attempted to understand the illness/difficulties as perceived by the user; come to an understanding and an agreement about the person's needs; imparted information about the proposed treatment; and offered alternatives where practicable (Chen, 1999). Overall there is a strong argument that the medication concordance paradigm constitutes a more appropriate approach than compliance or adherence as it is distinctly user-centred and engages the individual in her/his own recovery.

SUPPORTING RECOVERY

Despite some frustration with the process of finding the right medication and dealing with the side-effects of others, many service users indicate that medications can be helpful to their recovery (see Chapter 10: The Meaning of Recovery). Although some wish to manage their difficulties without medication entirely, for most service users the goal will be to take the least amount necessary to support recovery. It is vital, however, that one's assumptions regarding the likelihood of recovery, or at least 'symptom abatement', are considered. Although it is generally accepted that people are able to recover from depressive illnesses, schizophrenia is often viewed as a chronic illness with persisting or deteriorating symptoms and little hope for sustained remission and recovery of functioning. Countering this perspective, retrospective and prospective studies with both chronic and recent onset patients suggest that schizophrenia has a heterogeneous course and can be favourably influenced by comprehensive and continuous treatment. Also important can be personal factors such as family support and good neurocognitive functioning (Lieberman *et al.*, 2002). Lieberman *et al.* (2002) propose an operational definition of recovery from schizophrenia, that includes symptom remission; full- or part-time involvement in employment or education; independent living without supervision by family or surrogate caregivers; not being entirely dependent on financial support from disability insurance; and having friends with whom activities are shared on a regular basis (see Chapter 10: The Meaning of Recovery).

Bearing in mind the long-term nature of schizophrenia, each of the above criteria should be sustained for at least two consecutive years in order to satisfy the definition of recovery. While the reduction of symptoms and improvement of social functioning are essential elements of clinical recovery, Andresen *et al.* (2003) found that the definition of recovery used by service users was psychological recovery from the consequences of the illness. Four key processes of recovery were identified: finding hope; re-establishment of identity; finding meaning in life; and taking responsibility for recovery. Among the main elements of recovering from mental ill health are regaining social roles and identities. As mentioned, this may mean accessing education and training, getting a job, re-establishing family contacts and relationships. Effective management of medication should assist in facilitating the achievement of these outcomes in accordance with each individual's needs and desires.

CONCLUSION

Medication continues to be the main treatment approach in mental health care. It is clear from available evidence that efficacy in clinical trials is not always replicated in practice, probably as a result of service users' reluctance to continue prescribed medication. Factors that have been shown to influence medication concordance include the professional skills of the prescriber; the relationship between prescriber and user; and the perceived benefits and negative effects of medication. This chapter has proposed a framework for managing medication that is based on the values of partnership, rational prescribing, medication concordance and recovery. The very process of treatment requires that practitioners be skilled in developing therapeutic alliances, providing information that enables choice and shared decisions, making sound prescribing decisions and detecting and managing the negative side-effects of medication. These skills need to be underpinned by an appropriate level of knowledge of psychopharmacology, which includes a grasp of the available evidence on the effectiveness of psychotropic medication. On the whole, service users may find medication helpful but many want to be more involved in making decisions about how to use medication to best effect. Medication should thus be viewed as part of the broader package of care that supports a service user's journey to recovery.

CHAPTER 12
CO-MORBIDITY IN PHYSICAL AND MENTAL ILL HEALTH

Helen Robson, Carl Margereson and Steve Trenoweth

INTRODUCTION

Good mental and physical health are central to an overall sense of positive well-being. Indeed, how we think and feel is very much linked to our physical health (DH, 2001d). However, current systems of health and social care often dichotomize mental and physical health, resulting in unmet physical or psychological needs, or worse still, both. In this chapter, we explore the issue of co-morbidity, where there is both mental and physical ill health, a contemporary reality for health care workers in medical and mental health settings. We discuss how people with severe mental health problems have an increased vulnerability to a wide range of serious physical illnesses (Robson and Gray, 2007), such as coronary heart disease, diabetes, various infections and respiratory diseases (SCMH, 2003; Mentality/NIMHE, 2004); have poorer access to medical treatment and care; are less likely to be offered routine health checks such as blood pressure, urine, weight or cholesterol (SCMH, 2003; DRC, 2006); and are less likely to receive proactive advice on health promotion (Mentality/NIMHE, 2004; DH, 2006d). In this chapter, we also highlight changes required to the clinical practice of all health practitioners in an attempt to remedy this situation.

Contemporary Issues in Mental Health Nursing, Edited by J. E. Lynch and S. Trenoweth
© 2008 John Wiley & Sons, Ltd

THE EXTENT OF PHYSICAL CO-MORBIDITY

In 1934, the *British Medical Journal* published an article which linked mental 'illness' to poorer physical health status in people admitted to a psychiatric hospital (Phillips, 1934). By the 1980s, schizophrenia was described as a 'life shortening disease' by Allebeck (1989). Indeed, there is currently overwhelming and persuasive evidence that people with serious mental health problems have significantly poorer physical health when compared with the general population (SCMH, 1997, 2003; Harris and Barraclough, 1998; Cohen and Hove, 2001; Phelan *et al.*, 2001; Seymour, 2003; Stroup, 2004; DH, 2004c, 2006d), much of which goes undetected (DH, 1999a; Cohen and Phelan, 2001) or is poorly managed (Inventor *et al.*, 2005; DH, 2006a).

Moreover, there seems to be a relationship between medical and psychiatric/psychological ill health, in that the number of medical problems correlates with both the perceived physical health of the person and the severity of their psychotic and depressive symptoms (Dixon *et al.*, 2000). Furthermore, physical health problems tend to occur at a much younger age in people with serious mental health problems than in the general population, and the disparity is particularly pronounced in the 25- to 44-year age range.

The Disability Rights Commission (DRC, 2006) completed an 18-month investigation into the physical health inequalities experienced by people with mental health problems and those with learning disabilities. The report highlights the main physical health risks for people with schizophrenia, bipolar disorder and depression, and found that such clients are more likely to have diabetes, heart disease, respiratory disease and cerebrovascular disease. People diagnosed with schizophrenia and bipolar disorders are more likely to have breast cancer and hypertension, and are nearly twice as likely to have bowel cancer as others in the population. They also identified that these illnesses were more likely at a younger age and that people with serious mental health problems were more likely than members of the general population to die from such conditions within five years of diagnosis. With cancer, there is evidence that the survival rate in those with serious mental health problems is around 50% lower than the general population (Halbreich *et al.*, 1996). The phenomenon is not limited to the most severe forms of mental disorders, however. In a review of 152 studies, Harris and Barraclough (1998) found that over 27 forms of mental disorder were associated with an increased risk of premature death, with 60% of deaths due to natural causes.

Once people with mental health problems have illnesses such as coronary heart disease, they are less likely to survive them for more than five years (DRC, 2006). The risk of cardiac pathology manifested by sudden unexpected death has been reported to be three times as likely in patients with schizophrenia compared with the general population (Ruschena *et al.*, 1998; Casey *et al.*, 2004; Jindal *et al.*, 2005) and in people with serious mental disorders there is an increased prevalence of chronic obstructive pulmonary disease (Himelhoch *et al.*, 2004). On average, it is estimated that people with schizophrenia can expect to live for 10 years less than someone without a mental health problem (Mentality/NIMHE, 2004) and although suicide and accidental death contributes to some of this, death from poor physical health also remains a common cause. People with a diagnosis of schizophrenia also tend to experience, and have less access to, general health services (Mentality/NIMHE, 2004; DRC, 2006) and are less frequently hospitalized for their underlying medical conditions (Mentality/NIMHE, 2004).

RISK FACTORS

As a result of the overall poor medical care offered to this client group, the quality of life tends to be poorer whilst the mortality rates are higher than in the general population (Lambert *et al.*, 2003; Primhe *et al.*, 2005; DRC, 2006). The possible reasons for this are complex, and many explanations have been put forward to account for this heightened risk, such as the long-term use of antipsychotic medication for those diagnosed with schizophrenia (DH, 1999a; NICE, 2002a,b). Indeed, the side-effects of some medication used to treat mental health problems may cause physical symptoms or have an impact on existing physical conditions, such as diabetes (Mentality/NIMHE, 2004). However, much of the excess levels of illness and mortality are due to factors seemingly unconnected with their psychiatric or psychological problems (DH, 1999a). Unhealthy lifestyles, such as higher incidences of smoking, poor exercise and poor nutrition (Mentality/NIMHE, 2004), as well as social deprivation, social exclusion, poverty, poor housing and unemployment, have all been implicated as contributory factors to ill health (Mentality/NIMHE, 2004; DRC, 2006).

Some of the lifestyle factors which most influence the physical health of individuals with serious mental health problems were studied by McCreadie (2003). Body mass indices, smoking habits and quality of diet were examined and compared with those of the poorest socio-economic group within the general population. McCreadie found that those people diagnosed with schizophrenia had significantly poorer lifestyles in health terms than even those from the poorest groups in society. However, it appears that not one but several 'lifestyle' factors combined contribute to the poorer physical health of people with serious mental health problems. That is, independently, each risk factor is known to contribute to health problems, but when they occur simultaneously, as they often do in this group, the cumulative impact and compounded effect may account for the higher mortality rates. It is, therefore, necessary to be aware of a wide range of risk factors in order to fully respond to both the physical and mental health needs of this client group.

SMOKING

Smoking rates are consistently shown to be higher in people with serious mental health problems (McCloughen, 2003), with figures suggesting that they are twice as likely to smoke and indeed to smoke more heavily (20 per day or more) than other members of the population (Brown *et al.*, 1999). In this regard, there seems to be a large disparity between the general public and those with serious mental health problems (McCloughen, 2003). Indeed, Kelly and McCreadie (1999) reported that 68% of people diagnosed with schizophrenia who smoked were classified as being heavy smokers (over 25 per day in their study) compared with only 11% of the general population. Reasons offered for this phenomenon are many and varied, ranging from a hypothesis that smoking is a form of 'self-medication', as the nicotine is believed to interact with various neurotransmitters in the brain to help alleviate some of the psychiatric symptoms and the side-effects of medication (McCloughen, 2003). Other theories include the assertion that people with serious mental health problems smoke out of habit as it forms an important part of their routine, and that it offers a form of relaxation, pleasure and social contact (Robson and Gray, 2005).

Despite the very obvious and well-documented evidence that primary and secondary (passive) smoking has a deleterious effect on physical health (with associated increased risks of cardiovascular disease, respiratory diseases, cancers and diabetes; DH, 1998c, 2004d), smoking is felt to be part of the culture in mental health settings. Indeed, Stubbs and Gardner (2004) reported that 54% of mental health workers believe smoking is helpful in terms of creating therapeutic relationships.

DIET

A poor dietary intake is, of course, a major cause of cardiovascular disease, obesity, diabetes and some forms of cancer (DH, 1994b). However, while the Food Standards Agency (FSA) recommends that we eat at least five portions of fruit or vegetables each day, and at least one portion of oily fish per week (FSA, 2001), Brown *et al.* (1999) found, in assessing the diets of 102 people diagnosed with schizophrenia, that none of them were eating the recommended levels of fruit and vegetables.

Indeed, research studies have consistently shown that those with serious mental health problems have a poorer diet than the general population (Brown *et al.*, 1999; McCreadie *et al.*, 2003) in relation to the intake of higher rates of saturated fat and lower consumption of fruit and vegetables. Furthermore, McCreadie (2003) reported that in a sample of people diagnosed with schizophrenia, 53% demonstrated raised cholesterol levels. This finding remains consistent even where the diets are compared with those of the lowest socio-economic group in the general population, and therefore cannot be attributed solely to dietary restrictions necessitated by financial constraints.

Interestingly, there is also evidence that a poorer diet may adversely affect the symptoms of schizophrenia, and there is increasing evidence that a diet high in saturated fat, low in polyunsaturated fat and high in sugar is detrimental to the outcome of schizophrenia (Peet, 2004). Mellor *et al.* (1996), for example, identified negative correlations between dietary intakes of omega-3 fatty acids and the symptoms of both schizophrenia and 'tardive dyskinesia' (see Chapter 11: Supporting Recovery: Medication Management in Mental Health Care).

MEDICATION

A compounding risk factor of a poor diet is the apparent correlation found between antipsychotic medication and the risk of developing 'hyperlipidaemia', a contributing factor increasing the risks associated with cardiovascular and cerebrovascular disease. In an extensive study carried out by Koro *et al.* (2002), olanzapine was found to increase the likelihood of developing hyperlipidaemia by five times when compared with those not taking any antipsychotic medication. Other neuroleptics were demonstrated to increase the risks by approximately threefold. Despite this, there is evidence that this group of people are less likely than the general population to be prescribed medications to lower cholesterol levels (Redelmeier *et al.*, 1998). Furthermore, weight gain often accompanies the use of antipsychotic medication (Allison *et al.*, 2003), which may compound the risk for several physical disorders, such as Type 2 diabetes (Dixon *et al.*, 2004; Citrome and Yeomans, 2005).

EXERCISE

The potential risks of a poor diet within this group are increased by levels of inactivity. Brown *et al.* (1999) found that people with serious mental health problems took significantly less exercise than the general population, with around a third of the group admitting that they take no exercise at all. Physical activity would improve the overall health status of most people, by reducing the risk of cardiovascular disease, improving lung capacity and reducing the risk of many forms of cancer (Cormack *et al.*, 2004). It must be acknowledged, however, that the negative symptoms of serious mental health problems may have some influence on the uptake of physical activity, as do the side-effects of some of the medicines.

The potential positive gains of physical exercise can aid the person to overcome some of the barriers seemingly preventing such activity, by improving body strength, posture and flexibility. It has also been found to improve self-esteem, encourage social contact and improve sleep patterns (Daley, 2002). Indeed, a lack of physical exercise and a diet rich in saturated fats and sugar lends itself to obesity, which has been found to be a significant risk factor in the health of this group of people (McCreadie, 2003). Studies have found that 40%–62% of people diagnosed with schizophrenia are overweight or obese compared with 27% of the general population, and consistently demonstrate that obesity is more prevalent within females (Kendrick, 1996). Here, the use of antipsychotic medication is often implicated in the increased incidence of obesity in this group of people, particularly the newer (atypical) antipsychotics (Allison and Casey, 1999). However, an appreciation of the risks associated with the use of medication which might undermine the physical health status of an individual must be balanced against the possible gains for the individual in terms of their overall mental health and well-being.

MENTAL ILLNESS

Adults diagnosed with schizophrenia demonstrate an increased risk of developing glucose regulation abnormalities, insulin resistance and Type 2 diabetes mellitus (Lambert *et al.*, 2003). The evidence suggests that this is not simply due to the use of neuroleptic medication, but may be an independent factor associated with the illness itself (Peet, 2004). Indeed, those with such diagnoses, but not prescribed neuroleptics, have also been found to be insulin resistant (Ryan *et al.*, 2003). There may also be a genetic influence over this phenomenon, as Mukherjee *et al.* (1989) found an increased incidence of diabetes in the relatives of patients diagnosed with schizophrenia. Importantly, the risk of this metabolic profile developing into diabetes mellitus is considerably reduced by a healthy diet and lifestyle (Mann, 2002).

SEXUAL HEALTH

In younger people with mental health problems, there is increasing concern about their sexual health. Sheild *et al.* (2005) identifies that young people with a psychiatric disorder are at greater risk of contracting sexually transmitted infections, as they were found to be twice as likely as school-based peers to be sexually active and engaged in unsafe sexual practices (DiClemente and Ponton, 1993). They were also found to be at increased risk of contracting HIV and were twice as likely to be using intravenous drugs. Kessler *et al.* (1997) also argued that sexually active teenage girls with a mental health problem were more likely to become pregnant than those without such issues, and found an even higher trend for parenthood in the male teenage group with psychiatric diagnoses.

Of further concern is the finding that women with a diagnosis of a psychotic disorder have significantly lower rates of fertility from around the age of 25 than is seen in the general population (Howard *et al.*, 2002). This age-related finding may be due in part to the effects of neuroleptic medication associated with the treatment of psychosis, and the effect on increasing the concentration of prolactin in the blood which would naturally reduce the fertility rates in a woman. Howard *et al.* (2002) also note that the picture is very unclear as other studies have demonstrated lower fertility rates in women with first onset schizophrenia. This may well suggest that medication is not solely implicated with the lower fertility in that group. However, the use of antipsychotic medications and their impact on the endocrine system has been implicated in the increased risk of osteoporosis in this group (Halbreich and Palter, 1996).

DRUG AND ALCOHOL USE

Another very significant lifestyle factor affecting physical health in people with serious mental health problems is that of drug and alcohol abuse (see Chapter 10: The Meaning of Recovery). Reports suggest that 36% of this group will have some form of substance abuse problem over the course of a year (Primhe *et al.*, 2005), and up to 60% of people diagnosed with schizophrenia may abuse psychoactive drugs and other substances, which is clearly much higher than the general population (Citrome and Yeomans, 2005).

The physical implications of substance misuse include a poorer prognosis of mental health problems and an increase in the side-effects experienced by many patients taking neuroleptic medication, as well as an increased risk of violent behaviour and suicide (Vose, 2000). The increased levels of substance misuse may also go some way towards explaining the increased risk of hepatitis C and HIV/AIDS within this group.

SOCIAL AND ECONOMIC FACTORS

The social consequence of a diagnosis of mental 'illness' is consistently reported to have a significantly negative association with overall living conditions and other aspects of social life commensurate with the notion of 'citizenship' (see Chapter 8: Challenging Stigma and Promoting Social Justice). Those who experience mental distress and have a medical diagnosis of mental illness are more likely to be housed in areas where there are high levels of crime, unemployment and drug misuse, and are significantly more at risk of being, or becoming, homeless (Repper, 2000b). Around 30%–50% of homeless people have been found to experience mental health problems, and reports suggest that the impact of being homeless in terms of physical ill health include significantly higher rates of tuberculosis, skin diseases and respiratory problems, with the average life expectancy of rough sleepers being around 42 years (Griffiths, 2002).

DETECTION

Several issues can undermine the effective and proactive detection of physical illness amongst people with mental health problems. Indeed, several studies have indicated the overall poor rates of detection of physical illness amongst people with serious mental health problems. The generally poor rates of detection here seem to be related, in part, to the ability and responsiveness of professionals with primary and secondary services. However, there is also some evidence that the nature of mental health problems can lead to a lack of engagement with primary or medical services.

It seems that there exists a training deficit in specialist mental health practitioners' ability to identify and respond to the physical health needs of service users, both in in-patient and community settings (Dean et al., 2001; Phelan et al., 2001; DH, 2006d). Within secondary care services, Osborn and Warner (1998) argue that much more emphasis needs to be given to obtaining an in-depth medical history from the patient. Their findings demonstrated that a significant number of in-patients were not given a physical examination or an adequate assessment of their medical history. This is particularly significant as physical or somatic symptoms may be masked by, or indeed related to, psychological or psychiatric issues, and of course, vice versa. This also extends to a thorough assessment of the physical health effects experienced from the use of prescribed antipsychotic medication (see Chapter 11: Supporting Recovery: Medication Management in Mental Health Care). Conversely, there does appear to be evidence that psychiatrists and mental health workers in secondary care services have been rather quick in assuming that complaints of physical health problems by service users are psychosomatic or 'irrational' in nature (Jeste *et al.*, 1996).

Furthermore, many mental health practitioners and carers often seem to think, inaccurately, that people with serious mental health problems are uninterested in their physical needs (Mentality/NIMHE, 2004). There is also an assumption that people with serious mental health problems do not attend appointments or are non-concordant with treatment (DH, 2006d). However, service users, it seems, do not share this view (Dean *et al.*, 2001; Meddings and Perkins, 2002; McCloughen, 2003). Seymour (2003) found that mental health service users do have concerns about their physical health and would value helpful and effective health promotion information and advice, but this is largely lacking within existing primary and secondary care services.

There also appears to be an inability, or reluctance, amongst primary care practitioners (Seymour, 2003), and amongst nurses in a general hospital setting (Mavundla, 2000), to engage in the necessary depth of assessment required to elicit physical symptoms or perform a medical examination of those with serious mental health problems. However, the National Service Framework for Mental Health (DH, 1999a) requires better physical health care for people with mental health problems. Primary care services are required to provide a wide range of activities that include recognition and assessment of mental health problems and the provision of effective medical treatment and care.

Amongst general practitioners (GPs), there appears to be a lack of expertise and training in mental health issues (SCMH, 1997; Cohen and Hove, 2001; Phelan *et al.*, 2001; Seymour, 2003; Mentality/NIMHE, 2004). Indeed, the orientation of primary care is often reactive, and this does not fit well with patients who may be reluctant, or unable, to seek help. Short consultation times make it particularly difficult for GPs to undertake physical assessments, especially in vague or suspicious patients (Phelan *et al.*, 2001) or where there might be an impairment of social or interpersonal functioning, especially amongst those with chronic health needs (Seymour, 2003). That is, there is a concern that in primary health services, a lack of social skills amongst some service users and the stigma of a psychiatric diagnosis may make it less likely for this client group to receive optimum medical health care (Phelan *et al.*, 2001).

There is, however, some evidence that some people with mental health problems actively avoid contact with primary care services and appear to be less willing to disclose concerns about their health or to request health checks (Goldman, 1999; Phelan *et al.*, 2001; SCMH, 2003). It is also reported that people with serious mental health problems may sometimes be unaware of their physical health problems as a consequence of impaired cognitive functioning (Goldman, 1999) and that symptoms of physical illness may also be undetected or masked by the high pain threshold associated with the use of antipsychotic medications (Lambert, 2003). As a consequence, there may be less likelihood that medical help is actively sought or that physical symptoms are spontaneously reported during consultation (Phelan *et al.*, 2001; Seymour, 2003).

Within primary care services there may be an over-emphasis on the psychological and social issues surrounding a person's mental health problems. Indeed, there is considerable evidence that receiving a diagnosis of, for example, schizophrenia or bipolar disorder often means that physical health is overlooked or ignored or takes second place to their mental health care (Dean *et al.*, 2001; Friedli and Dardis, 2002). Furthermore, this 'diagnostic overshadowing' (Phelan *et al.*, 2001; DH, 2006d; DRC, 2006) can lead to a reinterpretation of physical symptoms in psychiatric terms (Seymour, 2003). As such, there have been calls for better medical screening and treatment of people with mental health problems (DH, 1999a). Taking a proactive stance to improving the physical health of those with mental health problems, it has been suggested, will necessitate comprehensive annual health checks (Seymour, 2003; DH, 2004a; Mentality/NIMHE, 2004; DRC, 2006) to screen for unmet needs and afford early interventions (DRC, 2006). Figure 12.1 provides a suggested framework for the annual health check.

Furthermore, there is a clear need to ensure people understand the effects and side-effects of their prescribed medication so people can decide the trade-off between relief from psychiatric symptoms and physical health risk (DRC, 2006).

The recent policy 'Choosing Health: Making Healthy Choices Easier' (DH, 2004c) and in particular the subsequent 'Choosing Health: Supporting the Physical Health Needs of People with Severe Mental Illness' (DH, 2006d) focus on supporting the development of programmes of health promotion for people with severe mental health problems. The latter document in particular describes examples of 'promising practice'; for example, the employment of a lead mental health nurse practitioner to coordinate health improvement programmes, signposting people to health-promoting services (e.g. healthy walking groups, smoking cessation, dieting programmes), ensuring referral and appropriate access to services.

So, whilst it is clear that there are some proactive steps being taken to improve the physical health of people with mental health problems (DH, 2006d), there still exists overall poor care in contemporary primary and secondary health services (DRC, 2006). As such, good physical health is seemingly a largely unmet need for this client group (Phelan *et al.*, 2001). Recent recommendations have been made for mental health nurses, who are in a strong position to respond proactively to the physical health care needs of their clients, to attain the skills required to improve the physical well-being of people with mental health problems (DH, 2006a). However, there seems to be a general lack of confidence and uncertainty of their role in relation to physical health needs of mental health service users (Dean *et al.*, 2001). This can often be exacerbated by the general absence of care protocols to offer physical health care in mental health settings or by mental health practitioners, and a clear organizational strategic vision which often results in care varying with the member of staff who happens to be on duty (Dean *et al.*, 2001; SCMH, 2003; Seymour, 2003).

- Calculation of body mass index, and/or body fat measurement and appropriate advice on healthy eating.

- Comprehensive blood tests (e.g. serum electrolytes/complete blood counts (CBC)/liver function tests (LFT) and so forth).

- Cardiovascular assessment, including blood pressure check.

- Assessment of levels of exercise and advice, if appropriate.

- Cholesterol-level monitoring and advice on preventing cardiovascular disease, if appropriate.

- Urine analysis for sugar, with fasting blood sugar if positive.

- Respiratory assessment, including peak flow readings.

- Smoking status, cessation advice, if appropriate.

- Annual influenza vaccination and other immunizations as appropriate.

- Regular preventative checks such as cervical smear, breast cancer and testicular cancer screening, and advice on self-monitoring.

- Advice on maintaining good sexual health and family planning with screening for associated infections, if appropriate.

- Assessment of alcohol use and other drug use with appropriate advice.

Figure 12.1
The annual health check

CONCLUSIONS AND RECOMMENDATIONS

The contemporary challenge for health care practitioners is to assist service users, who may well be difficult to engage (Primhe *et al.*, 2005), to meet their physical health needs (DH, 2006d). Not only do people with severe mental illness have higher mortality rates and poorer physical health, they are also disadvantaged in their access to medical care services. All of this points to widespread social inequalities amongst this group, which recent policy initiatives from the UK government seek to address (DH, 2004c, 2006d).

In primary health care settings, training for all staff (including health professionals and reception staff, clerical and administrative workers) about mental health issues may be required to assist the greater understanding of the needs of people with mental health problems and to avoid 'diagnostic overshadowing'. Primary care workers may also require basic training to increase their understanding of stigma and discrimination, and why people with mental health problems find it harder to engage with services. Central to this is the need for primary care workers to develop their skills and confidence in being able to communicate with, and respond effectively to the needs of, people with severe and enduring mental illness (Mentality/NIMHE, 2004; DRC, 2006).

Helping to improve the physical health of those with mental health problems will include appropriate and proactive health promotion advice and health education (such as smoking cessation advice, guidance on healthy diet and nutrition, sexual health, and weight management and exercise; DRC, 2006), and also requires the effective and comprehensive screening of physical health risk (DRC, 2006). There is also an apparent need to provide practical support for people who lack basic skills to help them use health information (DH, 2004a). Clearly, there is also a need for all health care practitioners to expand their skills, knowledge and clinical practice to be able to better respond to the complex needs of those who experience co-morbid physical and mental health problems (Inventor *et al.*, 2005; Robson and Gray, 2007).

CHAPTER 13
PHYSICAL ILLNESS: PROMOTING EFFECTIVE COPING IN CLIENTS WITH CO-MORBIDITY

Carl Margereson

INTRODUCTION

The previous chapter highlighted the contemporary imperative for mental health professionals to be aware of, and to be able to respond effectively to, the physical health needs of their clients (see Chapter 12: Physical Co-Morbidity in Mental Health). However, a significant proportion of individuals with ongoing physical and mental health problems will have difficulty with adjustment to, and coping with, the negative aspects of their health problems. Assisting people to cope with the effects of mental and physical ill health is, therefore, an important issue for mental health practitioners seeking to improve the overall health and holistic well-being of their clients. In this chapter, psychosocial influences on health behaviour and coping are explored, along with strategies which may assist in supporting health behaviour change. Consideration is also given to how the individual with co-morbid health problems may be facilitated to develop more control over his/her health and illness (see Chapter 10: The Meaning of Recovery). Implications for the role of mental health nurses are discussed.

Contemporary Issues in Mental Health Nursing, Edited by J. E. Lynch and S. Trenoweth
© 2008 John Wiley & Sons, Ltd

DEFINING COPING

Coping has been defined by researchers using both a 'trait' approach (emphasizing stable coping styles) and a 'process' approach (which emphasizes coping as a transactional phenomenon with coping efforts constantly changing to meet demands) (Penley *et al.*, 2002). Lazarus and Folkman (1984), for example, define 'coping' as the constantly changing cognitive and behavioural efforts used to manage specific external and/or internal demands that are appraised as taxing and that exceed the resources of the person. We can see from this definition that focusing on health behaviour alone is too simplistic, and it is important to remember the centrality of cognitions and beliefs in driving our emotions and behaviours. Emotions, in turn, are probably the biggest motivator of change, the biggest barrier to change and often the biggest reward of change (Anderson *et al.*, 2000) and need to be explored in therapeutic encounters. Two areas viewed as perhaps the most powerful predictors of initiation and maintenance of health behaviour change other than social influences are 'self-efficacy' and 'self-determination' (Gochman, 1997; Rollnick *et al.*, 1999; Miller and Rollnick, 2002), both key factors in self-regulation theory and subsequent clinical strategies, which will be discussed later in this chapter.

COPING AND HEALTH BEHAVIOURS

Over the years, 'coping' has become an important area of study for researchers interested in chronic illness. In encounters with mental health patients, professionals must be able to make an assessment of coping ability and determine which behaviours are health-promoting and which are potentially health-compromising. There is much evidence to suggest that health behaviours are implicated as co-factors in the relationship between psychopathology and immune function. Smoking, for example, appears to have synergistic effects with depression in reducing the effectiveness of natural killer cell destruction (Jung and Irwin, 1999).

Health *behaviour*, however, should not be seen in isolation. A number of theoretical frameworks have been developed over the years in an attempt to illustrate the complex mechanisms at play, not only in the development of pathological disorders, but also in the maintenance of these across the chronic illness trajectory where, at different stages, coping may be problematic. Cohen and Rodriguez (1995), for example, offer models to explain how, in individuals with physical disorders, the complex interplay of several pathways (biological, behavioural, cognitive and social) can result in negative affect. This model is seen as bidirectional, with negative affect also having a detrimental effect on the primary physical disorder through complex interplay of the same pathways. It is important, therefore, before discussing the concept of coping, that a range of possible psychosocial factors influencing health and health behaviours amongst clients with mental health problems is considered.

PSYCHOSOCIAL INFLUENCES ON HEALTH

A psychosocial factor is that which potentially relates psychological phenomena to the social environment and to pathophysiological changes (Hemingway and Marmot, 1999). There has been a tremendous growth in research exploring the effects of mental health on physical health and how such psychosocial factors can result in biological changes and disease (Marmot and Wilkinson, 1999). These factors can act in isolation or combine and exert effects at different stages of the life course.

An important psychosocial factor that most would agree is a major factor contributing to both the onset and course of physical and, indeed, mental ill health is that of 'stress' (Zubin and Spring, 1977; Herbert, 1997). Various psychosocial factors may result in excessive demand on individuals, and where coping resources are limited then stress can increase further the risk for poorer physical and mental health. Where disease has already been diagnosed, then stress may result in poor coping and possibly acute episodes. Of course, individual characteristics are likely to be relevant here, which Kuh and Ben-Shlomo (2004) refer to as 'personal capital', reflecting the accumulation of social and cognitive skills, self-esteem, coping strategies, attitudes and values. Coping with ongoing chronic stress may involve a range of negative emotions and the interplay of the psyche, neurohormonal activation and immune system is a major focus of study for a relatively new discipline called 'psychoneuroimmunology'.

Anxiety and depression are also associated with disturbed autonomic balance, poor adherence to medication and lifestyle advice (Lett *et al.*, 2004), the development of adverse cardiac events (Rozanski *et al.*, 2005) and an increase in proinflammatory cytokines. Cytokines are molecules released from many cells in the body enabling cells to communicate with each other and are involved in physiological regulation, although some have a more sinister role. Interleukin-6 (Il-6), for example, is a cytokine released in chronic stress which has been found to have a proinflammatory role in cardiovascular disease by promoting the production of C-reactive protein, an important risk factor for myocardial infarction (Papanicolaou *et al.*, 1998; Appels *et al.*, 2000; Kiechl *et al.*, 2001; Kiecolt-Glaser *et al.*, 2003). Ongoing difficulties with coping in chronic illness, particularly associated with failure to resolve negative emotional states, can therefore result in a continual chronic physiologic stress response.

A number of reports and authors have highlighted the importance of socioeconomic factors in explaining health inequalities, and poorer health is experienced by a number of different groups including those with mental health problems (Whitehead, 1987; Townsend *et al.*, 1988; DH, 1999d; Rasul *et al.*, 2001). Most would agree that both socioeconomic factors are important to consider in terms of health (Ebrahim and Smith, 1997). The risk of a chronic limiting illness, for example, is higher in those who are disadvantaged in the labour market, both in terms of their material rewards for their labour, or, indeed, unemployment or economic inactivity (Wilkinson, 1996). Furthermore, adults who are disadvantaged because of their socioeconomic position may not only consume a less healthy diet but may also smoke more and take less exercise (Irala-Estevez *et al.*, 2000) (see Chapter 12: Physical Co-Morbidity in Mental Health).

One area receiving a great deal of attention over the years is social support or more importantly, 'perceived' social support. This may be a key area in determining how individuals cope with ongoing health problems and in 'buffering' the impact of chronic stress. Received and perceived social support has been classified as being instrumental (helping with tasks), financial, informational (providing information), appraisal (help in evaluating a situation) and emotional (an affective restorative function) (Rozanski *et al.*, 2005). Perhaps the greatest challenge for all health professionals and society generally, is ensuring that there is effective social support which nurtures a feeling of 'belonging' and which helps to meet esteem needs.

There is now considerable evidence implicating depression, anxiety, social isolation, low perceived emotional support, hostility and work-related stress in the development of heart disease, with clustering of these factors possibly increasing risk further (Hemingway and Marmot, 1999; Rozanski *et al.*, 1999). These factors are also likely to impact negatively and increase risk further in a range of chronic disorders not only aetiologically but in terms of ongoing coping.

SELF-REGULATION THEORY

Individual appraisal of a given situation helps to shape health behaviours, and is influenced by our 'common sense' definitions of health threats. Such perceived threats are referred to as 'illness representations' by Leventhal and Nerenz (1983), and include beliefs regarding the causes and consequences of an illness, along with a perception that the individual can influence the outcome of their illness (Brownlee *et al.*, 2000). Accordingly, it is suggested that individuals construct a mental model on the basis of their representations of the perceived 'reality' of their condition (Maes and Karoly, 2005) (see Chapter 6: Truth, Uncertainty and the Mental Health Nurse).

Self-Regulation Theory (SRT) refers to a personal health management system, involving the self-monitoring and personal appraisal and evaluation of one's health status, with resultant changes in an individual's behaviour where they feel this is appropriate and necessary. SRT, therefore, represents an attempt by an individual to make personal sense of his/her current health issues. If 'self-regulation' is to be facilitated in mental health care then nurses must understand the individual's illness representations of illness/health. Individual appraisal will result in a decision being made as to whether something is perceived as a health threat or not. A meta-analytical review of the illness representation model (Hagger and Orbell, 2003) has shown that patients' perceptions of controllability/curability are positively associated with psychological well-being, social functioning and vitality, and negatively associated with psychological distress and ill health. For example, in a sample of individuals with chronic illness, Karoly and Ruehlman (1996) found that compared with individuals with no pain, men and women with persistent pain problems reported greater self-criticism, negative goal-related arousal and a poor perception and confidence in their own abilities to cope.

It is important that mental health practitioners do not dismiss an individual's 'common sense' interpretations of their situation, as no matter how implausible, these may influence their evaluation and subsequent behavioural responses. The idea that, in encounters with health professionals, patients present their problems as stories has led to the development of a narrative-based approach to care, particularly in primary care settings. Launer (2002) suggests that a narrative-based approach involves the search for better stories and offers a conceptual framework for understanding all the different discourses, including lay or folk accounts of the world.

SELF-REGULATION STRATEGIES

Coping strategies may be 'emotion-focused' or 'problem-focused' (see Figure 13.1). Problem-focused coping involves the individual taking active measures to modify the stressful situation, whilst emotion-focused coping may help to regulate the accompanying emotional distress. In most stressful situations, individuals will have at their disposal a number of preferred coping strategies based on personality characteristics (Shaw, 1999), and these are likely to involve both problem- and emotion-focused

Emotion-Focused Coping Strategies	**Problem-Focused Coping Strategies**
• Avoidance/disengagement	• Seeking information
• Repression	• Considering alternatives
• Denial	(costs/benefits)
• Projection	• Goal setting
• Venting feelings	• Selecting actions
• Intellectualizing	• Pacing activities
• Seeking emotional support	• Self-management

Figure 13.1

Emotion- and problem-focused coping strategies

approaches. Mental health practitioners need to be aware of, and be able to facilitate more effective, coping strategies where those being employed by the individual are perhaps causing further difficulties.

Recognition that self-determination is an important predictor in the initiation and maintenance of health behaviours has led to renewed interest in self-regulation strategies to promote health. Overall definitions of self-regulation tend to embody the basic ingredients of goal-setting, steering processes and strategies, feedback and self-evaluation (Zeidner *et al.*, 2000). Indeed, the setting of personal goals and the modification of individual behaviour towards the achievement of these goals is a vital component of self-regulation theory. Goals articulate a desired outcome or state, and, if realistic, possess the power to motivate individuals to move towards achievement. Cognitions, however, are also important determinants of goal selection, articulated in several social cognitive models (Rosenstock, 1974; Fishbein and Ajzen, 1975; Maes and Karoly, 2005). If health behaviour change is to be successful, then awareness of individual risk and vulnerability is important as are the social influences which may affect behaviour and goal achievement.

'Self-efficacy' is now considered a significant psychological construct in predicting behaviour performance and another important concept underpinning the self-regulation of health behaviours. Self-efficacy refers to the confidence an individual has in his or her personal ability to perform a task or specific behaviour, or to change a specific cognitive state successfully, regardless of circumstances or contexts (Bandura, 1997, 1998). Social cognition theory suggests that an individual's perceived self-efficacy is likely to prove fundamental to one's ability to set disease management goals (Bradley *et al.*, 1999). Indeed, Bandura (1996) draws a distinction between *efficacy expectations*, referring to the anticipatory belief that one is capable of executing behaviour required to produce an outcome, and *outcome expectancies*, which reflects an anticipatory belief that a specific behaviour will lead to certain outcomes. Accordingly, such beliefs will have a major impact on whether or not an individual will succeed with any behaviour modification designed to improve health status. Hence, the stronger one's perceived self-efficacy, the more proactive and persistent one's efforts will be to meet one's health goals.

Many of the problem-focused coping strategies in Figure 13.1 are important in self-regulation approaches and these are seen as important interventions in health care. Indeed, these interventions are particularly relevant today, with numerous health policy documents referring to empowerment, autonomy, responsibility, independence, self-direction, self-care and self-management.

SELF-REGULATION AND MENTAL HEALTH

Many studies have demonstrated the value of self-regulation in chronic illness, but samples have tended to involve patients with physical illness. There is no reason why, when promoting physical health, self-regulation approaches involving the selection of realistic goals to motivate behaviour change as outlined earlier, should not confer some benefit in individuals with severe mental health problems. Indeed, cognitive and affective health is necessary for the complex behaviours necessary in coping, not least in the utilization of care services (Fultz et al., 2003). Caution needs to be exercised, though, with regard to illness representations in those with severe mental health problems, as these may involve distorted cognitions. This is likely to be the case when psychiatric symptoms are severe, distressing or disabling. At such times it is unlikely that health-promoting strategies aimed at lifestyle modification to reduce risk of physical illness would be a major priority in any care plan. This is not different in those with physical disorders who experience an acute or chronic exacerbation of their condition requiring, for example, high dependency care because of compromised cardiovascular status. At such times, physical health promotion is not a priority and is left until homeostasis has been restored and symptom control optimized. However, the utility of self-regulation approaches in individuals with mental health problems needs to be tested further using appropriate research methodology (see Chapter 7: Where is your Evidence? Broadening the Scope of Professional Knowledge).

COLLABORATION IN CARE

With the rejection of medical paternalism, growing societal expectations that individuals take responsibility for their own health, and with self-regulation viewed as an effective strategy, there has been increasing momentum towards more collaborative care (see Chapter 3: User Involvement and the Micro-Politics of Mental Health Care). Certainly, if self-regulation is to be facilitated effectively in those with long-term conditions to promote physical health, then the partnership between client and health care provider must facilitate this process. In one study (Williams et al., 1998), diabetic patients whose autonomy was supported by health care providers tended to be more motivated to regulate their glucose levels, felt more able to do so, and showed improvements in HbA1c levels (an indicator of the average blood glucose levels over the previous six to eight weeks).

In promoting physical health in patients with mental health problems, collaboration is important not only between practitioner and client but also between the different sectors and agencies involved in care. Bandura (1998) suggests that health care systems can influence an individual's sense of perceived self-efficacy, either in a supportive or in an inhibitory way. Indeed, Bodenheimer et al. (2002) argue that for self-management programmes to work, a well-resourced and proactive professional team is required as is an informed, activated patient.

Four elements in particular are seen as enhancing collaborative management: (a) collaborative definitions of problems; (b) targeting of specific areas, goal setting and planning; (c) creating a continuum of self-management training and support services;

and (d) active sustained follow-up (Korff *et al.*, 1997). Equally, there should be shared goals, a sustained working relationship, mutual understanding of roles and responsibilities, and the requisite skills for carrying out respective roles (Punamaki, 1994; Rogers *et al.*, 2005).

Physical health in those with mental health problems needs to be monitored and checked regularly, but there is a debate as to which professional group should take this responsibility. The National Institute for Health and Clinical Excellence (NICE) (NICE, 2002a) believes that in clients diagnosed with schizophrenia the responsibility should lie with the GP. However, clients often engage with a number of health professionals across a variety of care agencies and all must take some responsibility in promoting physical health. Whilst the NICE guidelines outline both a range of physical health checks to be made and health promotion advice to be given, there are no details of how, why or when any of this should be undertaken (Citrome and Yeomans, 2005) (see Chapter 12: Physical Co-Morbidity in Mental Health). A number of client and provider issues may contribute to poor physical health, including staff having negative attitudes towards those with mental health problems and organizational design problems where mental health care and physical health care is often provided separately (Berren *et al.*, 1999).

Lessons need to be learned from experiences with individuals with physical disorders, where health-promotion strategies commenced in either primary or secondary care settings are often not communicated effectively so that continuation and reinforcement is not possible once the client is transferred/discharged. Communication at all levels is essential but as Thorne (2006) argues, communication has been seen as a 'soft' science and not a vital element in effective health care delivery. There is now increasing recognition of the key role which communication plays in health service improvement.

Redman (2005) suggests that health professionals have a strong responsibility to avoid harm, and by not providing the preparation for individuals to self-manage, or refusing to learn, is counter to this, with the consequence that the discrediting of patients' self-management skills could affect the provider–client relationship with erosion of trust and mutual alienation. Even where there is individual willingness to facilitate self-management, the infrastructure must support such interventions. Most health services in developed countries are experiencing acute financial difficulties and a lack of resources may work against professionals fulfilling their health promotion role effectively. Nurses may find this particularly frustrating and, it is argued, the inability to provide adequate self-management preparation is one cause of moral distress among nurses (Redman and Fry, 2000).

APPLICATION OF SELF-REGULATION THEORY IN PRACTICE: SUPPORTING SELF-MANAGEMENT

Health behaviour change may be necessary in a number of areas in those with both mental and physical health problems. Skills may be needed to monitor the effectiveness

of symptom control and understanding of the underlying disorder and the drugs prescribed will be important. Self-monitoring skills may involve the recording of physiological values, such as peak expiratory flow rate in asthma, as well as being able to
recognize deterioration and when appropriate action needs to be taken. Lifestyle modification may be necessary to reduce risk further and will necessitate a review of dietary
intake, alcohol and cigarette consumption and levels of physical exercise. It is important
that any action plan is realistic, as goals that are unachievable will only result in failure
and low morale.

The principles of self-regulation can be applied in a number of ways and with a
knowledge of risk factors underpinning health problems, practitioners working in
health and social care settings can have an effective role in health-promotion activities.
This could be one-to-one, where realistic goals are set and an action plan tailored to
fit an individual's day-to-day lifestyle. Motivational interviewing can also be used to
facilitate change and to promote recovery, and provides a useful framework with
guiding principles to achieve self-regulation (Miller and Rollnick, 2002) (see Chapter
10: The Meaning of Recovery).

One initiative that has gained in popularity is 'self-management', although this concept
has been open to a number of interpretations which makes comparison between studies
difficult. Some studies have interpreted self-management rather narrowly, simply referring to the teaching of self-monitoring skills to recognize early deterioration. For self-
management to be effective, strategies need to be built on sound self-regulation
principles, as outlined earlier. Apart from using self-management principles on a one-
to-one basis, they may also be incorporated into more formal programmes. Indeed, this
may be an issue for future 'psychoeducational' programmes (see Chapter 15: Enhancing
Effective Multidisciplinary Team-Working: A Psychoeducational Approach).

In 2001, a UK government report, 'The Expert Patient: A New Approach to Chronic
Disease Management for the 21st Century' (DH, 2001b), outlined how a more patient-
centred NHS could help people with long-term conditions maintain their health and
improve their quality of life. This was to be achieved with the Expert Patient Programme (EPP) based on the work of Kate Lorig (Lorig et al., 1981), who developed a
generic chronic disease self-management course which is now promoted worldwide.
Programmes run over a six-week period and are delivered by tutors who themselves
have a chronic disorder. Each weekly session is half a day and topics include relaxation,
management of symptoms and medication, as well as improving communication with
health providers. Although the pilot phase of the EPP was funded by the Department
of Health to April 2004, it is now supported from mainstream NHS funds and delivered
by Primary Care Trusts and other interested health and social care groups.

Most EPPs have focused on developing generic programmes with physical disorders,
but one preliminary study has identified the need for condition-specific programmes
(Kennedy et al., 2004). It is suggested that key stakeholders in primary and secondary
care would have greater confidence in programmes related more specifically to particular conditions. It is likely, for example, that a condition-specific course could effectively
meet the needs of individuals with mental health problems. However, Davidson (2005),

in reviewing the utility of self-management models in mental health, argues that those derived from physical illnesses cannot be implemented without changes. There are already good examples in mental health settings where self-management initiatives have been developed. This expertise needs to be shared so that where there is lack of under-standing regarding the needs of those with mental health problems, those with experi-ence of running user-led mental health initiatives can be involved in training, guidance and support. This will require increased awareness of self-management initiatives amongst health professionals, improved links with local agencies in the community and better networking with Primary Care Trusts. As with all programmes that have been developed in different settings, it is important that there is rigorous evaluation of their efficacy, effectiveness and transferability (Battersby, 2004). It may be that specific pro-vision is indeed necessary, but although prevention and well-being interventions are increasing generally, few services currently exist that are tailored to the needs of those with mental illness who already have serious physical problems (Jones *et al.*, 2004).

Although self-management programmes have a useful part to play, the ongoing role of practitioners in monitoring, feedback and reinforcement is crucial. Whilst the evalu-ation of self-management programmes has been positive, expectations must be realistic. Cardiac rehabilitation programmes, for example, which incorporate psychological and educational interventions (including motivational interviewing), have been effective in reinforcing health behaviour change and reducing risk following acute myocard-ial infarction. However, low participation rates have caused concern with as few as 25%–31% of eligible men participating, with even lower rates in women of 11%–20% (Melville *et al.*, 1999; Jackson *et al.*, 2005). Some of the factors contributing to low participation in this group include age, sex, culture, accessibility, depression and social deprivation, and these same factors may potentially affect participation in self-management programmes for those with mental health problems. In addition, most programmes are time-limited and additional health-promotion strategies are needed which will facilitate effective continuity of care across the various health and social care sectors. Continuity in terms of effective follow-up remains a problem, but one possible solution might be to make available 'client held' health-promotion action plans, which could be shared with appropriate professionals involved in care. The importance of ongoing social support should not be forgotten. Social support can have a significant impact on self-management in individuals with chronic illness but in an excellent review of social support, Gallant (2003) argues for further elucidation of the underly-ing mechanism by which support influences self-management and whether this rela-tionship varies by illness, type of support and behaviour.

CONCLUSION

Mental health nurses need to be aware that in those with severe mental health problems there is a higher risk of physical health problems. Ongoing review and monitoring is crucial, and this should not only focus on mental health problems. Effective assessments, including medical history-taking and physical examination, will enable new problems to be identified, and, where there is co-morbidity, early recognition of possible deterioration. An individual's subsequent coping behaviours, thoughts about their health status and emotional responses to ill health, whether physical or mental, need to be assessed and, where these are potentially health-compromising, appropriate strategies utilized to facilitate more effective coping. The success of any approach will depend on the knowledge and skills of the practitioner and where necessary this will need to be considered as part of the practitioner's ongoing professional development plan.

CHAPTER 14
RESPONDING TO THE NEEDS OF YOUNGER PEOPLE: THE BEREAVED ADOLESCENT

Yvonne Dexter

While compassionate care is important, compassionate but ill-informed care may be harmful (Royal College of Nursing, 2003, p. 12).

INTRODUCTION

Mental health nurses are amongst a range of health care professionals who may come into contact with bereaved adolescents. Responding to the needs of these young people is an example of how mental health nurses can develop their skills so as to be able to work in partnership with service users of all ages, their carers and other professionals to improve care and lead innovation in a range of new roles and organizations (DH, 2006a). This chapter will discuss responding to the needs of bereaved adolescents. It is a challenging task as the range of literature is wide and findings are often contradictory and inconclusive. Myths abound about the effects of loss and bereavement on children and young people, and debates exist about how to support them. Evidence about the effects of loss and bereavement on adolescents will be explored and the complexities of researching the issue will be highlighted. Interventions that have been developed to support bereaved adolescents will be discussed and placed in the context of adolescent health care in general.

Contemporary Issues in Mental Health Nursing, Edited by J. E. Lynch and S. Trenoweth
© 2008 John Wiley & Sons, Ltd

ADOLESCENCE, ADOLESCENT HEALTH AND SERVICE PROVISION

Adolescence is '. . . a transitional developmental period between childhood and adulthood characterised by more biological, psychological and social role changes than any other stage of life except infancy [and] a time when one's developmental and health trajectories can be altered dramatically in positive or negative directions' (Holmbeck, 2002, p. 409). It has been studied widely from different perspectives (Coleman and Hendry, 1999; Steinberg, 2002; Savage, 2007). Social scientists differentiate between early adolescence (10 to 13 years), middle adolescence (14 to 18 years) and late adolescence (19 to 22 years) (Steinberg, 2002). However, the end of adolescence seems elusive and ill-defined and there is a debate about whether the transition to adulthood is more stressful today than in the past (Jones, 2005; The Children's Society, 2006).

Since 1997, when it was identified that care of adolescents was given insufficient priority, lacked focus and had poorly developed services (DH, 1997b), there has been increasing interest in the health of this age group. Since this time, adolescent health care and possible interventions for improving young people's health has been increasingly examined (BMA, 2003). As such, there has been concern expressed about the overall health of this group and 'a general decrease in health-sustaining behaviour by young people, and an increase in potentially health-damaging behaviour' with a 'complex intertwining of factors which affect health behaviour' (Cater and Coleman, 2006, p. 25). One such concern, particularly regarding adolescent health, is the apparent increasing levels of mental health problems (BMA, 2006). The National Service Framework for Children, Young People and Maternity Services (DH, 2004e, 2006a) addresses the mental health and psychological well-being of children and young people. Its vision is to see:

An improvement in the mental health of all children and young people; That multi-agency services, working in partnership, promote the mental health of all children and young people, provide early intervention and also meet the needs of children and young people with established or complex problems; That all children, young people and their families have access to mental health care based upon the best available evidence and provided by staff with an appropriate range of skills and competencies (DH, 2004e, p. 4).

Indeed, adolescent health care services need to meet their specific and different needs and overcome barriers that may prevent young people from accessing them (Social Exclusion Unit (SEU), 2004b). This will need to be done by ensuring services and care delivery is youth-friendly, ensuring confidentiality, promoting respect for young people's views, providing information and ensuring expertise and continuity of care. It is also important to make services more accessible to groups of adolescents who have particular problems, such as looked-after young people (Royal College of General

Practitioners and Royal College of Nursing, 2002; World Health Organization (WHO), 2002a; Royal College of Paediatrics and Child Health, 2003; DH, 2005g).

BEREAVEMENT

Bereavement is a comparatively new area of research (Stroebe *et al.*, 2001). However, the literature on bereavement and bereavement care is developing and with it issues are being raised from differing perspectives (Wimpenny, 2006). One such issue is that of terminology. Terms in this area are difficult to define and are often used interchangeably. However, Strobe *et al.* (2001a, p. 6) affords some clarity as they define bereavement as 'the objective situation of having lost someone significant', whereas grief is often seen as an emotional reaction to the loss of a significant other through death, which can lead to psychological and physical health difficulties. Mourning, however, is 'the social expressions or acts expressive of grief that are shaped by the practices of a given society or cultural group' (Strobe *et al.*, 2001a, p. 6).

Various attempts have been made to explain grief, which has had an important influence on constructing policy and practice for bereaved people. 'Stage models' (e.g. Kubler-Ross, 1970) have been followed by approaches which reflect grief in terms of continuing bonds (Klass *et al.*, 1996), meaning reconstruction (Neimeyer, 2001) and movement between loss and restoration (Stroebe and Schut, 2001). The literature also reflects the problem of differentiating between those who adjust 'normally', those who experience 'complicated grief' and those who experience 'mental health problems' following bereavement. This, of course, has implications for diagnosis and subsequent intervention (Walter, 1999; Wimpenny, 2006). Indeed, 'the negotiation of normality between experts, popular culture and bereaved individuals is an ongoing feature of the social world of bereavement' (Walter, 1999, p. 165).

BEREAVEMENT IN CHILDHOOD AND ADOLESCENCE

Interest in child and adolescent bereavement has also increased in recent years, stimulating much debate (Corr and McNeil, 1986; Corr and Balk, 1996; Balk and Corr, 2001; Ribbens McCarthy, 2005, 2006). Importantly, links have been identified between mental health and loss in childhood and adolescence and subsequent vulnerability to mental ill health in later, adult life, such as depression (Black, 1996; Moore and Carr, 2000). Many key issues here, however, are fiercely debated and it is not at all clear that a cause–effect link exists between bereavement amongst young people and subsequent mental ill health. For example, on the one hand Black (1996, p. 1496) stated:

Controlled studies based on population samples have confirmed earlier clinical impressions that bereaved children have a significantly increased risk of developing psychiatric disorders and may suffer considerable psychological and social difficulties throughout childhood and even later in life

To this end, Black (1996) stresses the importance of counselling after bereavement in children, even though there are few good research studies to back up this claim. Harrington (1996, p. 822), however, responded:

Although psychiatric morbidity is increased in bereaved children . . . most of them do not develop important depressive conditions . . . Bereavement is painful but does not necessarily make children ill

Harrington (1996) suggests that children do not tend to experience loss due to bereavement as powerfully as loss through divorce or separation, and stresses the danger of simply applying models applicable to adults, such as bereavement counselling, to children.

Indeed, efforts are also made in the literature to demystify child and adolescent bereavement and the 'unproven assumptions about the impact of bereavement on children' (Harrington and Harrison, 1999, p. 230). The Work Group on Palliative Care for Children of the International Work Group on Death, Dying and Bereavement (1999, p. 443) examined '. . . some inaccurate myths that adults have generated concerning children, adolescents and death. These myths typify the outlooks of some adults and serve to deform relationships and interventions with some children and adolescents.' The concern is that such myths may provoke interventions which exacerbate the problems relating to grief (Boseley, 1999).

Adolescence and bereavement are indeed complex issues, and individual experiences are open to stereotyping, generalization and misinterpretation. Research into the subject is likewise complex and it has been suggested that there is little quality research in the area (Wimpenny, 2006). Furthermore, the conjunction of the disruptions of youth and bereavement are a 'double jeopardy' (Ribbens McCarthy, 2005, p. 1) requiring attention from policies and services for adolescents. Research evidence is contradictory and 'centralizes the question of whether young people do or do not constitute a distinct group in relation to issues relating to bereavement' (Ribbens McCarthy, 2006, p. 4). While this area has attracted some attention in recent years, it remains a little understood issue. There are major implications here for further research.

Adolescent bereavement research has tended to focus on the loss of parents (Balk, 1996; Worden, 1996) and siblings (Balk, 1983), with growing interest in the adolescerts' experience of loss of friends and peers (McNeil *et al.*, 1991), but minimal attention has been paid to the loss of a baby, miscarriage or abortion (Balk and Corr, 2001; Ribbens McCarthy, 2005). Likewise, little attention has been paid to friend and peer loss, and this is puzzling given the increased importance that peers have in adolescents' lives. Attention has also been paid to bereavement from different causes, for example, by suicide (Wertheimer, 2001) and violence (Salloum, 2004). However, the issue seems to be more complex than who died or how they died, and is likely to encompass considerations as to '... whether or not a particular bereavement is felt to be significant in the life of a young person ... [and] the meaning that relationship holds for the young person' (Ribbens McCarthy, 2005, p. 2).

Cross' (2002) unique study analysed written records of calls from bereaved children (mainly 11–16 years) to Childline over two years. It offers compelling and varied insights into what bereavement has meant for them. A disturbing finding was that the risk of abuse may actually increase after bereavement, raising implications for child protection practice. Indeed, the role of peers revealed in the literature is interesting in terms of both support and problematic relationships, from bullying and name-calling (peers being unsure how to respond, general withdrawal from friends, loneliness) to a sense of being different (Balk and Corr, 2001; Jessop and Ribbens McCarthy, 2005).

Adolescents' adjustment following bereavement partly depends on their understanding of the concept of death. Children's understanding of this concept has been widely studied. Early research focused on the link between concept acquisition and cognitive development and age (Kane, 1979), and suggested that full development of the concept occurred by age 7 or 8 years (Lansdown and Benjamin, 1985). More recent studies emphasize the role played by factors such as experience and culture in the development of understandings of death. Due to these factors, an accurate concept of death occurs as young as 6 years of age (Mahon *et al.*, 1999). Adolescents, however, appear to share the adult concept of death, but as Moore and Carr (2000, pp. 208, 210) caution:

While most adolescents recognize the inevitability of their own death at a cognitive level, the full emotional significance of this is not apprehended until adulthood, unless multiple bereavements or other traumatic events occur.

RESEARCH ISSUES

The consequences of bereavement for adolescents are unique due to the developmental challenges they are experiencing (Fleming and Adolph, 1986; Balk and Corr, 2001). Indeed, it is important to recognize that the development of adolescents, their health and illnesses occur within a changing developmental context (Holmbeck, 2002). Crucially, therefore, the quality of research on adolescents is likely to be advanced if such changes are recognized and studies focus on 'constructs, variables, and measures uniquely relevant to adolescents, thus making the study developmentally oriented' (Holmbeck, 2002, p. 410). Such a point has been echoed by Worden (1996, p. 90) who suggested that over time, '... the death of a parent does, indeed, affect adolescents' negotiation of the core issues facing them'. Furthermore, it is crucial to recognize that

. . . the life experiences of each young person have a unique influence in the development of that individual's brain and his/her current and future patterns of thinking, relating and behaving. The current understanding of the adolescent brain is pointing to the existence of a developmental period in which there is both increased vulnerability to negative environmental experiences and enhanced receptivity to positive, including therapeutic, life experiences – both of which carry long-term consequences for adult life (Young Minds, 2006, p. 5).

In terms of prevalence, it is difficult to establish how common adolescent bereavement experiences are (Ribbens McCarthy, 2005). However, in American studies assessing the prevalence of bereavement within college students, adolescent bereavement experiences were more common than previously thought (Balk and Corr, 2001). Indeed, Harrison and Harrington's (2001) extensive UK study found that the loss of a relative or friend was a common experience and was associated with depressive symptoms. However, in a cross-sectional study a causal association could not be established. A few adolescents felt the need for professional help.

The complexity of the nature of adolescent bereavement has implications for the research process. In bereavement research both quantitative and qualitative approaches are potentially valuable. Neimeyer and Hogan (2001, p. 113) advocate '. . . a stance of methodological pluralism, respecting both numbers and narrative and the distinctive forms of understanding that each can provide' (see Chapter 7: Where is your Evidence? Broadening the Scope of Professional Knowledge). Quantitative methods include psychiatric symptom scales, general purpose grief scales and specialized grief scales, but 'there is as yet no gold standard in the measurement of grief' (Neimeyer and Hogan, 2001, p. 114). Much quantitative research has focused on bereavement as a risk factor measuring personal outcomes (for example, physical and mental health) and social disadvantage outcomes (for example, educational qualifications, leaving home early, criminal and disruptive behaviour, employment and early sexual activity). Importantly, research seems to indicate some adolescents may not show any particularly negative effects of bereavement and there may be positive outcomes (Ribbens McCarthy, 2005).

Qualitative methods include grounded theory, content analysis, focus groups, ethnography and case study aiming '. . . less to generate incontestable "facts" than to discover and explore the unique and common perspectives of the individual being studied' (Neimeyer and Hogan, 2001, p. 105). Most adolescent bereavement research uses structured quantitative methods and as such many established qualitative approaches are hardly ever used, despite their advantages in offering 'real world' insights into the phenomena. For example, the ethnographic approach, which helps to understand social context and narrative analysis, may help to provide a longer time perspective and insight into adolescent experience (Ribbens McCarthy, 2005).

Furthermore, most studies are retrospective and cross-sectional. There is, however, a need for studies that use *longitudinal* designs to look at the trajectory of adolescent grief, pay careful attention to access and sampling (e.g. widely based community samples), define concepts clearly and develop frameworks and models (Fleming and

Adolph, 1986; Balk and Corr, 2001; Ribbens McCarthy, 2005). Control groups are important as some adolescents may experience adjustment difficulties during the transition to adulthood without experiencing bereavement (Fleming and Balmer, 1996).

There are obviously significant ethical issues in researching bereavement and youth issues. Key issues include recruiting participants, the timing of recruitment, obtaining informed consent, confidentiality, unanticipated disclosures, research–induced distress, protection from harm, avoiding pressure to participate and the training of researchers in the support of the bereaved (Cook, 1995, 2001; Parkes, 1995). A new orthodoxy has emerged in social science research advocating hearing the 'voice' of young people and undertaking research 'with' adolescents rather than 'on' them (France, 2004).

Some attention in the research literature has been paid to the issue of bereavement research as 'therapy' (Romanoff, 2001). That is, while 'Researchers are not in the role of therapist . . . it is important to recognise that interviewing individuals about emotionally painful issues of loss requires a variety of skills' (Cook, 1995, p. 118). In adolescent bereavement research, such skills of listening and asking questions sensitively are important. An illustration of this can be found in McNeil *et al.*'s (1991) case study, which explored the reactions of high school students 18 months after the death of a popular peer. They found that the students had hidden ongoing distressing feelings about the death, which emerged during the research process. They observed that there is an emotional impact on bereavement research participants which entails an obligation on the researchers to provide sources of support. Researchers may also feel the effects of the impact of such work for themselves, and may need to consider the emotional labour of this work.

INTERVENTIONS

Every Child Matters (ECM) is a radical new approach designed to change how services are structured, commissioned and delivered in order to respond more fully and effectively to children's well-being. It has introduced the 'Common Assessment Framework' – a standardized approach to conducting an assessment of a child's needs and deciding how their needs will be met, which can be used by practitioners across children's services in England. Indeed, bereavement may well be an issue that is identified during an assessment using this framework. Subsequent interventions are likely to be multi-disciplinary in nature. That is,

The wider ECM agenda is important in providing a framework within which mental health and psychological well-being . . . can be promoted. Everyone who works with children needs to have a clear understanding of what they can contribute to a child's mental and physical health and development. This means local children's services and Child and Adolescent Mental Health Services (CAMHS) teams engaging with each other to plan and develop patterns of joint working which reflect both their respective expertise and their shared responsibility (DH, 2006e, p. 3).

The identification and referral of young people needing intervention following bereavement is complex. Assessment is obviously a key issue, but as yet there is no consensus about who should be assessed, for example, should this be '... all children who experience bereavement or only those who show emotional/behavioural problems?' (Wimpenny, 2006, p. 28). Equally challenging is the issue of referral to services. Brown's (2006) UK study showed the extent to which young people may be unaware of services available to them with implications for facilitating adolescents' own direct access to services and providing accessible information. Furthermore, Griffiths (2003) identifies how adolescents with mental health problems may be hard to reach and that engaging them in therapeutic work can be difficult, self-referrals are rare, with reliance on family members and peers. As such, in order to promote the chances of being able to successfully work with such a client group, interventions '... should be characterised by confidentiality, choice and a determined effort to engage the adolescent's family' (Griffiths, 2003, p. 10).

Firm conclusions about adolescent bereavement are, however, elusive and, as such, there exists a debate about the suitability and effectiveness of interventions due to the wide range available, and indeed the varied aims they seek to achieve. Black (1996, p. 1496) suggests the interventions are important as they can

... alleviate the immediate distress of childhood bereavement and help prevent depression and other mental health problems in the future ... Primary prevention involves preparing the child for bereavement, supporting parents and caretakers after bereavement, explaining and talking openly with children about their experience, encouraging children's involvement in shared mourning practices and resumption of normal activities, and providing early professional help if needed.

Indeed, there are many possible psychological interventions – from cognitive behavioural therapy, social skills training, family therapy, interpersonal therapy and individual psychodynamic psychotherapy that are widely used to treat young people with mood disorders, but there is a need for more research to clarify which approaches assist in alleviating distress (Moore and Carr, 2000).

Resilience is another issue to consider in the health and social care of children and young people (Daniel and Wassell, 2002; Tusaie, 2004), as 'Resilient children are better equipped to resist stress and adversity, cope with change and uncertainty, and to recover faster and more completely from traumatic events or episodes' (Newman and Blackburn, 2002, p. 1). Individual, family and wider community factors have been associated with resilience in adolescence. These factors might explain different outcomes, positive as well as negative, in adolescents following bereavement. For example, Black (1996, p. 1496) identified that 'long term risks of bereavement in childhood are associated with inadequate physical and emotional care, particularly after the loss of a mother. Certainly, the outcome for a child is strongly related to the way that adult carers are able to cope with their own grief and the changes to their lives ...' Evidence suggests strategies to promote resilience in services for young people have significant potential (Newman and Blackburn, 2002).

The context within which such interventions for children and young people could take place has provoked much discussion. However, Rowling (2003, p. 2) advocates school as a safe place to 'confront, learn about and manage grief'. Death and bereavement can be normalized by inclusion of such issues in the curriculum, but seemingly there is reluctance by staff to teach this area, possibly because of a lack of training (Rowling, 2003). However, it is important to recognize that 'Some children, especially adolescents, may not view school as an appropriate place to deal with emotions . . . while others may want teachers to actively intervene. The overall message is that children's responses vary. While they need to be asked how they want it handled, often they are not consulted' (Jessop and Ribbens McCarthy, 2005, p. 49).

Dowdney *et al.* (1999, p. 354) found '. . . parentally bereaved children and surviving parents showed higher than expected levels of psychiatric difficulties' and 'service provision was not significantly related to parental wishes or to levels of psychiatric disturbance in parents or children'. Indeed, ongoing work at the University of Gloucestershire is looking at how bereavement services for children are organized, what they offer and how they are rated by the children using the service. However, the question of how to resource a service is interesting. Pressure on state funding makes it:

. . . difficult to justify diverting scarce resources from the treatment of children with established mental disorders to provide counselling for children at risk. Such a strategy would have to be supported by compelling evidence from randomised trials that counselling of bereaved children is an effective way of preventing mental illness, but no such evidence exists (Harrington, 1996, p. 822).

Indeed, specialist contact services are distributed unevenly across the UK and are provided mainly by the voluntary sector. The voluntary sector and some charities offer specialist help (for example, Daisy's Dream, 2002). Cruse Bereavement Care, for example, offers support, such as leaflets (Cruse Bereavement Care, 2004), a helpline and a website specifically for young people. In recent years, more specialist child bereavement services have been developed but there is 'minimum national debate and no agreed standards or guidelines' (Stokes *et al.*, 1999, p. 291), for example, Winston's Wish and Daisy's Dream, although the Childhood Bereavement Network has now produced guidelines for best practice. Such services provide a range of interventions including peer group activities such as camps, which allow adolescents to share experiences, overcome isolation and learn to contain and express emotions in safe environments (Stokes and Crossley, 1995; Rolls and Payne, 2004). However, there has been much political debate recently about the role of charities in service provision and the balance between state and voluntary sector funding. Charities are indeed 'good at filling gaps and inventing better practice' (Toynbee, 2006, p. 29). However, there are major implications for the careful selection, training, monitoring and supervision of volunteers.

The needs of children experiencing traumatic events are an important contemporary, and indeed global, issue and as such there is a need for international research and dialogue. Bereavement following a catastrophic event creates a particular risk of psychiatric disorder, and '. . . HIV infection, war, civil conflict, mass transport disasters, and violence are all likely to increase the number of children at risk' (Black, 1996, p. 1496). Various interventions have been developed here. Work with children and young people bereaved by AIDS (for example, by using 'memory boxes' in Uganda) is supported by UNICEF (UNICEF, 2007). Concern about children who have witnessed large-scale disasters, such as terrorist attacks, has increased in recent years (United States Department of Health and Human Sciences, 2007). Indeed, children bereaved by 9/11 have been at the centre of media interest and 'more thoroughly studied and the impact of the trauma on them more deeply analysed than in any previous disaster' (Pilkington, 2006, p. 18), and specific interventions and support have been developed for them. Further information on such interventions can be obtained from the 'World Trade Center' Family Center's website below.

However, further research is needed about vulnerable young people who are already at risk of poor mental health, for example, young offenders, adolescents following abortion and looked-after young people. Indeed, young offenders are a group for whom health care in the community remains inadequate (Mental Health Foundation, 2002; Commission for Healthcare Audit and Inspection, 2006). High levels of loss and bereavement have been identified as a risk factor in youth offending (Youth Justice Board, 2005). Questions are being asked about the needs of bereaved young offenders (The United Kingdom Parliament, 2004), but there appear to be limited specific interventions for them (e.g. grief awareness programmes) (Finlay and Jones, 2000), partnership working between Youth Offending Teams and Child and Adolescent Mental Health Services (Lake and Hall, 2005). Furthermore, bereavement issues following abortion is a little researched area, but studies examining whether teenagers are harmed psychologically by abortion suggest that they are not (Zabin et al., 1989; Pope et al., 2001). Zabin et al. (1989) found that teenagers who abort their pregnancy are significantly better off two years later, psychologically as well as socially and economically, than comparable women who choose to give birth to their child. However, there are clear implications for supporting young people going through this difficult experience.

There is clearly a need for ongoing debate and discussion about interventions, and a coordinated national strategy is required following a review of available evidence. It is important that all views about adolescent bereavement are considered, as this may help to frame the way services are developed, so as to avoid biases. There is certainly concern regarding the apparent medicalization of bereavement, as identified by Rowling (2003, p. 1), who suggests that the 'construction of grief in a "disease" framework distorts grief support'. There is a need to consider whether the development of specialist bereavement services for young people has been at a cost to general services. A balance is needed. Indeed, there is a much wider debate regarding interventions to support the experience of loss, described by Thompson (2002, p. 1) as 'a broad concept and does not relate solely to losses brought about by death'. Indeed, there is evidence to suggest that services should recognize the needs of young people experiencing losses that are not death-related, e.g. divorce, adoption and foster care, abuse, disability and ill health. The Office of the Deputy Prime Minister (ODPM, 2005, p. 1) highlights the needs of disadvantaged young people

. . . too often services will approach someone's problems as individual issues rather than looking at them as interlinked. As a result, individuals can find themselves pushed from pillar to post on unpredictable and repetitive journeys around different agencies and on a downward spiral of social exclusion. Such people will struggle to progress into independent, fulfilling adulthood.

Interventions and care of the bereaved adolescent is clearly a multidisciplinary, and possibly a multi-agency, issue. All professionals who come into contact with young people should be aware of how to respond to the needs of bereaved adolescents, to ensure 'youth-friendly' approaches. Professional education, therefore, at both pre- and post-registration levels, needs to highlight and address problems that may affect some adolescents after bereavement, a point reinforced by the National Institute for Health and Clinical Excellence (NICE, 2005a).

CONCLUSIONS

For Ribbens McCarthy (2005, p. 21) '. . . bereavement is 'a pervasive experience in the lives of young people' and as such 'bereavement . . . has a significance for major emotional and biographical disruption'. Illuminating this complex area and being able to effectively respond to the needs of bereaved adolescents is challenging. Whilst there is an increasing amount of research and interest being generated in this area, there still exists a lack of knowledge or, indeed, an overall consensus regarding the way forward. Contemporary emphasis in health care is being placed on a 'what works best' approach. However, as clearly identified by this field, there needs to be a blend of '. . . the best evidence from research with clinical expertise, patient preferences, and existing resources into decision making about the health care of individual patients' (Ireland, 2006, p. 177). It is, of course, challenging and complex to balance research evidence with professional expertise and patient choice in providing for the needs of bereaved adolescents. What is clearly urgently needed is 'to develop an interdisciplinary dialogue based on a constructive engagement between different perspectives and different professions' (Ribbens McCarthy, 2006, p. 5), as well as listening to the individual voices of young people and their families.

WEBSITES

Child Bereavement Trust (www.childbereavement.org.uk)
Childhood Bereavement Network (www.childhoodbereavementnetwork.org.uk)
Cruse Bereavement Care (www.crusebereavementcare.org.uk)
Cruse Bereavement Care's Youth Involvement Project (www.rd4u.org.uk)
Daisy's Dream (www.daisysdream.org.uk)
Every Child Matters (ECM) (www.everychildmatters.gov.uk)
World Trade Center Family Center (www.wtcfamilycenter.org)
Winston's Wish (www.winstonswish.org.uk)

CHAPTER 15
ENHANCING EFFECTIVE MULTIDISCIPLINARY TEAM-WORKING: A PSYCHOEDUCATIONAL APPROACH

John Cordwell and Lee Bradley

INTRODUCTION

Multidisciplinary team-working is the norm in contemporary mental health practice, but some argue that it fails to fulfil its potential to influence clients' experiences of care. As such, multi-professional collaboration should be nurtured rather than taken for granted, and opportunities for its enhancement may be particularly important. In this chapter we highlight the importance of multi-professional team-working with challenging client groups, and illustrate its significance to the care and treatment of clients who are considered to have 'dangerous and severe personality disorders' and are cared for within a high-secure setting. In so doing, we will draw upon and share some of our own clinical work in this area.

This chapter will also highlight how effective services and therapeutic interventions can be born out of open, supportive and collaborative multidisciplinary team (MDT) working, and the benefits this can have for teams and clients. We will draw upon some contemporary perceptions of MDTs and consider these with regard to the

Contemporary Issues in Mental Health Nursing, Edited by J. E. Lynch and S. Trenoweth
© 2008 John Wiley & Sons, Ltd

development of effective care and treatment plans. Furthermore, we will highlight how a multi-professional approach can be highly beneficial in the development and implementation of a 'psychoeducational programme' for clients with a diagnosis of personality disorder. All effective interventions for the clients are significant as they have been regarded as being difficult to engage with and difficult to provide therapeutic interventions for. The term 'personality disorder' is used in a generic sense to represent the clinical diagnosis as defined by the DSM-IV (the Diagnostic and Statistical Manual of Mental Disorders) (American Psychiatric Association (APA), 2000, p. 685) as:

An enduring pattern of inner experience and behaviour that deviates markedly from the expectations of the individual's culture, is pervasive and inflexible, stable over time and leads to stress or impairment.

THE PSYCHOEDUCATIONAL APPROACH

'Psychoeducation' can be defined as a process of educating individuals so as to improve their understanding and knowledge of their mental health problems. This includes focusing on symptoms, possible causes, psychological processes (thoughts, emotions and behaviours), and treatment options. Also important here is consideration of the implications that such problems may have for the individual's life, such as in their interpersonal functioning. The core elements to psychoeducation described within this chapter include assisting clients to increase their awareness and insights into their own psychological processes by teaching them about 'personality' in general and then their own identified problems and disorders.

The guiding paradigm is that the removal of knowledge deficits will increase treatment efficacy (Mericle, 1999). Research has also suggested that psychoeducation enhances progress within treatment and subsequent concordance (Rinder, 2000) (see Chapter 11: Supporting Recovery: Medication Management in Mental Health Care). Indeed, psychoeducation has been tried and tested within a range of forensic and other clinical settings, including use for socio-affective functioning (Stein *et al.*, 2003), attention deficit hyperactivity disorder (ADHD) in adolescents (Murphy, 2005) and reducing anxiety and depression for HIV/AIDS sufferers (Pomeroy *et al.*, 2000). Alongside this, positive research findings indicate the effectiveness of psychoeducation for the families of individuals who have experienced mental and physical health problems (for more examples see Rinder, 2000; Rusch and Corrigan, 2002; De Groot *et al.*, 2003; Van Deusen and Carr, 2004).

The psychoeducational approach per se is not a new treatment intervention, yet there is very little qualitative or quantitative research data that identifies or suggests even its efficacy with personality disordered individuals. However, one successful psychoeducation programme that has been established for a number of years with both positive and further promising outcomes has been run within a Regional Secure Unit in Leicestershire (see D'Silva and Duggan, 2002 for more details). Within our psychoeducation programme, the cognitive behavioural model was the theoretical process that supported the associated clinical work undertaken within both group and individual sessions. The basic underlying premise of the programme is that if the individuals learn to develop awareness and understanding of how and why they misperceive and misinterpret the world, they can learn skills and strategies that will help them to manage their problematic thoughts, emotions and behaviours. The actual changing and adapting of problematic beliefs, thoughts and emotions in order to modify behaviour is not within the remit of psychoeducation. Here, the process of psychoeducation is to complement and support other cognitive behavioural therapy (CBT) interventions, such as anger management for example.

Use of the psychoeducational process indicates that increased understanding of individual problems, aetiology, treatments and coping techniques can assist the CBT approach within in-patient (D'Silva and Duggan, 2002) and out-patient groups (De Groot *et al.*, 2003). This is promising because, compared with other approaches, CBT requires that clients have relatively high levels of knowledge and understanding of their problems. In order to decrease problematic and interpersonally difficult behaviours with this particular client group, the programme aims to aid individuals to develop further understanding into why their thoughts and emotions result in what can be highly problematic behaviours. The understandings that clients acquire from the programme can be used to support other therapeutic interventions that they may later be involved in.

Both group and individual aspects of the programme were developed from Young's Early Maladaptive Schema Theory (Young, 1994) and Beck's Cognitive Schema Theory of personality disorders (Beck, 1976; Beck *et al.*, 1990). These suggest that personality disorders may stem from understandings/perceptions that are formed through experiential learning in childhood and subsequently mould the ways in which individuals perceive themselves and their interactions with others. These beliefs inform the ways in which situations are remembered and understood. It was from this theoretical standpoint and the cognitive behavioural underpinning of our MDT process that the format and design of the programme were developed.

From a client-needs analysis, deficits were identified in clients' understandings and knowledge of personality disorder and the practical, social and treatment implications were considered. Unsurprisingly, these limitations were found both generally in the clients' understanding and knowledge of personality disorders and specifically in terms of their own individual personality disorder traits. The needs identified by the clinical team were to be met by having both group-based and individual elements to the programme. The group-based aspect of the programme focused more upon educational processes surrounding personality disorders, while the individual aspect addressed each clients' individual's diagnosis, traits and maladaptive cognitive/behavioural manifestations of the personality problems.

The aims of the psychoeducation programme were as follows:

Group Programme	Individual Programme
• Develop an awareness of personality and its origins. • Develop an awareness of personality disorders and their origins. • Group members to evaluate impact of personality disorders upon their lives. • Group members to evaluate effect of personality disorders on offending behaviours. • Develop an awareness of the functional link between personality disorders and problematic behaviours.	• Increase and develop awareness of care plans in relation to personality disorders and problematic behaviour. • Increase awareness of individual treatment needs to develop greater insight into individual diagnoses. • Identify and explore individual personality disorder diagnosis. • Encourage and develop insight into effects of individual personality disorders on social and therapeutic functioning. • Encourage development of links between disordered personality and offence behaviour (antecedents, behaviours, choices, consequences).

GROUP PROGRAMME

The group-based programme consisted of nine sessions, each between 60 and 90 minutes in length. The sessions included attention to the development of personality, the development of personality disorders and the diagnostic criteria for the 10 DSM-IV personality disorders (APA, 2000). Following this, the sessions covered how treatment needs are identified, formulated and addressed by the MDT. Individual and group-based tasks were used to facilitate understanding and learning through concepts such as perspective-taking and alternative idea generation. For example, the borderline personality disorder trait of 'feelings of abandonment' can be reviewed and used to incorporate thoughts and emotions in contexts such as therapy or the family environment.

The contents of the sessions included provision of an overview of the disciplines involued in the clients' care. This covered how the service as a whole provided their case treatment and it was here that the processes involved in needs assessment, risk assessment and risk monitoring were highlighted.

INDIVIDUAL PROGRAMME

The individual aspect of the programme was semi-structured in design to be both dynamic in approach and malleable in delivery. This method provides the freedom to tailor a programme to each client's needs while still attaining both programme and treatment integrity. Having a degree of flexibility allows for progress and affords facilitation by both ward- and non-ward-based staff. Therefore, the actual length of the programme varies according to levels of insight and progress and individual treatment needs. The individual aspect followed similar multidisciplinary themes to the group component of the programme. The implementation was coordinated by nursing and psychology disciplines, and the facilitation was conducted by all clinical disciplines. The format and schedule of the individual sessions were designed to match a one-hour-long framework which was considered ideal for both patient involvement and staff facilitation.

The process of the programme was progressive and modular as it was necessary to meet the aims and objectives of the sessions sequentially in order to move on within the programme. As such, the programme itself was divided into six 'blocks'. After the first, each was built upon the foundations of the preceding blocks (i.e. the aims and objectives for each block had to be satified in order to progress to the next block). The work in such 'blocks' included: familiarization and boundaries; personality disorder diagnosis and trait identification; core belief identification and formation; identification of problematic behaviours and behaviours that may interfere with therapy and care identified from MDT clinical notes; MDT treatment processes and interventions related to individual personality disorder diagnosis; and deciding action plans and identifying future needs.

It was integral to the structure and process of the sessions that all the clinical team members documented appropriate problematic behaviours/interactions within the MDT clinical notes. This was important because the sessions involved relating each individual's personality disorder diagnosis to problematic behaviours. Day-to-day behaviours were reflected upon in light of regard to previous problematic and/or anti-social behaviours and thinking patterns.

The care plans that were developed were reviewed with regard to individual personality disorder diagnosis. Clients were encouraged to reflect upon why the plans had been devised and what individual needs they addressed. As the care plans incorporated contributions from menbers of the multi-professional team, they assisted clients to understand how their treatment needs would be addressed by the team as a whole. The therapeutic programmes were subsequently reviewed with each client. This again aimed to cement the MDT approach to the provision of care and therapeutic interventions.

The last component of the individual programme involved clients identifying and developing 'action plans'. These aimed to highlight current and likely future needs or difficulties that the client would benefit from further work upon. 'Action plans' incorporated the MDT approach, both within the identification of needs and within the development of the strategies to tackle these. For example, a client who held a core belief of 'I will be abandoned' would be able to highlight common problematic thoughts associated with that core belief within a variety of contexts. This would allow the individual to recognise and identify with potential risky feelings and situations across all aspects of the therapeutic process, including being on the ward generally and within specific therapeutic interventions.

Alongside these 'action plans', post–programme case conferences were planned. These were similar to clinical team meetings and involved feedback for those providing direct clinical care for clients and information for those who were to be involved in future/ongoing care. This process assisted communication, appropriate decision making and the holistic approach to client care that is integral to the MDT philosophy.

MULTIDISCIPLINARY APPROACHES: POLICY AND DEFINITIONS

A key factor in the success of the psychoeducational programme described above was the ability of the MDT to work together. This is crucial if services are to be able to meet the requirement to continuously strive for improvements in the assessment and treatment of clients in the mental health care field. The National Service Framework for Mental Health (DH, 1999a), for example, specified not only the standards that services should be meeting but that they have the responsibility to monitor whether or not these are met through the process of clinical governance (DH, 1999e). Indeed, the 'NHS Plan' set out the aims for improving service delivery with a specific goal of breaking down the 'unnecessary boundaries' between staff, though it was also pointed out that the older and more hierarchical ways of working are giving way to more flexible team-working between different clinical professions (DH, 2000a). Underpinning the coordination of mental health services for individuals with mental illness and personality disorders is the Care Programme Approach (CPA) (DH, 1990, 1999c). This is the framework used to ensure that each individual's needs are assessed systematically, care plans/crisis plans are devised and risk assessments are undertaken. The emphasis within this approach rests on collaborative working across all disciplines involved in delivering health and social care in order to close gaps in care provision and improve standards.

Many national policies and recommendations for mental health services allude to how this should be implemented. However, while many of these implicitly state the importance of a multidisciplinary approach to delivering quality services within clinical care, few describe what is actually meant by the term MDT. It is a common term and one which would be difficult to avoid when working within mental health services, yet finding a clear definition can be extremely difficult. Leathard (1994), for example, found 50 possible meanings or interpretations.

Two descriptions for MDT are provided here. These have been chosen for their resemblance to current models of clinical practice and for their compatability with our working use of the term. Griffin (1989) described multidisciplinary team as the integration of the separate perspectives, knowledge or skills of the health care professionals involved, without the blurring of the disciplinary boundaries or loss of professional independence. A more intricate definition has been provided by Liberman *et al.* (2001, p. 1331), who suggest:

Teams must combine the expert contributions of professionals and para-professionals who can individualise a comprehensive array of evidence-based services with competency, consistency, continuity, coordination, collaboration and fidelity. A well functioning team contains specialists with expertise in critical areas, such as assessment and treatment of medical disorders and psychopharmocology, reliable diagnosis and ongoing assessment of the psychopathology of severe mental illness, functional assessment, management of substance abuse, skills training, family psychoeducation, and access to entitlements and benefits.

Although the importance of adopting an MDT approach to delivering mental health care is well established and reported, there appears to be relatively little research evidence as to its value. There is significant anecdotal evidence concerning its usefulness to be found within the literature. For example, Firth–Cozens (2001a) suggests that multidisciplinary teams make up the building blocks of health care and that every team is composed of different professionals with a variety of skills for the provision of safe and effective care. Two studies that have provided positive evidence for the value of multidisciplinary team-working are worthy of mention. A postal questionnaire of over 10 000 nurses, completed by Rafferty *et al.* (2001), suggested the value of team-work and its association with a range of positive occupational and organizational attributes, including job satisfaction, plans to remain in post and lower levels of reported burnout. In a study by Lowe and O'Hara (2000), 100% of the respondents provided examples of how services had improved since multidisciplinary team-working had been implemented. Efficiency, effectiveness and quality of service delivery were all reported to have benefited significantly.

Using a diverse professional team to develop the psychoeducation programme ensured it was comprehensive in outlook and in the skills available to draw upon and recognized as valid by all disciplines. Working difficulties between disciplines are encountered in most places from time to time, but one particularly pertinent issue here was the tension resulting from having structured therapeutic programme delivery away from in-patient wards. This issue was alluded to by Stanton and Schwartz (1954), who termed it 'the other 23 hours' (referring to the time spent away from specific individual psychological interventions). Cordess (2000) contributed to this discussion by highlighting that it is generally the forensic psychiatric nurse that would be with clients for the 'other 23 hours'. The design and development of the psychoeducation programme reflected a desire to reduce perceived separateness and distance and to generate a more unified and integrated service. For example, expertise shared on aspects including knowledge of personality disorders, knowledge of the clients on the ward and the practicalities of implementing new programmes was found to be extremely valuable to the overall effectiveness of the programme design. Also, this MDT approach appeared to have a positive impact on professional relationships and the promotion of respect between those involved in the programme development. This issue may be particularly relevant when treating and caring for those with diagnoses of personality disorder. Sometimes there are increased complications due to factors including paranoid or antisocial traits, where some may experience spells of erratic mood and become interpersonally distant and difficult to engage with. It is therefore crucial that assessment, treatment, decision making, and evaluation are all founded upon sound collaborative, multidisciplinary team-working (Robson *et al.*, 2005).

In addition to benefits to the clinical team, it has also been noted that clients' experiences of being cared for by a multidisciplinary team are positive. Overall standards of care are thought to have improved with MDT working, but more specifically it has been suggested that when clients know that they are being looked after by a team they may aquire a sense of confidence or reassurance similar to that which may be gained from having a second opinion about a serious a spect of health care. This may reduce suspicions that treatment is based on the opinion of only one clinician (Carter *et al.*, 2003) and may be especially beneficial for clients' interpretations of decisions that impact upon their treatment types and durations (it may even raise questions pertaining to their human rights, e.g. regarding detention under mental health legislation).

There are other advantages to an MDT approach in the treatment of individuals with a diagnosis of personality disorder, especially those who have complex needs and require frequent risk assessments, and continual engagement if they are to remain in treatment. These clients may provoke powerful counter-transference reactions and an MDT approach can make the monitoring of these feelings easier and offer individuals some protection against over-involvement (Bateman and Tyrer, 2004). Indeed, this feature was particularly relevant to the delivery of the sessions within the psychoeducation programme where multidisciplinary clinical supervision was designed and implemented to monitor these potential problems.

Noak (1995) commented on the fact that individuals with personality disorders pose some of the most frustrating work for mental health staff, while Swinton and Boyd (2000) highlighted the challenges that may be faced by nursing staff who are involved in delivering care around the clock. These authors continue by also suggesting that it should be the responsibility of the MDT as a collective of professionals to ease the psychological distress of staff teams to optimize the treatment and the care delivered. Evaluation of having both an MDT delivery approach and an MDT supervisory process in place suggested that the management of the programme was both effective and efficient.

Where concerns regarding MDT working have been documented, they seem to be of a more obviously interpersonal nature. Humphries (2005), for example, suggests that there may be problems in relation to: professional and/or personal statuses and roles; team aims and objectives; leadership and effective management; and disagreements over working practices and boundaries. Robbins and Finley (2000) further highlight issues including: misplaced goals and objectives; policy and procedural issues; personality types; and leadership problems. As such, when it comes to working in a multidisciplinary manner, considerable emphasis needs to be laid on proactively developing team-working skills and addressing sources of tension and conflict. Indeed, Burke *et al.* (2000) identified key pillars of MDT practice to include role definition, clinical responsibility and accountability, and understanding between the professions. Effectiveness is aided by agreed goals and plans, effective communication styles, clear team roles and competent leadership, and mutual support and education (Firth-Cozens, 2001b). Brown (1986) and Wilson and Pirrie (2000) support this view and, in relation to education, suggest that personal commitment, common goals, clarity of roles and communication, and institutional support are the most important factors encouraging MDT working.

EVALUATION

From the outset of developing the psychoeducation programme, the MDT had clear understandings of what was to be achieved and structured plans as to how the goals were to be reached. Each individual within the team had a sound grasp of her/his role and specific areas of responsibility within the programme. There was a recognized needs deficit in the treatment offered at the time, and an identified knowledge deficit within the client group regarding diagnosing key features of these and their impacts upon interpersonal conduct and relations. To aid the whole process, the programme's treatment manager (a forensic psychologist) and the authors (from nursing and psychology disciplines) would ensure regular MDT meetings were held to discuss progress and offer guidance where necessary.

Communication was aided by sharing ideas and problem-solving strategies. Also, using a transparent and collaborative approach throughout the developmental stages of the psychoeducation programme, the clients were consulted and individuals' opinions and feedback were incorporated into the design. These processes are among the most important required to implementing an MDT service, and, especially, the concept of therapeutic practice within that service. It is integral to effective and efficient intervention delivery that the structure, format and process of the therapeutic intervention mirrors that of the host multidisciplinary team philosophy. This concept should also be reflected within the aims and objectives underpinning the given treatment intervention.

It is important that MDTs and the care they offer are not regarded by clients as either hierarchical or dependent upon one discipline. Historically, there has been some division between nursing, psychology and other disciplines, and forensic settings have been no exception. This has been especially marked according to working hours, where comparison has been made between 'ward-based staff', especially nurses and Health Care Assistants who work shifts, and those who work office hours and do not spend virtually all of their time in one ward/clinical area. This contrast is apparent to clients as well as staff. A focused approach to MDT working can allow these supposed barriers to be broken down and a more effective and productive form of collaborative practice developed. Previous work that the authors participated in demonstrated how potentially negative role perceptions could be addressed and altered (Cordwell et al., 2004).

As well as providing positive benefits for clients, the programme has assisted clinicians in other ways. According to feedback from both the initial training and the facilitation, some staff members have aquired significant increases in their understanding and knowledge of personality disorders and effective therapeutic processes.

CONCLUSION

The psychoeducation programme described in this chapter was part of an initiative that aimed to cement clients' understandings of their problems and how they could be helped to address these. Both aspects of the psychoeducation programme were devised, developed and implemented by nursing and psychology disciplines. This collaboration was inherent throughout the design and delivery of the programme and the monitoring of its integrity, and within the supervision of those delivering the sessions.

The psychoeducation programme has been assessed for treatment impact and efficacy. Due to a paucity of similar treatment interventions specifically developed with individuals who have personality disorders, it is important to evaluate and research it further. Initial empirical investigations into its efficacy and impact suggest that the programme has helped participants to develop awareness, knowledge and understanding about themselves and the problems they may have. This increased understanding and insight is evident within clients' understandings of which problematic aspects are common to them and their interpretations and perceptions of others. This, in turn, reflects positively in their ability to relate their increased awareness and knowledge to other therapeutic interventions (Cordwell and Farr, 2007). Overall, these findings are encouraging and potentially important given that these clients are among those considered to be likely to pose very serious risks to others at this time in their lives.

Though it continues to develop, the programme is an example of a positive treatment intervention for clients who are regarded as difficult to engage. Multidisciplinary team-work has been crucial to this and it is encouraging to note that there is some indication that it, and resistant to participation in therapeutic interventions within any substantial sense, can be beneficial even to clients who have had little previous benefit from services.

SECTION 3
RISK ISSUES

- A Systemic Approach to Violence Risk Assessment and Management (Charlie McGrory and Steve Trenoweth)

- No Euphemisms: The Use of Force in Mental Health Care (Jonathon E. Lynch)

- The Psychological Impact of Restraint: Examining the Aftermath for Staff and Patients (Gwen Bonner)

- Masculinity as a Risk Variable in Physical and Mental Ill Health (Steve Trenoweth and Jonathon E. Lynch)

- Some Considerations for Mental Health Practitioners Working with Patients who Self-Neglect (James Matthews and Steve Trenoweth)

Virtually all contemporary references to mental health nursing and mental health care mention the notion of risk. Indeed, the concept of risk is a contested and sometimes controversial one. Clinical risk assessment and clinical risk management have become routine elements of practice in many areas, and no contemporary book in this area could omit mention of the theme. In this section, the authors offer some discursive, critical and thought-provoking chapters which underpin contemporary approaches to risk. Many chapters ask us to consider such issues in a broader political, interpersonal or systemic context. Also given for consideration is the issue of 'self-neglect', which does not usually feature in mental health texts, despite its clinical prevalence and the significant impact it has on an individual's health and well-being.

The section includes attention to all broad aspects of risk: from assessing and managing risk of harm to others, risk of harm to self and risk of self-neglect. In the first chapter, it is argued that assessing risk of violence in mental health service users is neither a simple nor a discrete matter. Professionals can and do become involved in the dynamics inherent in assessment processes: their perceptions, anxieties, strengths and weaknesses colour not only their interpretations of what is apparent and what they infer but also the care and experiences service users subsequently receive. This input from professionals also influences the ways in which individual service users perceive and respond to their circumstances.

Managing the risk of harm to others in in-patient settings has been influenced to an extraordinary extent by the manual restraint of service users over the last 10–15 years. Although there have been numerous different approaches to this across the country, it is fair to say that in many mental health services relatively little serious attention was devoted to assessing the general suitability of restraint course contents for vulnerable people. Some of the results of this are taken up in two chapters that are both essentially about restraint as risk management, but with different foci and perspectives. The introduction and arguably the continuation of sanctioned restraint training cannot be considered in isolation from socio-political contexts. Coordinated team-restraint training entered institutions during a period of comparative social unrest. However, today's political climate remains somewhat tough, somewhat punitive (see Chapter 4: Compassion), which has implications for psychological traumatization of staff and service users alike.

Being 'male' is a variable often implicated in a wide variety of risk events, particularly violence and suicide. However, in the chapter 'Masculinity as a Risk Variable in Physical and Mental Ill Health' we consider what it is about being male that is so risky, or more accurately, why certain types of 'masculinity' may be harmful to your health. Suicide is challenged only by road traffic accidents as the major cause of death of young males. However, many of those young men who take their own lives were not in touch with mental health services prior to their deaths, and, to compound the tragedy, may have spent their last few days and weeks suffering in silence due to a fear of being seen as weak or vulnerable, thereby apparently enacting social roles and perceived obligations. That is, the expression of different types of masculinities may make the difference between life and death.

CHAPTER 16
A SYSTEMIC APPROACH TO VIOLENCE RISK ASSESSMENT AND MANAGEMENT

Charlie McGrory and Steve Trenoweth

INTRODUCTION

Today, much emphasis is being placed on attempting to understand the nature and aetiology of aggressive and violent behaviour in mental health care services (Allen, 1997), so as to ensure effective organizational and professional responsiveness (Dale *et al.*, 2006). In this chapter, we explore the complex issue of violence risk assessment and attempt to challenge the current orthodoxy, which seems to attribute the cause of violent behaviour to factors that stem from 'within' an individual. Instead, we suggest that for a risk assessment to be fully comprehensive, consideration must also be given to contextual, social, interpersonal and environmental factors, which may have an impact on the aetiology of violence. Furthermore, we argue that the accuracy of risk assessment may be influenced by the assessor's anxiety at both conscious and unconscious levels. To this end, we suggest that a 'systems' approach to the risk assessment of violence is more appropriate, and discuss how such assessments may be compromised by confusion over the 'primary task' in mental health care. We discuss the implications for the clinical mental health nursing role.

Contemporary Issues in Mental Health Nursing, Edited by J. E. Lynch and S. Trenoweth
© 2008 John Wiley & Sons, Ltd

VIOLENCE AS AN INTRAPERSONAL PHENOMENON

The 'intrapersonal' perspective of violence seeks to identify relatively stable factors within individuals, their history and experiences, which are most commonly associated with future violent behaviour. To this end there have been several calls, not only from the medical literature but also increasingly from the nursing literature (for example, Mason, 1998), for more precise and systematic methods to measure those dispositional, historical and clinical features, apparently reflective of a violent individual (Wenk et al., 1972), which may be triggered by a particular context (Steadman et al., 1994). Such a model often supports a 'technological' approach to risk assessments, which assist in the scientific capturing of patient data to identify the violent person. Once identified, strategies can be implemented to reduce and contain an individual's risk behaviour.

Central to this approach is the development of risk assessment 'tools', such as the Violence Risk Appraisal Guide (VRAG) (Harris et al., 1993), which collate the relatively stable demographical or clinical data from population studies that are statistically associated with a heightened risk of violence (Doyle and Dolan, 2002). The capturing of such data, it is thought, affords the identification and discrimination of high-risk people from within groups or populations. Thus, for example, young men who have a history of violent behaviour, experience acute symptoms of mental illness or are under the influence of drugs and/or alcohol are perceived to be of a heightened risk of becoming violent (NICE, 2005b). In addition, the most common behaviours of patients which are statistically predictive of short-term violence seem to be confusion, irritability, boisterousness, verbal and physical threats, and property damage (Almvik and Woods, 2003).

The 'intrapersonal' model seems to be echoed by professional and government bodies, for example, in 'Recognition, Prevention and Therapeutic Management of Violence in Mental Health Care', published by the United Kingdom Central Council for Nursing and Midwifery (UKCC, 2002) (the forerunner to the Nursing and Midwifery Council (NMC)) and the recently published 'Violence: Clinical Guidelines on the Short Term Management of Violent/Disturbed Behaviour in In-patient Settings and Emergency Departments' (NICE, 2005b). In the latter guidelines some reference is made to the avoidance of provocation and the importance of the initial use of de-escalation techniques to defuse aggression, and the need for self-awareness amongst assessing and intervening practitioners. However, there is much emphasis placed upon the assessment of those demographic and clinical factors of the individual that are likely to give rise to violent or disturbed behaviour. Consequently, much emphasis is also placed upon the physical responses to control the violent person and, in particular, the use of rapid tranquilization, restraint and seclusion (see Chapter 17: No Euphemisms: The Use of Force in Mental Health Care). This rather reinforces the perception that all violent behaviour is a function of the individual, and as such it is the individual who needs to be controlled if 'his/her' violent behaviour is to be contained or managed.

VIOLENCE AS AN INTERPERSONAL PHENOMENON

The intrapersonal approach, however, has been criticized for its tendency to perceive people with mental health problems as 'objects' of risk (Roberts, 2005), who are to be prevented from becoming a nuisance or a danger to society (Godin, 2000). Concerns have also been expressed that this approach is a process of:

. . . codification, commodification and aggregation. In the mental health care setting this can mean attempting to control the actions and behaviours of consumers and clinicians to best meet the fiscal needs of the organization (Crowe and Carlyle, 2003, p. 19).

Indeed, there seems to be a tendency in the health care literature, particularly from medical studies, to portray violence as stemming solely from *within* the individual. Here, violence is often seen as a function of a personality trait (Barratt, 1994) or of an individual's history (Monahan, 1988). Recently, within this approach, violence has been seen to stem, at least in part, from a genetic mutation or other biological abnormality (Moosajee, 2003), or is seen to be a pathological medical symptom of an underlying 'disease'. It has subsequently been suggested that adherence to a medical model ideology can have a significant impact on the care process and lead to authoritarianism rather than a nursing model based on cooperation (Morrison, 1990; Chin, 1998). Indeed, it has been argued that the '. . . politicisation of mental illness has led to the medicalisation of dangerousness' (Chin, 1998, p. 66) and, as Aiken and Tarbuck (1995, p. 169) argued:

If the prevalent ideology is based on the medical model where 'cure' rather than 'care' is valued and client behaviours, especially assaultive behaviours, are [. . .] seen as symptoms of an illness rather than as the result of environmental factors such as lack of personal space, then the resulting norms and staff behaviours may reflect an authoritarian and inflexible model of care, in which blanket security policies stifle individualised care.

Some authors feel that an intrapersonal, medical model approach oversimplifies the phenomenon of violence (Lipscomb and Love, 1992). They argue that violence and aggressive behaviour do not occur in a vacuum, but is in fact a complex event that may arise from the dynamism within an interpersonal encounter (Lowe, 1992; Lowe *et al.*, 2003). Indeed, as Dobash and Dobash (1984) argue, the impression given by some research into violent behaviour is based on the assumption that:

. . . all violent events involve two males squaring off in some sort of adolescent contest of honour . . . researchers see violent episodes as some sort of gun fight at the OK Corral (Dobash and Dobash, 1984, p. 285).

The intrapersonal approach may be useful in identifying overall trends of violence within populations, and in identifying socio-demographic and clinical factors most commonly associated with violence. However, such an approach may be insufficiently sensitive to the complex interplays and heightened emotional contexts within which violent behaviour often occurs. Indeed, demographic data in itself may be of little assistance to the nurse in making assessments of imminent risk in potentially violent clinical situations (Davison, 1997), particularly if they are already working with 'high-risk clients', such as in forensic settings. That is, it might not be helpful for nurses to know that violence is statistically associated with young males who are acutely unwell and have a history of violence and substance misuse problems, when they are working with the same client group.

Those who see violence as an 'interpersonal' phenomenon, however, stress the importance of changeable environmental and contextual factors in the assessment of violent, or potentially violent, behaviour (Johnson and Webb, 1995). As such, factors such as noisy, poorly ventilated environments, overcrowding, a lack of privacy, low staffing levels and high sickness rates, poor relationships, the high use of bank and agency staff, poor leadership, poor information and a lack of social support can also be seen as areas to consider in the aetiology of violent or aggressive behaviour (Dale *et al.*, 2006). Furthermore, unlike observations undertaken in sterile laboratory conditions, risk assessments involve a perceiving individual who is attempting to understand and make sense of clinical events (Trenoweth, 2003; Bowers *et al.*, 2007a,b), whose actions may increase or decrease the display of violent behaviour and who may be personally affected by the risk, either emotionally or, indeed, physically.

SYSTEMS THEORY

In a discussion of both patient and staff views on the causes and management of aggression, Duxbury (2002) and Duxbury and Whittington (2005) propose a range of models to account for episodes of violence. The 'internal' intrapersonal model, described above, identifies the patient's 'disease' as a significant risk variable leading to aggression. Such a model may be inherently attractive because of the relative ease of collecting clinical and actuarial data, and its 'locating' of violence in the 'other'. The 'external' model, however, recognizes the effects of the environment, both built and social in terms of unit design and its organizational activities. The 'situational model' notes the effect of negative staff–patient relationships, certain staff being prone to assault, limit setting and controlling practices arising from organizational demands, which seem to be related to episodes of violence (Mulvey and Lidz, 1984, 1995; Duxbury, 2002; Lowe *et al.*, 2003; Duxbury and Whittington, 2005).

The 'situational model' may be amplified by relation to 'systems theory' (Bertalanffy, 1973; Roberts, 1994; Hinshelwood and Skogstad, 2000). This approach recognizes that a living organism survives by exchanging various materials with its environment, converting materials needed for survival into nutrients and excreting what is not required as waste. It is suggested that this process requires certain properties, most notably a 'boundary'. The boundary must be sufficiently robust to maintain inside from outside, while at the same time permeable enough to allow the transfer of materials across it for it to be an 'open' system. Open systems can be characterized by a potential for growth, development, change and learning – an adaptive process which assists living creatures to meet the demands of their environment. In a complex organism, such as the human body, a number of such open systems will operate simultaneously (Roberts, 1994). However, where the boundary becomes impermeable, the organism becomes a 'closed' system and will not survive as it is incapable of meeting the demands of the environment. An extreme form of a closed system in mental health care was the 'total institution' described by Goffman (1961, p. 11) as 'a . . . place where a large number of like-situated individuals, cut off from wider society for an appreciable period of time, together lead an enclosed, formally administered round of life' (see also Barton's (1976) discussion of 'institutional neurosis').

The boundary in a complex organization requires management of the processes to ensure the requisite output arises from the input and conversion process. For example, in a factory this may include the intake of raw materials from the environment and the subsequent production and output of manufactured goods. This would require the identification of materials needed, the procurement of such materials in timely fashion, the availability of trained staff and requisite technology to convert materials, and the subsequent infrastructure to export manufactured goods to the market place. The conversion or throughput of materials and their return or export to the environment, may be viewed as the 'primary task' the factory or organization has to complete to ensure its survival.

Within mental health care, people in mental distress may be seen to be 'inputted' through (or imported across) the boundary by their referral to secondary care services, the response to which is their treatment and care (conversion), leading to an improvement in the health and social functioning of the individual and the community as a whole (outputs). However, this may not be as straightforward a process as it first seems. For example, attempts to achieve the 'primary task' in mental health care may be particularly confusing, as it may not be clear if the system exists to treat, cure, control or care for the individuals who enter the system (Bott, 1976; Bott-Spillius, 1990). Furthermore, practitioners may also have different definitions of the primary task (Roberts, 1994), or perceive that they lack the ability to respond effectively and meaningfully to clients' needs, due to the complexity of a client's psychological needs or problems, and a perceived lack of a capacity to 'heal'.

Similarly, the conversion process may not assist the client to improve their overall well-being, as practitioners may become focused on controlling 'madness' and 'restraining' an individual's potentially violent behaviour to the detriment of responding to their health or social care needs (Clulow, 1994; Morrall, 1998). As a consequence, there may be a discrepancy between the stated aims of mental health services on the one hand, and the actual outputs of mental health care on the other. The resultant danger of a vagueness or confusion surrounding the primary task and the practice of mental health care services, then, may be the development of a closed system incapable of evolving or of effectively responding to the needs of individuals or the community or a system. Indeed, the 'primary task' of mental health nursing practice may be equally confusing. There are potential discrepancies between the requirement of forming therapeutic alliances to assist the client to improve their overall health and well-being on the one hand, and the protection of the public on the other. As such, mental health nurses are required to take positive and therapeutic risks to assist in promoting the overall health and well-being of their clients (UKCC, 1998; NMC, 2004b), whilst simultaneously containing and managing their own personal anxiety about violence (Bowers *et al.*, 2007a), the anxieties of the organization (by working within various policies and protocols), and the anxieties of society (by working within legislative frameworks).

CONTAINING ANXIETY

The violent situation is a complex clinical event, which potentially poses a number of professional challenges for the mental health nurse. Assessments of risk are often made in highly stressful situations, and often have to be made rapidly. In emergency situations, the nurse has to make an immediate decision about the appropriate course of action based on the available information in the current situation as well as their previous knowledge of the patient, which may be supplemented by information supplied by other staff who are offering assistance at such time. Risk assessment, then, may be an inexact 'science' (Doyle and Dolan, 2002), characterized by much uncertainty (see Chapter 6: Truth, Uncertainty and the Mental Health Nurse).

Not only is violence, or the threat of violence, an event likely to pose a professional challenge for the nurse, but it may also represent a personal challenge in that it is likely to provoke anxiety (Lowe *et al.*, 2003). Indeed, the impact and non-somatic effects of violence, such as fear, anxiety, guilt and post-traumatic stress, can be profound and long-lasting (Prins, 1981; Boettcher, 1983; Lanza, 1983; Dobos, 1992; Whittington and Wykes, 1992; Poster and Ryan, 1994; Needham *et al.*, 2005) (see Chapter 18: The Psychological Impact of Restraint: Examining the Aftermath for Staff and Patients). Such personal challenges and clinical experiences can have a profound influence on the assessing individual's perception and judgement, and the subsequent quality/accuracy of their risk assessments.

In systems theory, a variety of strategies may be developed, both at an individual and organizational level, to contain resultant anxiety. That is, it is possible nurses may attempt to deal with their own anxiety feelings, at both conscious and unconscious levels, by the use of various 'defence mechanisms'. For example, if a nurse was unable to contain or tolerate their own angry or aggressive impulses, there might be a denial of such feelings, and the subsequent projection of these impulses onto patients who are then viewed as dangerous. This defensive manoeuvre in turn may create a view of 'good' staff (who are perceived as rational, sane and do not have such violent impulses) and 'bad' patients (who are perceived as irrational, insane and prone to violence).

Indeed, there seem to be many systemic areas of concern for contemporary mental health care, which may further increase levels of anxiety amongst staff and service users alike. In addition to staffing issues mentioned above, in-patient clinical environments can be busy and poorly designed (Cleary and Edwards, 1999), where there exists an increasing use of substances and a lack of planned therapeutic or structured activity (Gijbels, 1995; Gijbels and Burnard, 1995; SCMH, 2005; Dale *et al.*, 2006). As a consequence, many service users have reported feelings of a lack of security and safety whilst receiving care in mental health settings (see Chapter 2: Rebuilding Lives: A Critical Look at the Contemporary Role of the Mental Health Nurse), whilst some have reported physical abuse and sexual harassment (Dale *et al.*, 2006). Furthermore, the increased level of violence which mental health nurses are exposed to (Stephen, 1998; Lowe *et al.*, 2003), without sufficient psychological support, has been linked to a number of strategies to cope with anxiety that may further undermine the development of a therapeutic relationship (see Chapter 18: The Psychological Impact of Restraint: Examining the Aftermath for Staff and Patients). For example, an assaulted member of staff may seek to escape from, or avoid, clinical situations for fear of further assaults. The outcome of such avoidant behaviour may be a decrease in staff–patient interaction (Whittington and Wykes, 1994). While such distance may afford short-term protection against the psychological pain and distress of 'difficult' clinical situations, it concomitantly appears to undermine the nurses' ability to undertake risk assessments of violence, for as Benner (1984) argues:

A 'distanced' observer is less likely to notice subtle changes in patients . . . a certain level of commitment and involvement is necessary for expert performance (Benner, 1984, p. 164).

In clinical mental health nursing terms, the emotional and physical distance, and subsequent lack of a therapeutic relationship with service users, may have an impact on the quality of risk assessments. That is, while avoidant behaviour may contain his/her own personal anxieties about violence (Whittington and Wykes, 1994), the nurse is subsequently left to rely upon the observations and second-hand clinical information from other members of the care team. As a consequence, the nurse's ability to employ personal knowledge, experience and clinical insight to critical thinking regarding risk is compromised in their ability.

Defences against anxiety can also be understood in terms of the Kleinian psychoanalytic anxiety-defence model of individual psychology (Klein, 1946, 1959). For example, Cameron *et al.* (2005) argued for the adoption of 'object relations theory' as a means to improve talking–listening encounters. This approach recognizes that while we relate to others, they may have properties which can be influenced by our internal world and external reality. Such an approach influenced the work of Jaques (1955), and led to the observation and understanding that cohesion, whether in groups, organizations or institutions, is used as a defence against 'psychotic anxiety' – that is, the anxiety which is characterized by persecutory beliefs that others are aggressive, attacking and denigrating, and that one's 'self' is vulnerable to exposure. The observation was made initially in industry and subsequently elsewhere by workers at the Tavistock Institute of Human Relations (Roberts, 1994). Within health care, Menzies (1959) made the connection that the individual uses the social system of an organization to defend against the unconscious experience of psychotic anxiety raised by dealing with illness, death and dying. The anxiety is provoked by the demands of the nurses' role in achieving the primary task required of them in the intimate care and contact of others, and the conflicts that inevitably arise in defining the task and its achievement.

In her seminal study of general nursing practice, Menzies (1959) highlighted how the defences against anxiety caused by caring for damaged people can become fixed in the social system. Central to these defences are the processes of splitting (for example, locating aggression within the other), denial (of one's own aggressive impulses) and projection (of one's own violent impulses onto others), which was discussed by Miller and Gwynne (1976) in their study of the long-term care of the disabled.

A SYSTEMS APPROACH TO RISK ASSESSMENT AND MANAGEMENT

A systems approach to risk sees:

. . . the degree of danger that an individual represents to himself or others varies markedly as a function of a number of variables (Megargee, 1976, p. 5).

As such, a risk assessment may require consideration of multiple domains (Monahan, 1988) and may involve a wider appreciation of violence than the study of a 'decontextualized' individual. Therefore, it is crucial when undertaking risk assessments that the contextual, interpersonal, situational and systemic factors which extend beyond the individual at risk, are also examined. Indeed, an awareness of the general environment and ensuring the safety and protection of others is seen by qualified nurses as an important part of their professional role (Powell *et al.*, 1994; Gijbels and Burnard, 1995). The National Institute for Health and Clinical Excellence (NICE) guidelines for 'schizophrenia' (NICE, 2002a) also point to the importance of ensuring that clinical environments are suitable to meet the needs of those who are acutely unwell, and that factors that can lead to frustration, such as overcrowding, lack of activities, poor communication between patients and staff, are also addressed. There are, of course, many implications for undertaking such assessments, not least in the complexity and detail of observations that are required, and the knowledge and understanding of the context within which such behaviour occurs. Furthermore, the assessor needs to be able to consider what situational factors might motivate or inhibit violent behaviour, the systemic pressures on the actions of individuals within such contexts, and how individuals overall function *in situ*.

Indeed, such an approach is described by Megargee (1976), who proposed formulae by which an assessor could judge the likelihood of violence by considering: an individual's motivation to become violent (M_x); the individual's past history of being reinforced for violent behaviour (H); factors within the situation that may facilitate violence (S_f); factors which inhibit (I) violent acts (a) against a victim (x) ($I_{a.x}$); and factors within the situation which may inhibit violence (S_i). Megargee (1976) suggested that when the inhibitions were stronger there would be less likelihood of violence ($M_x + H + S_f < I_{a.x} + S_i$), and where factors leading to violence were stronger than inhibitions, violence would be more likely ($M_x + H + S_f > I_{a.x} + S_i$).

However, such an approach does not seem to consider the perceptions of risk, or the fears, anxieties and emotional context of the observer (Blom-Cooper *et al.*, 1995; Ryan, 1998). In a study by Trenoweth (2003), all participants considered the support by colleagues to be invaluable in situations of perceived imminent, or potential, violence. This, it appeared, was more due to the perceived quality of the skills and personal attributes of nurses rather than the numbers of available staff. Moreover, this variable seemed to affect *how* the violent situation was perceived by individuals, that is, the presence of adequately trained, skilled staff in the nursing team was associated with a reduced level of perceived personal risk and anxiety. An attribution or assessment of risk, then, may also be influenced by the presence or non-presence of suitably skilled staff, which suggests, as Tardiff (1988) does, that:

. . . *a patient may be viewed as more dangerous than he actually is because of staff anxiety that is projected onto the patient* (Tardiff, 1988, p. 543).

Similarly, clinical areas with trained and experienced staff working well together, with good leadership and high morale, tend to be less violent (Royal College of Psychiatrists, 1998) (see Chapter 15: Enhancing Effective Multidisciplinary Team-Working: A Psychoeducational Approach). Indeed, as Benner (1984) noted:

Patient care is much too demanding and complex to be accomplished by any one team member. It was evident that expert nurses recognize the team as an integral part of their own effectiveness as they are in the business world (Benner, 1984, p. 151).

Indeed, many studies have highlighted difficulties associated with staff who are inexperienced, inadequately trained, rejecting, hostile, unprofessional and authoritarian (Lipscomb and Love, 1992), which may lead to the creation of tough environments within which violent behaviour is more likely (Morrison, 1990) (see Chapter 17: No Euphemisms: The Use of Force in Mental Health Care and Chapter 19: Masculinity as a Risk Variable in Physical and Mental Ill Health). Such findings have clear implications for the training and personal/professional development of less experienced staff, and the need for cohesive and supportive team-working in undertaking assessments of, and responding to, clinical risks.

The systems approach to risk in clinical nursing practice emphasizes the quality of the nurse–patient relationship. The literature attests to the value of the nurse–patient relationship in the provision of overall nursing care (Benner, 1984; Rew and Barrow, 1987; DH, 1994a, 2006a; Doyle, 1996; Olsen, 1997), described most poignantly by Benner (1984, p. xxii) as a '. . . a kaleidoscope of intimacy and distance in some of the most dramatic, poignant, and mundane moments of life'. Indeed, the Mental Health Nursing Review Team (DH, 1994a, p. 18) offered the following guidance to mental health nurses:

In responding to the variety of mental health problems, mental health nursing draws on a range of core skills that are grounded in the therapeutic use of self within the central relationship with the client . . . Nursing responses and interventions should be founded upon a sound understanding of the individuals in their care

Within a systems framework we may argue that one's knowledge of one's patients, and the development of a clinical relationship, will have an impact on personal perceptions of violence due to the level of anxiety we experience. As such, the level of anxiety that we experience may be lessened and more reality-based, as opposed to an anxiety which, in systems thinking, may be described as 'psychotic'.

INFLUENCES ON THE PRIMARY TASK

The mental health nurse has potentially a great deal of access to patients' lives (Lewis and Webster, 2004) and is ideally placed to undertake a contextualized, systemic assessment of risk based on a sound knowledge and understanding of their patients (Allen, 1997; Buchanan-Barker and Barker, 2005), and the subtle interactions and possible tensions between individuals and their relationship to the organization. Likewise, nurses are best placed to assess and manage the overall physical quality, and psychological climate, of the clinical environment.

There are, however, possible difficulties within contemporary mental health nursing that may affect the development of therapeutic relationships and undermine systemic assessments of risk. In the current climate of mental health nursing, large amounts of nursing time is apparently spent in activities other than nurse–patient contact or providing direct patient care, such as administrative and clerical duties, considered by nurses to be the least satisfying aspects of their work (Nolan *et al.*, 2007). Higgins *et al.* (1999), in their study of a wide range of acute in-patient services, report for all grades of qualified nurses a decrease in direct patient contact and an increase in administrative duties, arguing this is as a result of the devolution of managerial duties to wards. This is echoed by a report in community services (Garcia, 2006). In consequence, nursing care is often delivered by unqualified staff, employed on a casual basis (Ford *et al.*, 1998).

There has also been, in recent years, a reduction in bed capacity, leading to an increase in occupancy rates and a perceived concomitant rise in levels of aggression (Lowe *et al.*, 2003) and level of acuity amongst people requiring in-patient admission (SNMAC, 1999). To this end, staff may be too busy to develop or build a therapeutic relationship with their patients (Pollock, 1988; Gijbels, 1995; Gijbels and Burnard, 1995; Cleary and Edwards, 1999) and so are unable to affect early intervention in potentially violent situations. As Ryrie *et al.* (1998) argue:

Against this back drop it seems difficult to reconcile professional directives which recommend that a majority of nursing time is spent with patients responding to their needs (Ryrie et al., 1998, p. 849).

Indeed, the situation has led SNMAC (1999, p. 20) to report that: 'A great deal of evidence now supports the conclusion that levels of stress experienced by nurses working in in-patient settings are unacceptably high.'

In such a climate, there is also a danger that the work of a mental health nurse will become reactionary or ad hoc rather than planned, structured and therapeutic (Gijbels and Burnard, 1995; Ryrie *et al.*, 1998). The apparent hand-over of direct, hands-on care to junior, often unqualified grades employed on a casual basis (Ford *et al.*, 1998), leaving the senior, qualified staff to deal with the administrative, organizational and managerial aspects of care, may create a distance from patient contact (Ryrie *et al.*, 1998) and may also deny the nurse the benefit of developing and subsequently using their knowledge of, and relationship with, the patient in potentially violent situations.

Some of the wider influences on tasks in mental health nursing care are the media portrayals of the mentally ill as violent and dangerous (Wilson *et al.*, 1999; Cutcliffe and Hannigan, 2001; Nolan *et al.*, 2007) (see Chapter 8: Challenging Stigma and Promoting Social Justice) and the subsequent perceived need for mental health services to 'control' such risks on behalf of society (Doyle and Dolan, 2002; Crowe and Carlyle, 2003). The policy of detailed enquiry and reports on episodes of violence is epitomized by the reports on Christopher Clunis (Ritchie *et al.*, 1994) and Andrew Robinson (Blom-Cooper *et al.*, 1995), among others, which may help mental health services to improve their practice. However, such reports appear also to have fuelled media interest in, and crticism of, mental health care (Laurance, 2003), with the possible consequence of increasing fears about the performance of the primary task and increasing confusion about what this may be. For example, such reports repeatedly seem to identify similar failings to communicate effectively, monitor patients and misjudgements of threat posed at every level by organizations, professional groups and individuals, such as the recent Barrett Inquiry (NHS London, 2006).

The succession of media comments and reports identifying perceived failings of organizations, professional groups and individuals leads to a growing sense of failure to meet the primary task and increased efforts at controlling the behaviour of others, staff and patients in order to minimize the high levels of anxiety that are raised (Allen, 1997). This may be manifested by the development of ever more detailed policy and procedure to regulate the interaction in the system. In systems theory, this often leads to the adoption of successive defensive actions in an attempt to contain and lessen such anxiety. For example, the development of policies, procedures and attempts to routinize and simplify work and attempts to avoid the possibility of blame and complaint if errors or oversights occur (Alazewski *et al.*, 1995) (see Chapter 6: Truth, Uncertainty and the Mental Health Nurse).

For the individual nurse, this will inevitably fuel personal anxiety, affect capacity to manage work loads for fear of being blamed for adverse events (Nolan *et al.*, 2007) and, most essentially, lead to an inability to think about the care of an individual patient in the face of conflicting demands beyond the adoption of defensive practices (RCN, 1999; Evans, 2006). Indeed, there often seems to be confusion regarding the role of mental health nurses and a lack of clarity about their primary task. This has led to the development of conflicting tasks, which are seemingly required of the mental health nurse, such as the potential conflict between therapeutic and custodian roles, with consequent anxieties raised at conscious and unconscious levels. As a consequence, nurses express disquiet in responding to violent or aggressive behaviour (Nolan *et al.*, 2007). Indeed, there seems to be some evidence that nurses' anxieties (especially fear and anger) can be linked to the choice, and employment, of measures to respond to aggressive behaviour, with a suggestion that more anxiety leads to more strongly coercive measures such as physical restraint and seclusion (Bowers *et al.*, 2007a,b).

Such anxieties and moral ambiguities may not be addressed or resolved, but rather spread around the structures of, and individuals within, the organization (including doctors, nurses and, indeed, patients) (Lützén and Schreiber, 1998). Indeed, this may contribute to an understanding of the very different views on the causes of violence expressed by patients and nurses. That is, while the contemporary clinical portrayal of violence appears to follow an internal/intrapersonal model, which views mental illness as a precursor to aggression, it seems that patients hold an interactional/interpersonal stance in which staff behaviour, such as poor communication, contributes to aggressive episodes (Duxbury and Whittington, 2005).

Onyett (2004) and Bowles and Jones (2005) outline the notion of 'whole systems working' and suggest that this could be defined as one in which all component parts are in place and in balance to meet the needs of patients. However, Bowles and Jones

(2005) suggest such a situation may not be in place in mental health practice, which may lead to difficulties for mental health workers in caring for patients. As such, frantic efforts may be made to affix blame and fix *parts* of the system (such as individuals, professional groups or departments) rather than address failings of the *whole* system (that is, how the various parts of the organization fit together).

It may also be that this approach may never materialize, being based on a 'phantasy' of the possibility of designing a perfect system to deal with madness/mental illness. It may also fail to recognize the inherent challenge posed by working with individuals who are severely damaged. Hence, institutional and personal anxiety may lead to an over-reliance on the production and prescription of policy dictated by authority. This may create or reinforce the conditions identified by Main (1990), in which the hierarchical promotion of knowledge, seen as the 'right' way, can prevent learning and restrict thought by individuals who become unable to resolve the inherent anxieties in the nature of the work.

CONCLUSION

An intrapersonal approach to risk assessment considers factors within an individual suggestive of violence. It is our contention, however, that a risk assessment which solely adopts such an approach oversimplifies the phenomena and is likely to be incomplete, as it may not consider or identify the important contextual issues that may underpin the violent situation. That is, in seeking to identify the relatively static demographic or clinical features of the 'violent individual', the intrapersonal approach may be unable to capture the contextual subtleties or dynamism of violent situations. Furthermore, we suggest that risk assessment is a complex, emotionally charged activity, and as such an appreciation needs to be made of the nature of 'anxiety' and the implications that this may have on the outcomes of assessments, and the subsequent strategies identified to manage risks. Some strategies, we suggest, may be a reflection of the need to contain personal or organizational anxieties rather than as a direct response to the clinical needs of the client. As such, organizational and other systemic pressures may add to anxieties by creating expectations regarding the role and function of the nurse, which may conflict with their perceived professional duties, and subsequently restrict their clinical decision making.

Indeed, there seem to be many influences on the nurse's ability to fulfil their 'primary task' which, in any case, may lack clarity. What is clear, however, is the need for support for those who are required to respond to violent situations, as anxiety may affect the ability to respond to crisis situations (Bowers *et al.*, 2007a). While the impact and effects of violence on the individual can be profound, and long lasting (Prins, 1981; Boettcher, 1983; Lanza, 1983; Dobos, 1992; Whittington and Wykes, 1992; Poster and Ryan, 1994) (see Chapter 18: The Psychological Impact of Restraint:

Examining the Aftermath for Staff and Patients), research also indicates that social support may assist the nurse to reflect upon, and learn from, such situations (Benner, 1984). Furthermore, strategies that focus on the system as a whole, and assist nurses to deal with the effects of violence on themselves, both real and imagined, may afford a renewed willingness to engage in therapeutic relationships with patients, recognizing and assessing the potential risk for violence and aggression arising from 'systemic' pressures.

CHAPTER 17
NO EUPHEMISMS: THE USE OF FORCE IN MENTAL HEALTH CARE

Jonathon E. Lynch

INTRODUCTION

The words 'use of force' are rarely mentioned in in-patient mental health care settings, but there can be no doubt that registered nurses and health care assistants (HCAs) – and sometimes other employees – use physical force on clients at times. Much of the available literature and guidance refers to the 'management' of clients' aggression, though critics have argued that such terms are not only misleading but disingenuous (Bartlett and Sandland, 2003, p. 392). This chapter will include the term *use of force* when considering physical interventions used on clients, because these are the words used within 'the rules' set by the outside world. The force used by nurses often reflects the contents of 'aggression management' or 'control and restraint' courses, or ones with similar titles that share common origins. As well as possessing different names, course contents vary in manual techniques and underpinning ideologies, so in order to consider the array of programmes taught to nurses, the term *team restraint* will be used for convenience. For the following discussion, *force* is considered to be any intentional physical contact that is coercive or restrictive in nature.

The use of force will always be contentious in mental health care, because clients are considered vulnerable (United Kingdom Central Council for Nursing, Midwifery and Health Visiting (UKCC), 1998), and nurses and others are required to afford them some protection. Parenti (1978, p. 71) suggests that those detained in any total institu-

Contemporary Issues in Mental Health Nursing, Edited by J. E. Lynch and S. Trenoweth
© 2008 John Wiley & Sons, Ltd

tion 'must be placed at the lowest end of any index of power'. In in-patient settings, power and authority are clearly – though sometimes unavoidably – unbalanced and although efforts to reduce this are making progress, it has to be acknowledged that the social exclusion and marginalization that many clients experience has led some to be discredited when accounts of controversial incidents have been contested (Box and Russell, 1975). Sayce (1995, p. 143) argues that the law institutionalizes society's mistrust of psychiatric patients: in 1986 the House of Lords ruled that juries should be warned about the danger of subjecting secure hospital employees to criminal prosecution on the unsupported evidence of a single patient. Clear practices and robust regulatory structures are therefore essential for the protection of individuals who are vulnerable to poor treatment (from peers or staff) yet may not be taken seriously if they complain. However, nurses and other staff can be subject to physical attack and have responsibilities to maintain safety, so use of force is unavoidable at times. As they are also vulnerable to allegations of malpractice, especially if there were no witnesses to an incident, transparent use of force can assist nurses who act in good faith.

Coping with aggression has remained a prominent theme for over a decade in health care, and recently created bodies have assumed lead roles in this. The most recent and important guidance is Clinical Guideline 25 (CG25), titled *Violence*, produced by the National Institute for Health and Clinical Excellence (NICE) (2005b). Aimed mainly at in-patient mental health care settings, its contents are based on evidence that was available when it was produced. 'Physical interventions' are mentioned as possible options if others have failed, though there is some concern about the lack of evidence concerning their effectiveness (NICE, 2005b, p. 7). [Readers are later advised (pp. 42–43) to read guidance on all 'other interventions' alongside the *Code of Practice* for the Mental Health Act 1983 (Department of Health and Welsh Office (DH&WO), 1999), a wise tip given its significance as a standard for inquiry reports.] The National Health Service (NHS) Security Management Service (SMS) has developed a training curriculum – *Promoting Safer and Therapeutic Services*, which focuses on mental health and learning disability care settings – and explaining the use of 'reasonable force' is one objective of SMS's more generally applicable *Conflict Resolution* syllabus. The National Institute for Mental Health in England (NIMHE) (2004b) has developed positive practice standards to support the management of aggression and intends to accredit trainers. Together, these appear to offer significant resources for nurses, yet others can also benefit from improvements in this area. Some clients' accounts seem to indicate that nurses' use of force makes in-patient care a very unpleasant (and lasting) experience. The ubiquitous term of today is 'service user', which implies choice, respect and meaningful involvement in decision making. While it is indeed quite right that these matters become further established in mental health care, it is arguable that realities such as clients' experiences of force, receipt of unwanted medication and denial of free movement mean the term 'service user' is sound in ideology but questionable in some instances. The word *client* is used here, though this, too, is not without its critics.

FORCE, MENTAL HEALTH AND MATTERS OF OPINION

'Aggression management' and 'control and restraint' courses are run in many NHS Trusts and private hospitals, and local policies often use the same words. While it is reasonable for many trainers to have moved away from the name 'control and restraint' – because they do not teach prison course contents and because the word *control* in particular can be problematic in mental health care – 'aggression management' and similar terms are rarely used outside health care and have been known to cause amusement when they are. Some nurses believe that outsiders don't really know much about mental health care, so their views are unimportant. This is not necessarily inaccurate, but it may be rather naïve. Dismissing or ignoring others' views can serve to separate nurses and mental health care from society, as the disparaging of wider perspectives promotes an 'us and them' mentality and supports an estranged occupational culture. This is potentially problematic and stands in sharp contrast to the social inclusion ethos inherent in mental health care today. Clarke (1999b, p. 37) urges caution over 'the manner and speed by which enclosed communities [can] become laws unto themselves'. A subsequent 'hermitage morality' may, he adds, redefine clients 'as less worthy of the basic decencies'. Practising consciously and transparently can complement professionalism and support relationships with clients, especially for those who may be suspicious or anxious about in-patient care. It could also prove valuable should it be necessary to account for actions, whether this is to managers, clients' relatives or even inquiry teams or courts. And for some nurses this will be necessary.

Relatively little attention has been devoted to clients' experiences of force. Some of them undoubtedly know a great deal about the use of force in in-patient settings though, and studies indicate that there is much to be learned about their perceptions (Haglund *et al.*, 2003). A small study by Kumar *et al.* (2001) indicated that nurses' use of manual restraint – referred to by clients as 'being jumped' – could be upsetting to witness and painful to receive. Perceived as 'violence perpetrated by staff', clients considered it punitive. In Sequeira and Halstead's (2002) study, clients also perceived punishment and felt anger towards nurses. Although some felt safe through the 'containment' involved, restraint evoked traumatic memories for some victims of earlier sexual abuse. Bonner *et al.* (2002) studied the subjective experiences of restraining nurses and restrained clients and found evidence of trauma and distress among both groups. Small studies are inevitably restricted in the extent to which their findings can be generalized, but some offer valuable evidence with important implications. It is also notable that clients' views accord – at least in general negative terms – with recipients' perceptions of force in other institutional settings (see Jameson and Allison, 1995; Lord Carlile of Berriew, 2006).

The things that people read, watch and hear influence their opinions and attitudes, especially towards people and places that they do not encounter personally. News media can be particularly influential and their references to mental health care rarely include positive events (see Sayce, 1995). Many focus on violent acts by mentally unwell people. Perhaps it should come as no surprise then that in the community many people with mental health problems are marginalized and some are abused by citizens. There is also evidence of a marked willingness on the part of law enforcement agencies to use force on mentally ill people at times (Skolnick and Fyfe, 1993; Green and Ward, 2004). As Muir (1977) remarked, 'irrational' people can induce immense anxiety as they may be unperturbed by sanctions and risks that would deter most others. Familiar to many thousands of students of social sciences and law, Steven Box (1989, p. 12) asserted that 'governmental control agencies' effectively abuse their power but are protected by a fog that allows them to evade the consequences. He includes 'special prison hospital staff' in this 'when they brutalize and torture persons in their protective custody'. Box provides no reference for this claim, but it would appear that it is a swipe at forensic mental health nurses. While many nurses will be unmoved personally by his claim – because 'that doesn't happen here' – it is undeniable that mental health care has witnessed some dreadful events involving use of force, even if very serious incidents are uncommon. Inquiries have been undertaken, but criminal and even disciplinary proceedings have been rare.

Could it be that large organizations produce such fragmentation of responsibility that no *individuals* seem to be to blame, even when there are terrible results (Baumeister, 1999)? Or is it more likely that State employees are protected from repercussions as long as there is no *overt intent* to harm others? Having vulnerable people in one's care can mean that certain omissions can be as serious as actions. Cynical perspectives can lead to assumptions that those who express difficulties are always attempting to deceive or manipulate. Physical or mental health problems may then be overlooked. Attitudes such as these are unprofessional and unacceptable. They are not only likely to facilitate negative experiences, but may increase the chances of serious incidents. Bowling and Phillips (2002) allude to these matters when discussing the deaths in custody of men from ethnic minorities. At the time of writing, the government is attempting to save the Corporate Manslaughter and Corporate Homicide Bill. If it becomes law, the 'controlling minds' of companies (certain directors or senior managers) could be prosecuted if it is alleged that company negligence has led to fatalities. The proposal to exclude deaths in custody (i.e. police cells, prisons and mental health units/hospitals) from the provisions has invited some criticism, and this matter will certainly be worth following.

Certain 'outside' opinions of mental health care may appear unrealistic or uninformed, but comments and opinions on highly controversial matters are best assimilated, not ignored. Indeed, these perspectives can contribute to clients' overall protection. Possessing insight into the somewhat suspicious ways in which some see mental health care can assist nurses to bolster relevant standards of care and provide greater clarity for practices. These could be crucial factors when either ambiguous or very serious situations arise and questions are asked.

FORCE AND REGULATION

Information about law and the use of force in mental health care has improved significantly over the last decade (e.g. Paterson and Tringham, 1999; Wright *et al.*, 2002 – guidance for the Learning Disabilities field may also be useful, for example Lyon and Pimar, 2004). Their contents will not be repeated here, but some key points will be highlighted and other examples of the regulation of force will be considered.

Subjecting a person to unwanted physical contact is illegal unless specific justification exists (Davis, 2003, p. 74), so a basic understanding of law is essential to nurses' practice. To be lawful, force must be 'reasonable in the circumstances', though use on vulnerable individuals can be especially contentious. Hoggett (1996, pp. 134–137) outlines five principal legal justifications for 'measures which might otherwise be unlawful' in mental health care settings. They are if: valid consent is given; used for medical treatment under the Mental Health Act 1983; it is a necessity; harm is being prevented; or required for ' "detention" and discipline'. So force can be used either for the administration of treatment or to contain clients who appear to pose threats to their own safety or that of others. Clearly, there are overlaps at times, but it is equally clear that clients are not subjected to force only if prescribed treatment is administered or if they attempt to cause harm. It may be judged necessary if a patient is experiencing a manic episode, for example. If she/he seems to have lost physical control this could lead to extreme distress, to exhaustion and possibly even to life-threatening circumstances; however, physical intervention itself could also lead to life-threatening circumstances (see Paterson *et al.*, 2003a). There are other examples, of course, such as if a client is in such immense distress that she/he experiences a chaotic, personal state of crisis. Whether physical interventions are termed safety maintenance or control, Bartlett and Sandland (2003, p. 392) state that the law sees them as part of 'treatment'. However, a key point is that if nurses have only been trained to use aversive interventions then these are likely to be used. Perhaps sight has been lost of the purpose and the variability of mental health care in in-patient settings. 'Aggression' has come to dominate the agenda so much that methods taught for its management are applied unquestioningly to situations for which they may be inappropriate.

Covering England and Wales, Section 3(1) of the Criminal Law Act (CLA) 1967 states that a person may use such force as is reasonable in the circumstances in the prevention of crime, or in effecting or assisting, or in the lawful arrest of offenders or suspected offenders or of persons unlawfully at large. What is *reasonable* will vary from situation to situation, so decisions about using force must be made by each individual and be accountable for her/his actions. Force should be necessary, or if it comes to light that it was not necessary then the *belief* that it was necessary should have been a reasonable one, with a defensible rationale. Overall, actions should be proportionate in degree and duration to the harm being prevented (Gostin, 1986) and be unlikely to escalate the level of violence (Eustace, 1990).

If Section 3(1) were to be relied upon to justify force, it would be essential that a crime was being prevented (or an individual detained lawfully). As Wright *et al.* (2002, p. 68) point out, it would not apply 'in the minority of cases where the patient is insane within the meaning of the McNaughton rules (because such a person is deemed incapable of committing a crime due to the absence of *mens rea*)' (meaning literally 'guilty mind' – the mental element of a crime). Hence, common law might offer legal justification if force had to be used in such cases. This allows use of force to prevent a breach of the peace, to act in self-defence (or to defend others), or to 'confine a person who is insane' (Bartlett and Sandland, 2003, p. 395). Common law is also important should nurses intervene physically in emergencies involving informal clients (see Bartlett and Sandland, 2003, chapter 7). Card (2006, p. 771) states that a person who uses force with a common law defence is usually engaged in the prevention of crime, in which case the individual also has the defence under the s.3(1)CLA 1967. For practical purposes then, common law and statutory defences overlap, though Gostin (1986, p. 147) suggests that mental health care staff are 'well advised not to rely upon' these to justify force when mental health legislation can be utilized.

Section 127 of the Mental Health Act 1983 is conspicuous by its absence from much mental health care education and training. Titled 'Ill-treatment of patients', this makes it a criminal offence to ill-treat or wilfully neglect a client. One might have thought that this was sufficiently important to warrant mention on all team restraint courses and official guidance. The Mental Capacity Act 2005 may be of particular significance for clinical nursing with certain clients. Section 6 makes explicit mention of restraint and sets out basic guidance on what is permitted. Section 44 creates a new criminal offence of ill-treating or neglecting a person who lacks mental capacity (see also Department for Constitutional Affairs (2007)).

If an allegation of unlawful use of force ever progressed to a criminal court, it would be up to others to decide whether or not the force that had been used was reasonable in the circumstances. This would then be a question of fact, not of law. Gostin (1986, p. 147) states that those using force in emergencies are 'not expected to make . . . fine calculation[s]', but they are of course accountable for their actions. Force used by a solitary person who was attacked suddenly – and who acted instinctively – may well be considered different from incidents in which more than one person acted and their actions were preconceived.

Having to attend any court could be an unpleasant experience. One might claim that actions were undertaken in good faith, that reasonable care was taken and that the force used was within the law, but others may attempt to paint a different picture. This is the territory of trained legal professionals. Paid to represent and to influence opinion through persuasion, these advocates are invariably partial and frequently determined. As Pannick (1992, p. 2) puts it, they will illuminate 'anything other than the central weaknesses of a client's case'. For Hadfield (2006, p. 179), the competitive nature of legal arguments renders lawyers less concerned with 'the truth' than with manipulating and editing witnesses' accounts. Emitting confidence, the language they use is of course quite likely to be in keeping with that of the law. If representing a person who has 'used force', they may refer to actions that were reasonable in the circumstances, proportionate to the harm that they sought to avoid and unlikely to escalate any existing levels of violence (Eustace, 1990). If arguing against, the word *force* may be preceded by 'excessive' or 'unnecessary'. Amid the brief direct references that English law makes to the use of force, there is no mention of the words found in policy and incident documents in mental health care, and these differences may be very interesting to the sophisticated rhetoricians who seek to destabilize the arguments of 'the other side'.

Mental health care's lack of direct reference to use of force lounges in contrast to that provided for prison and police employees. In prisons, the policy on 'use of force' is covered by Prison Service Order 1600. Currently there are two *Control and Restraint* manuals. One pertains to basic training and is issued on CD-ROM to governors and local instructors. The second, an advanced training manual, is a restricted document covering 'tornado response', staff and procedures for managing concerted disorder or other incidents requiring use of protective equipment. This blatant paramilitary feature is one example of how different prison and mainstream mental health care practices really are, despite common ancestry. (See Woolf and Tumim's (1991) report for further examples and Jameson and Allison (1995) for some prisoners' perspectives.)

Schedule 1 to the Police (Conduct) Regulations 2004 contains a Code of Conduct for officers. English and Card (2005, pp. 278–279) suggest that this still works like the previous 'Discipline Code', in that what might now be termed 'failure to meet the appropriate standard' for one or more of the Code's 12 paragraphs continues, in effect, to be a disciplinary offence rather than a failure to meet a performance objective. Breach of the principles could ultimately lead to dismissal. Paragraph 4 is headed 'Use of Force and Abuse of Authority'. Officers must never knowingly use more force than is reasonable, nor should they abuse their authority. English and Card (2005, p. 747) state that it:

must be emphasised that if the force used to prevent a crime [. . .] is unreasonable in the circumstances, it will be unlawful and the person using it will not have a defence to the charge of battery or of another offence against the person.

Nurses' use of force seems to be increasingly considered alongside that of police and prison officers (Police Complaints Authority, 2002; House of Lords/House of Commons Joint Committee on Human Rights (HL/HC JCHR), 2004). Why then do we have euphemisms when the guidance available to them contains the words that matter in law? 'Force' may seem incongruous for health care, but it is up to nurses to forge a distinct professional identity and to situate within it occasional safety-oriented and treatment-oriented uses of force on clients. Some fields of clinical practice require possession of a range of restraint skills, certain of which are undeniably restrictive and/or aversive – e.g. for coping with determined physical assaults – while others are inherent in the care of mentally unwell people when they experience immense distress and/or inner chaos. Open discussions on the rationales for restraint could benefit clients and nurses (Sequeira and Halstead, 2002, p. 15), yet so could more thorough and open consideration of the realities of nurses' work and incorporation of this into education and training programmes.

TEAM RESTRAINT: TRAINING AND PRACTICE

For those unfamiliar with them, team restraint systems usually involve three people (or four if on the floor) holding/restraining a client by using set techniques and procedures. These are learned on short courses – typically five working days. Course contents often include restraining a client who is sitting or standing, taking her/him to the floor, standing up from the floor, walking and going through doorways, etc. Many also include de-escalation from restraint (to no restraint), and procedures for releasing and leaving a client in a seclusion room. The most contentious elements of those courses that contain them are pain-compliance techniques. That is, the infliction of pain, usually to wrist joints, to force a client to comply with nurses' requests – e.g. to stop trying to harm someone. NICE CG25 makes explicit mention of pain-compliance techniques, stating twice that the:

deliberate application of pain has no therapeutic value and could only be justified for the immediate rescue of staff, service users and/or others (NICE, 2005b, pp. 8, 45).

In other words, inflicting pain on a client is only acceptable as a distracting or controlling method if someone is being hurt or appears to be in imminent danger of being hurt. In an earlier document, NIMHE (2004b, p. 31) implied that NICE would offer further guidance on 'use of pain', but NIMHE's explicit page on the subject is possibly of more value than NICE's bullet points. With guidance marked by brevity, nurses' professionalism must dominate their use of force nationwide. NICE CG25 was potentially crucial to this because professionals are 'expected' to take its contents 'fully into account when exercising their clinical judgement' (NICE, 2005b, p. 2). While the document's generally uncritical acceptance of pain-compliance techniques has disappointed some, NIMHE and NICE have at least opened the door for further consideration of this nationally. The Nursing and Midwifery Council (NMC), its predecessor the UKCC and the Department of Health fell short of addressing this thorny issue explicitly.

Most team restraint training courses in England and Wales can be traced back to the *Control and Restraint* programmes which were introduced to prisons in the early 1980s. Their contents were derived from close-quarter martial arts skills, such as attacking joints and pain-compliant restraint (e.g. see Morris *et al.*, 1996), and these were apparently modified further before their introduction to some secure mental health services later that decade. From there they spread into mainstream services. One problem was that the lack of regulation and standards allowed stark variations and inconsistencies to emerge (see Lee *et al.*, 2001). At one extreme, obviously client-centred and professionally justifiable course contents were taught and used in practice; at the other, 'heavy-handed' procedures championed 'no nonsense' approaches. Although nurses and HCAs were the main users of team restraint skills, nurses and the key bodies failed to embrace and take ownership of them nationally. Where ownership was taken in hospitals/NHS Trusts, this was due to local professionalism and initiatives.

The clients' experiences of force referred to earlier might suggest that *laissez-faire* approaches to the regulation of force effectively allowed in more aversive experiences than would have been the case if greater responsibility for contents had been taken initially by leading bodies. Many courses failed to offer a suitable range of options for use in clinical settings – the poorest portrayed clients in simple terms, as 'violent' bodies to be controlled. 'Breakaway' techniques featured in most programmes, offering skills for escaping if grabbed/held by a client. Some were extreme and likely to be excessive for most clinical situations. Others were so unlikely to be used that teaching and practising them was a waste of time. Post-training analyses later complemented the abundant anecdotal evidence that many skills had been lost quickly or were unlikely to be required (see Parkes, 1996; UKCC, 2002; on team restraint skills retention see Tarbuck *et al.*, 1999). This is not surprising given research evidence about acquisition and retention of psychomotor skills and their viability under stressful conditions (e.g., Siddle, 1995).

Importantly, nurses' professional responsibilities and accountability were overlooked on some courses. The ability of some trainers to situate and discuss issues that are key to nurses has to be questionable. Principal among these are the NMC's *Code of Professional Conduct*, sustaining therapeutic relationships with clients, the effects of mental ill health on behaviour and perception, the Mental Health Act 1983 and effects of psychotropic medication. Nurses should be able to expect that those training them to use some of the most contentious interventions they will ever undertake are well versed in their professional *raison d'etre* and responsibilities. Having non-nurse trainers was unavoidable in the early days of team restraint training, but it is not now. There is some irony then in the reflections of nurses who consider some of the early trainers who did not have nursing backgrounds to have offered more professionalism, greater sensitivity to clients' experiences and more humanity in their courses than some later exponents who were nurses! Let us now consider how the time at which *Control and Restraint* was introduced to prisons may have influenced the occupational culture within which it was institutionalized before it entered health care settings.

BC&R: THE SOCIO-POLITICAL CONTEXT

Prison *Control and Restraint* did not emerge from nowhere. It could be argued that the rejection of its predecessor, *Minimum Use of Force Tactical Intervention* (MUFTI), plus the socio-political climate of the time, created pressure for regulated and controllable, but nonetheless robust, use of force. The 1970s and 1980s were difficult years in political terms, and key events prompted the development of specific methods for dealing with 'problem' groups. The 1970s witnessed serious disorder in British prisons (see Evans, 1980; Adams, 1994), that in Hull in 1976 being particularly significant. There are minor inconsistencies in the literature about when MUFTI teams were first used, but there seems to be some consensus that they were created after the Hull riot (Adams, 1994, p. 157). However, their existence was not mentioned publicly prior to when they intervened at London's Wormwood Scrubs prison in August, 1979. It was after this that major concerns were raised about the force used on prisoners (who claimed to have been demonstrating peacefully). Fitzgerald and Sim (1982, p. 21) assert that the Home Office initially denied that anyone had been injured but later conceded that over 50 prisoners had been (see Cavadino and Dignan, 2002, p. 196). Although the MUFTI team was congratulated publicly on its professionalism at one point (Fitzgerald and Sim, 1982, p. 21), Adams (1994, p. 158) states that the 'crude violence of MUFTI' was superseded by the 'more sophisticated' *Control and Restraint* training.

In 1981 widespread disorder erupted on British streets. This recurred on a smaller scale several years later and a policeman was murdered by rioters in London. Another key event was the miners' strike of 1984, when somewhat desperate strategies were employed by the Conservative government, including highly criticized policing styles. In sum, these events – plus the seemingly persistent conflict in Northern Ireland – rendered the role of government highly demanding. Under pressure to quell very visible disorder, the government's response was essentially a tough one that asserted a willingness to 'fight'. There is too little space here to do justice to the complexities, but the key point is that in response to political needs, law, authority and policy were utilized to situate the 'problems' within others and to forge apt solutions to these. This is not to suggest that no one was culpable for the episodes of disorder that occurred, rather that approaches based on a 'you're the problem, we'll solve it' perspective rarely achieve lasting and satisfactory resolutions. As authoritarian, centralized approaches to conflict were being cemented, it was no coincidence that prison *Control and Restraint* was developed and introduced, nor that there were paramilitary features in procedures and training. As evaluation indicated its success in prisons (Brookes, 1988), *Control and Restraint* was adopted in some secure mental health care facilities. It is unclear whether it was initially intended that these methods should eventually enter mainstream services. After they had become established, it is notable that in the third version of the Code of Practice for the Mental Health Act (DH&WO, 1999, paragraph 19.9) the words 'control and restraint' were omitted/removed from guidance on training. In the full guideline on *Violence* (NICE, 2006b, p. 26) (i.e. the source document for CG25), NICE states that the word 'restraint' was avoided due to its association with *Control and Restraint*. However, 'restraint' is (inevitably) used in the definition of NICE's preferred term, 'physical interventions' (*ibid*), and there is a strong case for openness about practices even if the *Control and Restraint* term and its 'order maintenance' notion are rejected.

POST-C&R?

Many clinical nurses work with a wide range of clients and situations so they should be equipped with a range of practical interventions. In order to meet their professional requirements, courses should offer a force continuum or hierarchy. These have existed for some time in other contexts, where employees may be required to use force (Alpert and Dunham, 2004). For incidents in which clients use physical aggression, three contextual concepts of force may be useful starting points: force used when alone and attacked by a client (one-to-one); force used when assisting someone else who is being attacked; and force used as part of team restraint procedures. Each can have a guiding continuum covering different levels and types of force. For the use of team restraint on clients who are acutely unwell and chaotic (but not trying to hurt anyone), it may be necessary to have a discrete continuum or at least distinct acknowledgement of this within the team restraint continuum. Restricting options too much can be problematic. As much anecdotal evidence testifies (and as can perhaps be inferred from clients' experiences), the exclusion of lower levels of force from many early courses meant that some nurses only had harsh methods at their disposal. This did not meet their needs as accountable professionals. However, excluding higher-level/more aversive force also reduces options and might increase the chances of nurses or clients being injured in the more extreme situations that occur from time to time. Having said that, it is interesting to hear how nurses who are not taught pain-compliance techniques cope with extreme situations.

Techniques that achieve the desired 'results' in training are not necessarily destined to do so in clinical situations. The mental states and determination exhibited by some clients cannot really be experienced in training and there is anecdotal evidence that pain-compliance techniques may fail to distract or allow control. The Royal College of Psychiatrists (1995, p. 6) commented that these techniques might become:

particularly problematic and hazardous where the patient's perception of pain is altered (as might occur with learning disability, autism or various psychiatric states).

Some clients' pain thresholds may be influenced by alcohol or illicit drugs, which are not uncommon in many settings, even if forbidden officially. In these instances, continued and determined 'application of pain' may cause injury, a matter for which the person inflicting pain will presumably be accountable. Nurse–client relationships may also be damaged.

Force continua for one-to-one situations should of course be acceptable professionally and legally, yet it should be acknowledged that professionalism and legality do not always tally. Some nurses encounter extremely serious threats to their safety from which they are unable to escape. On these occasions, the force required may actually lie beyond the parameters of professional practice, but then these are not normal professional encounters. The unpleasant reality is that strikes might be all that could possibly assist someone who is alone, unable to escape and believes her/himself about to be harmed very seriously. If life seems to be at stake, a nurse cannot be expected to 'be a nurse' – she/he has the human right to do what is necessary to stay alive and the legal right to use force that is 'reasonable' in those particular circumstances, though not on any health care training syllabus. Willis and Gillett (2003, p. 75) state that striking clients is 'severely frowned upon', and so it should be, but training and guidance should be explicit about very serious situations even if options for the extreme end of a force continuum are not offered.

There are obvious benefits in having the use of force suitably professionalized, through centralization and regulation. It is perhaps ironic that if health care services (which exist to care for patients/clients) had been as rigorous as the prison service was in regulating what went on in its territory, course contents and practices might have been suitably amended and kept in check. The duty of *care* that nurses owe to clients is more distinct than that owed by prison and police officers to inmates and suspects, respectively. Losing sight of this poses the risk that nurses' use of force will be subsumed in a broad State agents' manual on force. This alliance seems apt not only to news media but also to key authorities. The Mental Health Act Commission and the Department of Health are two of the 14 organizations represented on the *Forum for Preventing Deaths in Custody* (HL/HC JCHR, 2007); the others are all either linked to police or prison services or interested in observing and monitoring these. Other commentators that refer to use of force in mental health care alongside prisons and police custody contexts include the Institute of Race Relations (1991) and INQUEST (2004). There is much we can learn from others' initiatives (e.g. see the Prison Service violence reduction strategy; Butler and Drake (2007) on 'respect' and the 'decency agenda'). Nevertheless, nursing's own identity and skills for practice are essential requirements for us, and it is arguable that this crude aggregation is unhelpful. Questionable euphemisms are used to proclaim that 'what we do is different', but some clients and some 'outsiders' are unconvinced. So are some insiders. What else should be inferred from the disinclination of other disciplines to partake in team restraint practices and training even when local policies state otherwise? Their claims that 'non-therapeutic interventions' are not in their remits mean that nurses and HCAs are often the only ones to use force on clients in health care.

An improved focus on use of force should be clear about accepting the mandate, yet be specific to the needs of nurses who provide unique care to clients. This may exist already in many places through local policies and training initiatives, but a more sharply defined, more clearly sanctioned and better publicized national strategy could help expand and solidify a distinct nursing/health care ideology and enable greater openness and consistency. Indeed, consistency of practice appears to be very important to NICE, especially on contentious matters. Take the 'observation and engagement' of in-patients, for example. NICE has insisted on consistent practices across England and Wales (NICE, 2005b, p. 37).

FORCE AND PAIN – SENSITIVE TOPICS

If pain-infliction is only justifiable for someone's 'immediate rescue', NICE (2005b, pp. 8 and 45) is presumably saying it is not acceptable when no one is in immediate danger. So, for example, restrained clients who offer 'passive resistance' may not be creating situations in which it is justifiable to apply pressure to their wrists. This may seem straightforward, but the institutionalization of previous training and practices cannot be overlooked. While these may be inherited rather than intentionally hostile, the persistent disinclination of some trainers to acknowledge the recommendations/ guidance of the UKCC (the previous governing body for nurses) (UKCC, 2002) and the Royal College of Psychiatrists (1998) is worrying. Regulation of training contents and health care focused standards may have been promised but certain quarters of the variable terrain may prove difficult to penetrate. NIMHE and SMS are national bodies with solid profiles, and the time does appear to be right in that many Trusts have made remarkable progress in implementing clinical governance strategies and other significant changes. Influencing de facto practices remains a tall order though, and is only likely to be achievable over years rather than months and through active regulation. But some practices do need to change.

The Human Rights Act, 1998 brought into statute law further protection from abuses of power by the State. Article 3 states that no person shall be subject to torture or inhuman or degrading treatment or punishment. Article 1 of the United Nations *Convention Against Torture and Other Cruel, Inhuman and Degrading Treatment or Punishment, 1987* defines torture as:

- any act by which severe pain or suffering, whether physical or mental, is intentionally inflicted on a person for such purposes as obtaining from him [*sic*] or a third person information or a confession; or

- punishing him for an act he or a third person has committed or is suspected of having committed; or

- intimidating or coercing him or a third person;

- when such pain or suffering is inflicted by or at the instigation of or with the consent or acquiescence of a public official or other person acting in an official capacity;

- but not including pain or suffering arising only from, or inherent in or incidental to lawful sanctions.

The last point suggests that the legality of actions may enable some pain or suffering to be situated outside the definition and underlines the general importance of law to claims to legitimacy for use of force. (Interesting discussions have occurred on the international political scene recently following attempts to redefine torture and 'severe pain'; e.g. see Luban, 2006.) However, while the threshold for torture may be high, the fact that pain-compliance techniques do not sit comfortably outside this definition is potentially problematic, especially when some clients feel they are treated badly and some outsiders are highly critical of in-patient care. Some nurses intentionally inflict physical pain on clients' wrists, even if not to acquire information. Is mental suffering ever *intended*? We would hope not. Is pain ever applied to punish clients? That seems to be what some of them perceive. Punishment is obviously not within nurses' professional remits, yet NICE felt it necessary in the legal preface of CG25 (NICE, 2005, p. 12) to state that 'punitive action' should not be undertaken by staff. NHS nurses are effectively public officials, and private sector facilities are considered to be public authorities when exercising powers of detention (HL/HC JCHR, 2004, p. 11). In summary, pain-infliction in health care is a complex and contested subject that warrants comprehensive 'guidance' from the uppermost authorities.

Mental health care settings are hardly unknown to the international literature on torture and inhuman treatment (Stover and Nightingale, 1985; Green and Ward, 2004). Although it seems unlikely that critics could equate the force common to many mental health care settings here with that of torturers, it does not require much imagination to see how parallels might be drawn. Studies suggest that many torturers are ordinary people who do extraordinary things (Conroy, 2001; Green and Ward, 2004, p. 140). Their vocabularies are 'rich in euphemisms' (Cohen, 2001, p. 107). Baumeister (1999, p. 316) describes how torturers 'play' with words, and 'present the shocking and horrific as mundane and ordinary'. It is not suggested here that nurses routinely torture or abuse their clients, rather that if there is a place for pain-inflicting techniques in team restraint procedures in particular, there must be greater appreciation of their potential for harm.

In 1997 a group of expert advisors recommended to the Home Secretary that prison restraint methods could cause injury to under-18s as their bones and joints had not developed fully. It was also contended that previous experiences of physical or emotional abuse, which are not uncommon among young offender populations, could be exacerbated by robust physical contact during detention. Hence, it was argued, by approving these practices, the Home Office could be rendered liable to future legal action. The group's report is not publicly available, but pain-compliant methods were subsequently stopped in secure training centres (see HLPR, 2002).

It is remarkable how few nurses challenge pain-inflicting techniques on professional grounds. Critical approaches do exist in practice and in the literature, but the very notion of hurting clients intentionally does not seem to be a major concern for the majority. Nursing lecturer Brodie Paterson takes issue with one of the tenuous lines heard on some team restraint courses. Imagine a situation where nurses are restraining a client with her/his wrists flexed and the claim that 'if it hurts when she/he struggles then she/he is causing it, not me'. Paterson (2005, p. 20) asserts that such pain is not effectively self-inflicted:

. . . in that if the [client's] struggle can be reasonably anticipated then placing [her/him] in a situation where such struggles will result in pain is effectively still care giver inflicted and therefore remains deliberate.

The ethical responsibilities that are integral to professional health care should compel nurses to address unconvincing arguments, which expose not only unprofessional attitudes towards clients (Morrison, 1990) but also a cynical rejection of accountability. Tarbuck *et al.* (1999, p. 237) reported that the phrase 'the therapeutic use of pain' was not uncommon in the late 1980s. There is also anecdotal evidence of restraint trainers stating: 'Think "comfortable pain" – you're comfortable and he [client] is in pain'. How would 'outsiders' interpret these phrases, or terms such as 'juice', used casually in some areas to refer to the application of 'pressure' (i.e. pain) to clients' wrists? The suitability of courses should be assessed not only by lists of contents and the efficacy of techniques, but by the attitudes that are instilled and the feasibility of continuing professional *relationships* following the use of force.

It is unfortunate that there is no clear lead from nursing when the implications of use of force are greatest for us. In an inquiry report, Prins (1993, p. 76) and colleagues (including a very senior nurse) suggested that only registered nurses be trained to use restraint so that such force would be subject to the principles of the NMC's Code of Professional Conduct. Some might dismiss this as unrealistic, because a 'nurses only' restraint policy would exclude HCAs and they constitute the majority of staff in many units. Another view is that it implies that HCAs – who are not subject to professional regulation – cannot be trusted to use force and pain-compliance techniques. The Royal College of Psychiatrists (1995, pp. 15–16) may also have had professional regulation in mind when suggesting that restraint should only be taught by registered nurses, and that prison courses were inappropriate for health care. Conceptual and practical clarity are long overdue, and nurses must lead on this.

FORCE AND HARM IN MENTAL HEALTH CARE

In the early 1990s the *clinical risk* notion applied to mental health was the inverse of that for most others in health care. In those, the 'risks' to be assessed and managed related to *professionals* harming clients/patients accidentally while undertaking clinical care. In mental health care, the risks were posed by clients – risk of direct harm to others or to self or, receiving less attention, the risk of self-neglect. However, it is naïve to assume that no members of staff ever cause harm to clients, whether accidentally or intentionally. Professional disciplinary hearings and occasional removals from professional registers offer compelling testimony to the latter, though criminal prosecutions are rare.

Sim (2004, p. 116) argues that a consensus has been built around the essential benevolence of certain State institutions and employees and that 'simultaneously socially constructing these . . . as living in perpetual danger . . . has been central to this process'. Focusing on police and prison officers in particular, Sim (*ibid*) suggests that:

[t]he hegemony concerning the 'truth' surrounding the dangers [they face], while contested and contingent, nonetheless operates as a powerful, ideological mechanism for securing the legitimacy of the criminal justice system and the wider definitions of social order that this system upholds and defends.

In deconstructing data on the victimization of other agencies' employees, could Sim have a point for mental health care? He is open to criticism for what may seem like a cold appraisal of attacks on police and prison officers, yet his paper is thought-provoking. Sim claims that poor health and safety structures are more of an issue for them than violence from suspects and inmates, respectively. Controversially, he points to figures suggesting that on-duty police officers are more likely to be killed in traffic accidents than they are to be murdered and most assaults on them are not sufficiently severe for courts to imprison perpetrators (Sim, 2004, pp. 122–123). Sim also cites figures concerning assaults and deaths in prisons before concluding that prisons are more dangerous for prisoners than for staff.

If harm in in-patient settings were to be assessed, how would that inflicted on nurses and other disciplines compare with that experienced by clients? Emotional harm is of course difficult to measure, but it does appear that some in both staff and client groups experience this: most may be minor but some is not (see Chapter 18: The Psychological Impact of Restraint: Examining the Aftermath for Staff and Patients). Records might indicate that staff collectively experience more minor and more serious physical injuries than clients, whether through direct victimization or attempts to avert other incidents. At the most serious and disturbing end of a harm continuum, deaths of staff are very rare but each is a disaster.

In a preliminary survey, Paterson *et al.* (2003a) set out to identify clients' deaths that were associated with restraint in UK health and social care settings. They located 12 deaths that had occurred approximately over the preceding 20 years; nine appeared to be in mental health care. At least one occurred before team restraint training became common, and reference is not made to whether or not the staff present in the others had received training. (Another point to be considered with restraint-related deaths in the last 20 years is whether the methods used at the time were the same as those taught or were employed as they were taught – see Paterson *et al.* (1998) for an example of an apparent modification.) Other deaths have occurred after physical altercations between nurses and clients, but if not reported as 'restraint related' they would not appear in searches using this criterion. For example, in a fairly well-known case in 1988, Joseph Watts died following a struggle and administration of intramuscular medication (Institute of Race Relations, 1991, p. 42). Mr Watts' death did not appear in Paterson *et al.*'s (2003a) search results. Overall, the number of client deaths is small, but each is a disaster.

The latest report from the *National Confidential Inquiry into Suicide and Homicide by People with Mental Illness* (University of Manchester, 2006) included 249 cases of homicide by current or recent clients in incidents that occurred between April 1999 and December 2003. These constituted 9% of the homicides in England and Wales in the period and worked out at 52 clients committing homicide per year. Fifteen were in-patients at the time, though only three occurred on wards and one in the hospital grounds. The information is not broken down to allow identification of the victims of ward-based incidents but of the 15 victims, eight were cited as family members or either current or former partners, six as friends or acquaintances, and one as a prostitute. Comparing deaths of staff and clients in in-patient facilities may be methodologically problematic, as one would not necessarily be comparing like with like (regarding time spent in the area, numbers in each population, etc.). However, if the number of staff killed by clients in a given period was less than the combined numbers of clients killed by other clients plus clients whose deaths were restraint-related, it would suggest that, at the extreme end of a harm continuum, in-patient facilities were more dangerous for clients than for staff.

CONCLUSIONS

Overall, coordinated approaches to the use of force in mental health care have not made a positive start. The successes of team restraint practices have been publicized less than the problems and serious incidents, so more substantial enquiry into efficacy must be undertaken and findings disseminated. Force-related deaths may never be stopped entirely, but guidelines on physical care and observation during restraint (NIMHE, 2004b; NICE, 2005b) must be taken seriously in all settings. Perhaps the clinical risk notion in mental health care should be revisited and reformulated.

It would be interesting to research force-related deaths in the long histories of our hospitals and to find out whether they were becoming more or less common. This is a complex matter and clients' vulnerability to force may differ according to periods in time. The effects of psychotropic medication (introduced around 50 years ago) could be relevant to some incidents, as some can cause cardiac conduction abnormalities, reduce cardiac output and lower blood pressure (Royal College of Psychiatrists, 1993, pp. 9–10). It has been estimated that around one death per week results from neuroleptic medication (Cobb, 1993, p. 19). When force is used, medication administered intramuscularly to a client who resists may be especially problematic. Unexpected movement may make it difficult to locate the correct site and accidents are more likely. Physiological arousal will facilitate a faster absorption rate due to the greater blood flow to the muscles, and clients will subsequently require relatively intense monitoring and support. There may also be a greater chance of the needle entering a blood vessel as these invariably dilate at these times (see Prins, 1993, chapter 13 for theories concerning the death of a client who apparently struggled at administration). Inserted needles have been known to snap during struggles, leaving part in the muscle (Mason and Chandley, 1999, p. 199). It is notable that on the rare occasions that injecting resistive/struggling clients is mentioned, the advice is to do so with caution (Royal College of Psychiatrists, 1997, p. 29; Holmes *et al.*, 2001, p. 49) and/or avoid it if possible (e.g., Prins, 1993, p. 47). Reviewing deaths of detained patients reported to the Mental Health Act Commission (Bannerjee *et al.*, 1995, cited in RCPsych, 1997, p. 13) suggested that 'the risk of sudden cardiotoxic collapse in response to neuroleptic medication given during a period of high physiological arousal should be widely publicised'. This does not seem to have happened. The Maudsley guidelines have for some time advised against injecting struggling/resistive clients with Clopixol Acuphase (zuclopenthixol acetate) (most recently, see Taylor *et al.*, 2005, p. 318 who cite risk of intravasation and oil embolus). Holmes *et al.* (2001, p. 47) advise similarly because of the potential effects on the myocardium (the heart's muscular tissue). Psychotropic medication assists countless clients but it can cause harm. So can restraining them to administer it.

Illicit drugs may also pose risks that are exacerbated by restraint. Cocaine is a recognized concern (Wetli and Fishbain, 1985), though the mechanisms associated with fatalities are complex and uncertain (RCPsych, 1997, p. 15). It may be worth considering as a possible extra risk factor when physical interventions are used on (inexplicably) psychotic individuals who do not have histories of mental ill health (see also Pollanen *et al.*, 1998 regarding unexpected deaths and excited delirium). The risks of positional asphyxia have been recognized for some years but were apparently not raised on team restraint courses uniformly. When a factor appears to increase the risk of fatalities it must be relevant to training and practice (Wright *et al.*, 2002, p. 54), and without effective regulation only good networking and research awareness can inform practices (see Wright *et al.*, 2002, pp. 54–58 for a useful summary of risk of death during restraint). Perhaps the use of force and manual restraint would have been further researched beforehand (and, in mental health care, better regulated) if prison inmates and mentally unwell people were not seen as inevitably at the undesirable end of a 'rough–respectable' continuum (Scraton and Chadwick, 1987). As Paterson *et al.* (2003b, p. 17) concluded, potentially dangerous procedures should be 'eliminated from practice before, rather than after tragedy'. Some clients die due to use of force in health care; their families' lives are damaged irreparably. Nurses who have clients die literally in their hands will never forget this. It is important that support is provided for those who view clients in positive terms, act in good faith and strive to provide quality care. And when the most serious events occur, should responsibility lie solely with those present – even when there was no known intent to harm, recklessness or incompetence – or is a wider, institutional responsibility more appropriate? If so, this should not necessarily be restricted to one organization. The history of *laissez faire* approaches to mental health care may mean that all the major bodies, including nursing, must hold up their hands. Team restraint training has improved in most places, but this must be truly harnessed so that unambiguously health care oriented practices can be established nationally. As the main users of force and with immense professional accountability, nurses must lead on this and be the main beneficiaries of standards. These benefits can then be passed on to clients.

CHAPTER 18
THE PSYCHOLOGICAL IMPACT OF RESTRAINT: EXAMINING THE AFTERMATH FOR STAFF AND PATIENTS

Gwen Bonner

INTRODUCTION

This chapter aims to examine some of the complex issues related to the aftermath of restraint in in-patient mental health settings for staff and patients. A background discussion related to the historical context of restraint will be considered, followed by a discussion of current contemporary issues related to the nursing management of incidents which involve some form of physical restraint. The psychological impact of restraint for patients and staff will be considered, particularly in reference to acute mental health in-patient settings and a discussion of how aspects of trauma and Post-Traumatic Stress Disorder (PTSD) can inform understanding of the impact. A framework for post-incident review will be offered as a way of moving forward some of the issues discussed, as well as an approach to addressing some of the ambiguities that nurses may struggle with in trying to manage the psychological aftermath of restraint. Because of the additional complexities unique to children, adolescent and elderly care, this discussion excludes these groups; however, it is likely that the issues raised may apply to these settings.

Contemporary Issues in Mental Health Nursing, Edited by J. E. Lynch and S. Trenoweth
© 2008 John Wiley & Sons, Ltd

HISTORICAL CONTEXT

The physical restraint of people with mental health problems has a long history. Documented methods of restraint date back to the 1700s, with shackles, chains and manacles being common forms of managing the 'mad'. Indeed, the 'attendants' at the Bethlem Hospital allowed spectators to view the mayhem at a cost of one penny (Jones, 1972). As well as the view that mental illness was symptomatic of immorality at this time, there was also an increasing belief that insanity had physiological causes. The theory of the brain being the organ of the mind was being established, and the search for treatments and cures began in earnest. These cures included 'aquatic shock treatment', which involved pouring cold water, usually over the head, of patients who required calming (Scull, 1993). Another form of treatment was the 'tranquillizer chair' that restricted all body movement, the underlying theory being that blood flow would be reduced to the brain resulting in a sedative effect (Scull, 1981). The use of restraint, however, remained the dominant model of treatment intervention. The shackles and chains of the 1700s were replaced with restraining gloves, sleeves and waistcoats in the 1800s. Seclusion was introduced in the form of leather or padded cells, which according to the 1871 Annual Report by the Medical Superintendent, contributed to the tranquillity of the dormitories (Gilland, 1871).

The 1900s were dominated by physical treatments such as 'deep insulin therapy' for psychosis and 'modified insulin therapy' for neurotic disorders. Both involved inducing coma by the administration of insulin over a period of days or weeks depending upon the severity of mental disorder. Electroconvulsive therapy was used routinely and is still in use today, albeit as a carefully selected option following a number of first line treatments (NICE, 2004). Opiates, barbiturates, bromide and chloral hydrate were the main drugs of choice for challenging and aggressive behaviour, and their use continued well into the 1970s. The 1950s heralded the advent of psychotropic medication as we know it today in the form of 'Chlorpromazine', which effectively treated symptoms of psychosis for many psychiatric patients, the result for some being freedom from the institutions and reintegration to the community (see Chapter 11: Supporting Recovery: Medication Management in Mental Health Care). Little has been documented which considers the psychological consequences of historical treatments for patients, and there is an absence of historical literature that considers any psychological effects that nurses may have experienced in the aftermath of the daily challenges that they faced within the asylums.

The nursing role, therefore, has evolved alongside such developments – from 'attendants' on the insane to modern practitioners working alongside and in collaboration with those experiencing mental health problems (Nolan, 1993; DH, 2006a). This is in part due to changing professional understandings about the nature of illness over this time, but also due to the development of concomitant treatment options.

CONTEMPORARY ISSUES

The role of the mental health nurse has also developed as a result of a greater understanding regarding the needs, wants and wishes of those with mental health problems. This is seemingly reflective of changing societal attitudes regarding the rights of individuals to be listened to and to be heard (see Chapter 2: Rebuilding Lives: A Critical Look at the Contemporary Role of the Mental Health Nurse and Chapter 3: User Involvement and the Micro-Politics of Mental Health Care). In the late 20th and early 21st centuries, rigorous approaches to researching and understanding mental health and illness have also developed and continue to evolve (see Chapter 7: Where is Your Evidence? Broadening the Scope of Professional Knowledge). Research evidence is easily accessible to health care staff, and a clear agenda in education and practice has been set for staff to become evidence-based practitioners in order to provide the best possible cost-effective care to service users. However, the contemporary challenge is for nurses to be able to synthesize and clinically apply the increasing research base relating to the management of violence and aggression in mental health care to provide comprehensive, consistent and therapeutic management of untoward incidents in mental health settings (UKCC, 2002; NICE, 2005b).

There have been a number of social policy changes in recent years, which seem to have had a direct influence on the levels of violence and aggression on acute in-patient wards. The psychiatric hospital closure programmes have resulted in a major shift towards community care (Leff, 2001), while acute in-patient facilities are increasingly used to 'contain' the most disturbed individuals who are unable to be cared for in the community. Bowers (2005) highlighted that one of the main reasons for admission in present times was in relation to perceived 'dangerousness', and the necessity for some form of containment to prevent harm to self or others.

There are a variety of clinical and nursing responses to violence, but the most dominant model in UK mental health care for responding physically is *Control and Restraint* (C&R) (see Chapter 17: No Euphemisms: The Use of Force in Mental Health Care). C&R was originally developed by the prison service in 1981 and expanded into health and social care in the mid-1980s, following recommendations made within the Ritchie Report (1985) that training in C&R should be provided for nursing staff in special (high-security) hospitals. Techniques were subsequently modified for less secure environments. Other methods, such as breakaway skills, have been developed and are mandatory in most UK Mental Health Care Trusts. However, the efficacy of breakaway training is questionable. For example, Rogers *et al.* (2006) audited 47 staff in a medium-secure unit and found that none of the sample had used breakaway in the preceding 12 months, 40% were unable to break away within a 10 second period, and 60% did not employ correctly taught techniques. Indeed, according to Wright (1999), there is a lack of research into the efficiency and safety of the methods used for C&R in general, and more recently Paterson *et al.* (2003a) highlighted that training techniques are costly to provide and their use can result in serious injury and death. Duxbury and Paterson (2005) have further emphasized the lack of empirical evidence related to therapeutic value of physical restraint and continued concerns over appropriate training methods. There is also some evidence that incidents of aggression were at their highest when staff absences were high (Bowers *et al.*, 2007c), suggesting that when staff were on leave from the clinical area to attend training in C&R, untoward incidents were increased.

Restraint is frequently used as an intervention to manage violence and aggression, and there is a growing body of associated literature. While much emphasis has been placed upon the negative impact of such interventions in the literature, there have also been counterarguments that consider the use of restraint as a positive method of containment, which may not necessarily be to the detriment of those involved (Paterson, 2005; Bowers *et al.*, 2007a,b). However, the impact of using physical methods of restraint remains under-researched. Current research has tended to focus upon the prevention of aggression by considering what factors may contribute to the cause, and influence the escalation of, aggression within in-patient units. There also seems to be a widespread belief amongst nurses that violence can be anticipated (Bonner and Wellman, in press). This is indeed a complex issue, and environment and staff attitudes are seen to play a great part in the escalation of situations (Sheridan *et al.*, 1990; Whittington and Wykes, 1996; Wright, 1999). However, bearing in mind the changing in-patient population and the heterogeneous nature of violence and aggression, it is unrealistic to believe that all aggressive situations can be prevented.

At any one time on a generic acute admission ward the in-patient population is often over 100% bed occupancy. Individuals are unlikely to be admitted unless they are very 'disturbed' and unable to be 'contained' within the community setting. Unfortunately, acute in-patients' environments have been described as anti-therapeutic (Cameron *et al.*, 2005), with staff shortages and high use of casual and temporary staff and a lack of satisfying activity and poor engagement (Ford *et al.*, 1998), which further compounds feelings of boredom and irritability. Tempers can often be frayed on both sides. It is no surprise that these circumstances spark aggressive incidents, which require use of physical restraint as a way of controlling aggression and violence.

While the evidence base related to contributing factors of violence and aggression continues to expand, there remains a paucity of research related to the aftermath of restraint. Very little is known about what the psychological effects of being involved in restraint incidents may be for patients or staff in these settings. Recent guidelines from the National Institute for Health and Clinical Excellence (NICE, 2005b) recommend that a post-incident review should take place following an incident involving restraint, which should consider events leading up to the incident, contributing factors to the escalating situation, and any changes which need to be made as a result of the event. In some clinical areas post-incident review is integrated within the process of managing incidents, yet in other areas such review happens on a seemingly ad hoc basis, if at all. There is a belief that aggression is 'part of the job', as is the physical harm that may befall the participants involved in aggressive episodes. However, it is clear that the psychological consequences of being involved in restraint can be very significant and far-reaching.

THE PSYCHOLOGICAL IMPACT OF RESTRAINT FOR IN-PATIENTS

The psychological and emotional impact of being restrained is difficult to measure. While the assessment of the antecedents, targets and physical harm resulting from aggression or violence can be measured (for example, by using the Staff Observation of Aggression Scale (SOAS) (Palmstierna and Wistedt, 1987) or the more recent revised version of this scale – SOAS-R (Nijman *et al.*, 1999)), the psychological effects and personal impact of violence and aggression are subjective and are therefore more difficult to define. Within the general population, exposure to traumatic events can have severe psychological consequences, particularly the risk of developing PTSD. NICE (2005c) guidelines for PTSD acknowledge it as common and suggest that around 25–30% of individuals who experience a traumatic event will go on to develop PTSD. In light of these figures it would make sense that physical confrontation in psychiatric settings, such as restraint, would have similar effects upon individuals involved. Indeed, the experience of restraint may well be perceived as a traumatic event, and in the author's current study (Bonner, 2007), which examines the psychological aftermath of restraint for staff and patients, strong negative emotions such as fear, humiliation, loss of control and anxiety were described by a number of the participants. In the same study, 40% of patient participants warranted further screening for PTSD after application of the Trauma Screening Questionnaire (Brewin *et al.*, 2002), which measures indicators for trauma symptoms. Despite the connections described here, there is very little research evidence which examines the links between restraint and subsequent PTSD.

PTSD is a disorder that can occur following exposure to a traumatic incident where the individual either experiences or witnesses an event that is perceived by the individual to threaten death or serious injury. This may be a one-off untoward event or ongoing systematic trauma, such as domestic violence or childhood sexual abuse. PTSD is characterized by symptoms which include anxiety, flashbacks, avoidance of stimuli associated with the trauma and numbing of general responsiveness (APA, 2000). For patients, there is a growing research base which identifies that PTSD can be missed in the in-patient setting, and some research suggests that around 40% of the in-patient population may have an undiagnosed PTSD (Mueser *et al.*, 1998b; McFarlane *et al.*, 2001). Psychological trauma has been identified as a factor which contributes to severe mental health problems (Coid *et al.*, 2003; Koss *et al.*, 2003) and the experience of psychiatric hospitalization can be a trauma in itself (Jackson *et al.*, 2004).

There are some studies which have found that the experience of restraint can reawaken memories of previous traumatic encounters for patients (Brase-Smith, 1995; Gallop *et al.*, 1999; Bonner *et al.*, 2002; Sequeira and Halstead, 2002; Bonner, 2007). These memories have included previous experience of rape being likened to being restrained, as well as other violent encounters outside of the mental health setting. If the experience of restraint does retraumatize the patient, this is likely to make PTSD symptoms worse. If, as some studies suggest, PTSD is undiagnosed, staff may well misinterpret symptoms for other pathology. The result is inappropriate treatment for the patient. There is research to support that patients often have a long history of abuse and trauma (Cascardi *et al.*, 1996; Craine *et al.*, 1988), therefore we may again be introducing further trauma to exacerbate existing symptoms. In terms of the Stress Vulnerability Model (Zubin and Spring, 1977), these further stressors which are introduced may tip the precarious balance of the mental state for already vulnerable individuals. Individuals who have previous histories of vulnerability may be less likely to cope with restraint situations and fare worse than individuals who have previously been able to adapt to difficult and challenging life events.

THE PSYCHOLOGICAL IMPACT OF RESTRAINT FOR STAFF

Richter and Berger (2006) found that 17% of staff met criteria for PTSD at baseline following an assault by a patient. Caldwell's (1992) study found that 10% of staff who had experienced a work-related trauma qualified within DSM-IIIR criteria for PTSD and 61% of staff had PTSD symptoms but did not meet full criteria for clinical diagnosis. The author's current study (Bonner, 2007) found that 7% of staff participants who were interviewed following an experience of restraint warranted further screening for PTSD, and a further 67% had sub-clinical trauma symptoms. In this study, similar to patients, 57% of staff described reawakened memories of previous traumatic encounters including previous violent restraint incidents, and other incidents such as assault outside of the hospital setting, during a recent experience of restraint.

For staff, team cultures influence reporting of psychological distress (see Chapter 15: Enhancing Effective Multidisciplinary Team-Working: A Psychoeducational Approach and Chapter 16: A Systemic Approach to Violence Risk Assessment and Management). For example, in some units where managing aggression and violence is an everyday occurrence, the prevailing ethos may be that to admit to feeling shaken or upset following an incident shows some sign of weakness and inability to manage the role. If the psychological impact has caused symptoms of PTSD, the nurse is susceptible to flashbacks, hyperarousal and avoidance behaviours, which may influence his or her reactions to incidents in the clinical environment. If a nurse is working in a psychiatric intensive care unit where aggressive incidents may be common and they are experiencing these symptoms, there may be a reduced readiness to assist colleagues should an incident arise. Conversely, in teams where post-incident review is encouraged in a non-threatening way, nurses report that this is helpful to them in terms of managing their distress, and in considering how they may or may not manage subsequent incidents of restraint (Bonner *et al.*, 2002; Lee *et al.*, 2003; Bonner and Wellman, in press). Indeed, positive attitudes towards the decision to restrain may have an impact upon the subsequent psychological effects of these methods. Bowers *et al.* (2007a), for example, found that student nurses who reported optimistic attitudes towards patients with personality disorders viewed containment methods more positively, and further reported that decisions regarding containment are made with safety for patients being at the forefront of the decision making process (Bowers *et al.*, 2007b).

Other research suggests that nurses who choose to work in mental health care may, themselves, be mentally vulnerable (Little, 1999). They may, therefore, be at a higher risk of subsequent psychological injury following traumatic experiences of restraint. Resilience has been identified as a factor in the study of trauma (Herman, 1992), which can influence whether the individual will experience post-traumatic symptoms, and this may also be a factor in the aftermath of restraint. In Werner's (1989) longitudinal study, certain characteristics were identified in relation to the ability to withstand adverse early environments. These characteristics included high sociability and communication skills, as well as a strong sense of having the ability to control their destiny. In the author's current study, 50% of staff interviewed in the aftermath of restraint reported that good teamwork, with particular emphasis upon communication, was helpful in constructively addressing the management of restraint. Although these findings were in relation to team working, the nurses who reported these more positive findings rated individually lower on trauma screening scales than their colleagues. Good communication and a feeling of control was identified in this study as factors, both individually and within the team, which may prevent adverse psychological effects following incidents of restraint for staff.

ADDRESSING THE AFTERMATH OF RESTRAINT – A WAY FORWARD

Despite developments in preventing incidents of violence and aggression from happening, a small number of untoward events are likely to continue to require physical interventions (see Chapter 17: No Euphemisms: The Use of Force in Mental Health Care). The after-effects are complex and cannot be ignored. It is therefore necessary to think about how the aftermath can best be managed. The World Health Organization (Sethi *et al.*, 2004) suggest a public health approach to violence prevention, and Paterson *et al.* (2007) discuss use of a public health promotion model in managing violence. They suggest that tertiary health promotion approaches (which should consider organizational issues, the review of care of the aggressive individual, and actions of staff) can promote positive outcomes for the patient and provide flexible supports to staff.

The NICE (2005b) guidelines on Prevention and Management of Violence advise that some form of post-incident review should take place within 72 hours of an event occurring. This should be aimed at any individual involved, including witnesses of the event. While this would appear to be fairly straightforward direction, some caution must be made before implementing such guidance. In the specialist area of PTSD, an approach to managing the aftermath of trauma, such as natural or manmade disasters, was that of 'Critical Incident Stress Debriefing' (Mitchell, 1983). This was a method of reviewing events systematically with individuals soon after the incident. Vivid 'reliving' of the event was encouraged as a method of facilitating resolution and preventing further psychological sequelae. This model of debriefing has, however, now been discredited as having neutral or, in some studies, harmful effects (Rose *et al.*, 2004), and NICE (2005c) guidelines for PTSD advise that this approach is no longer indicated for addressing the aftermath of trauma. Indeed, Rose *et al.* (2004) found that re-exposing participants to feelings of helplessness and terror soon after the event potentially increased the trauma.

The NICE (2005c) guidelines for PTSD suggest that 'watchful waiting' should be considered, and that individuals should allow natural healing processes to take place for at least four weeks before any intervention would be necessary. This introduces some conflict to the reviewing of events following restraint. Where NICE (2005b) guidelines for Prevention and Management of Violence advise that a review within 72 hours is indicated, NICE (2005c) guidelines for PTSD advise that Critical Incident Stress Debriefing should not take place, and that some time is necessary following the event for the individual to process the trauma naturally. Whether restraint can be identified as a trauma is subjective, however, it is clear that the complex factors discussed earlier may make certain individuals in both staff and patient groups more likely to experience restraint as traumatic.

Some distinction must be made regarding best practice in light of these conflicts. First, evidence suggests that PTSD is common within in-patient units and currently re-experiencing of the trauma through Critical Incident Stress Debriefing should not be used following restraint. Second, it is clear from discussion earlier in this chapter that some form of non-threatening post-incident review would address the current neglect in this area, as well as address the issues raised in NICE (2005b) guidelines for Prevention and Management of Aggression. An unambiguous distinction between 'debriefing' and 'post-incident review' must be made to address the aftermath of restraint for patients and staff. The Thames Valley University (TVU) Post Incident Review Framework (Figure 18.1) offers a way forward in addressing the aftermath of restraint for both.

This format offers a simple guide for practitioners to consider events which may have led up to the incident, factors of relevance during the incident, and issues for

Guidance note: the prompts in brackets are to assist the person conducting the review

I'm interested in what happened on *(date/time of incident)* **when** *(outline brief details of incident)*

Can you describe to me what happened?

Can you describe to me anything that was happening before this or which led up to it?

Can you describe to me how you were feeling before *(use patient/staff member's words to describe the incident)*

How did you feel during *(use patient/staff member's words to describe the incident)*

Was there anything that you found <u>helpful</u> during *(use patient/staff member's words to describe the incident)*

Was there anything that you found <u>unhelpful</u> during *(use patient/staff member's words to describe the incident)*

How did you feel after *(use patient/staff member's words to describe the incident)*

Was there anything that you found <u>helpful</u> afterwards?

Was there anything that you found <u>unhelpful</u> afterwards?

Do you think that there is anything that the staff or anybody else could do to help prevent something like this from happening again?

Is there anything else that you would like to tell me about *(use patient/staff member's words to describe the incident)*

Sometimes during an upsetting incident, we remember other upsetting incidents from our past. Did this happen to you during the incident that we have been talking about?

Do you have any questions that you would like to ask me or is there anything else that you would like to talk about?

Figure 18.1

Thames Valley University (TVU) Post Incident Review – A Framework for Practice

future practice following the incident. The format is simple to use, and when evaluated in a recent study (Bonner and Wellman, in press), 97% of staff participants and 94% of patient participants agreed that it was a useful framework for reviewing incidents involving restraint in practice. This framework has been designed bearing in mind concerns related to Critical Incident Stress Debriefing, and is not a framework for dramatic review through systematic 'reliving' of the trauma. Rather, it is offered as an option which staff may wish to use to consider the aftermath with colleagues, patients and any other witnesses or participants involved in the incident in a non-threatening, flexible way. However, it may not always be appropriate to use and discretion should be made. For example, if individuals are angry and hostile, timing must be considered. It may be that more than 72 hours are necessary before considering the events, and this should be discussed within the nursing or multidisciplinary team.

The post-incident review is also an opportunity to identify early indicators for PTSD. The use of the Trauma Screening Questionnaire (TSQ) (Brewin *et al.*, 2002) is an option which can supplement the review to identify early indicators for PTSD. The TSQ is a simple 10-point yes/no checklist which highlights trauma-related symptoms. Bearing in mind the natural processes that have been discussed, the TSQ is not indicated for use within four weeks of a traumatic event, but can be a useful indicator for further screening for PTSD. An educational approach should be used in explaining that individuals, both patients and staff, may experience anxiety, numbness, fear, guilt, sadness, anger, tiredness and preoccupation following the event, and that this is a natural process. This can be done following the post-incident review and a supplementary leaflet outlining some of the common feelings and reactions can be helpful for individuals to look at subsequently.

ETHICAL ISSUES

While restraint was historically a common method of managing the mentally ill, as mental health care has evolved the use of restraint has become a thorn in the side of humanistic care, an ideology which has often been cited as an important underpinning for contemporary nursing practice (Playle, 1995). If the nurse aspires to the role of carer, nurturer, therapist, then the use of restraint within this role is apparently in conflict with the underlying humanistic philosophy. To question what nurses find helpful during and following restraint is to acknowledge that this is an aspect of their work that is worthy of investigation. In making this explicit we are inviting the nurse to confront this aspect of their role in depth. This may create feelings of discomfort within the nurse who, according to Marangos-Frost and Wells (2000), may well view restraint with a sense of dread. There is also a sense of intrusion into a situation of conflict where nursing decisions have been made, and post-incident review may highlight areas of practice that were poor and could have been managed more effectively.

The culture of nursing has historically been that of blame, where any indiscretion brought to management's eyes is duly met with punishment. However, the Clinical Governance agenda (DH, 1999e) espoused a change in culture where mistakes are remedied through supportive intervention. Using a sensitive approach to post-incident review can address these issues and facilitate change in a positive way. The main areas of risk for patients would be from the risk of reminding them of memories of recent untoward incidents and from the release of distressing emotions surrounding these incidents.

In the evaluation of the TVU Post Incident Review framework (Bonner and Wellman, in press), 94% of patient participants reported that the review had been helpful to them and none of the patients interviewed became distressed when reviewing the events. On the contrary, they had valued the opportunity to review incidents of restraint. Caution must still be taken, however, and necessary supports mobilized should staff or patients become distressed. If the review is causing distress it should be stopped, for both staff and patients. It may be that symptoms of PTSD become evident following an incident of restraint. As discussed, watchful waiting would be indicated; however, if symptoms continue, further screening and specialist intervention for PTSD may be necessary to supplement current treatments for patients. Staff who have been involved in an incident which has been upsetting to them should be given some time out if necessary. This may be for a short break away from the clinical area, or if necessary some time at home to allow emotions to settle. Watchful waiting would again be indicated and further interventions facilitated if required. In the author's current research, staff who felt valued for their efforts had a much more positive outlook towards the aftermath of restraint. If staff require further support they should be encouraged to contact their GP, occupational health services or staff counselling if available. In turn, GPs, occupational health services and staff counselling should be aware of referral systems for specialist PTSD services should they be required. NHS organizations should be aware, at the highest levels, what their support systems are able to offer and a clear message given to their staff regarding what is available to them (see Chapter 16: A Systemic Approach to Violence Risk Assessment).

CONCLUSIONS

Until recently, the psychological impact of restraint had been uncharted territory, but through research and consideration of other models of distress, such as PTSD, some insights into the consequences of restraint can be made and suggestions for treatment and interventions suggested. The suggested post-incident review format (Figure 18.1) is a promising and potentially helpful way to consider the impact of restraint, as well as to detect early warning signs for PTSD and activate early interventions if necessary. Every staff participant interviewed in the author's current study reported that they have used restraint as a last resort and did not want to use restraint if it could possibly be avoided. Until such time as alternative methods are identified, restraint will continue to be used on a small number of occasions to contain potentially dangerous situations. It is therefore important to continue researching the effects of this intervention to develop our understanding of the impact of restraint, as well as the efficacy of post-incident review, in preventing psychological harm.

CHAPTER 19
MASCULINITY AS A RISK VARIABLE IN PHYSICAL AND MENTAL ILL HEALTH

Steve Trenoweth and Jonathon E. Lynch

INTRODUCTION

A substantial body of evidence seems to demonstrate that men have higher rates of physical health problems (Courtenay, 2000; Payne, 2004), increased rates of suicide (DH, 2002b; University of Manchester, 2006), and violence and drug/alcohol misuse (Möller-Leimkühler, 2003). Being a man, it seems, is harmful to your health and well-being. Increasingly, however, explanations of possible links between one's biological sex and a range of risk- and health-related behaviours have begun to take into account issues of *gender* (that is, the social and cultural construction of identities *arising* from one's biological sex) (Courtenay, 2000; Payne, 2004). So, what is it about being 'male' that is so 'risky'? In this chapter, we explore how masculinity may be a theme that underpins health behaviour, and discuss implications for physical and mental health care and nursing practice.

CONSTRUCTION OF GENDER IDENTITY

A contemporary view of gender identity sees notions of 'masculinity' and 'femininity' stemming not purely from one's biology, but as socially constructed, reflective of widely

Contemporary Issues in Mental Health Nursing, Edited by J. E. Lynch and S. Trenoweth
© 2008 John Wiley & Sons, Ltd

held cultural norms and ideals of typical 'male' and 'female' characteristics (Soulliere, 2005). Furthermore, a number of constructions, and expressions, of 'masculinities' can be identified rather than a universally agreed concept (Winlow, 2001), and hence the roles and 'normal behaviours' of men tend to vary across human societies (though most people in what are known as the developed countries are familiar only with societies that are somewhat similar to their own). Like all identities, masculinities can be considered 'invented categories' (Weeks, 1991). They are the end products of attaching attributes, dispositions and ways of behaving to men (who are willing to accept them) and are located within time and place (Nixon, 1997; Courtenay, 2000). As societies and cultures expect conformity to a socially defined range of normative behaviours and attitudes, any transgression of the rules may be followed by social penalties and sanctions (Jewitt, 1997) (see Chapter 8: Challenging Stigma and Promoting Social Justice).

As such, societies appear to ascribe different and specific qualities to men and women. For example, in Western industrialized societies, stereotyped masculine qualities are associated with aggression, dominance and visible resilience, whereas feminine qualities are often seen to be associated with caring, submission and passivity. However, criticism has often been raised against such over-generalizations. Kulis and Nieri (2007), for example, distinguish between 'positive masculinity' (protectiveness, honour) and 'negative masculinity' (aggressiveness, domination). Further distinctions can be made between 'positive feminine' (nurturing, empathic) and 'negative feminine' (passivity, dependence). 'Masculinity' may thus be seen as part of a range of identities and seemingly does not simply stand in polar, categorical opposition to 'femininity'. Further distinctions can be made between the cultural forms of 'ideal' masculinity and those which are *perceived* by society to be less than ideal. 'Hegemonic masculinity', for example, may be constructed as the culturally dominant, 'ideal' masculine type, often reflective of the most powerful social group (Courtenay, 2000), which provides normative attributes and rules of behaviour against which all other forms of masculinity are judged and subsequently subordinated (Connell, 1995). 'Hegemonic masculinity' in Western societies is seen to be indicative of dominance, achievement, competitiveness and sexual and sporting prowess (where risk, pain and injury are glorified), and means that men are socialized into assuming that they must present themselves as both emotionally and physically strong; must hide and contain their feelings; and must not show signs of vulnerability or weakness. Such a display of hegemonic masculinity is seen to give one positional prerogative and power within the community, affording the subordination of other forms of masculinity – which may have feminine qualities, and which can lead to mockery, pressure and violence (Royo and Món-Catalunya, 2002) or to which the stigma of being homosexual may be attached (Connell, 1995; Jewitt, 1997; Payne, 2004; Souillere, 2005) (see Chapter 9: Homophobia in Mental Health Services).

Socially and culturally constructed views of 'hegemonic masculinity' and masculine ideals are seen to be reinforced and perpetuated by mass media portrayals, especially in film and television (Soulliere, 2005), both in terms of behaviour and visual representations (Jewitt, 1997). Televised professional wrestling, for example, emphasizes hegemonic masculinity with its recurrent themes of aggression, violence, emotional restraint, heterosexuality, dominance, achievement, success, competitiveness, toughness, risk-taking and courage (Soulliere, 2005).

GENDER INFLUENCES ON HEALTH AND RISK BEHAVIOUR

Men, it has been argued, live in a 'harness' brought about by conformity to their gender roles – hypersensitive to how others perceive them and overly concerned with their status within their community (Goldberg, 1977). It would not be surprising if resultant stress from such pressures led to both physical and mental health problems. In this section we examine some of the evidence which appears to relate gender and health.

GENDERED PHYSICAL HEALTH

There is, indeed, much evidence to link hegemonic masculinity with premature death due to physical health problems, such as coronary heart disease and cancers (Courtenay, 2000; Nicholas, 2000; Möller-Leimkühler, 2003; Payne, 2004; Hunt *et al.*, 2007). There are, of course, many influences on physical illness, such as social and environmental factors, injury, genetic influences and so forth. Gender is one such influence, which may interact with other variables to increase or decrease the likelihood of a physical health problem (Payne, 2004). Hence:

Many sociocultural factors are associated with and influence health-related behaviour. Gender is one of the most important of these factors (Courtenay, 2000, p. 1386).

As such, the aetiology of physical illnesses is likely to be multi-factorial (see Chapter 13: Physical Illness: Promoting Effective Coping in Clients with Co-Morbidity).

Courtenay (2000) argues that health-related beliefs and behaviours can be a demonstration of the way in which gender is constructed, enacted and defined. For example, gender can be associated with health behaviour choices, as men have higher rates of smoking, excessive use of alcohol, unprotected sex with large numbers of partners and appear to make unhealthier lifestyle choices (Goldberg, 1977; Payne, 2004; Kulis and Nieri, 2007), such as a poor dietary intake. 'Real' men, it seems, eat foods high in fat and low in vitamins (Payne, 2004). Ironically, then, the 'hegemonic' masculine goals of achieving 'ideal' masculine physical frame (i.e. muscular and trim, a notion reinforced in mainstream entertainment media (Sparks, 1996)) are incongruous and unrealistic considering such high-risk unhealthy behaviour. Payne (2004) suggests this may lead to anxiety regarding one's size and shape, as this itself may be far removed from the hegemonic ideal.

Indeed, this seems to extend not only to a set of behaviours which increases the risk of physical health problems and accidents, but also to engagement in a range of behaviours which actively undermines health. For example, it seems that women tend to engage in far more health-promoting behaviours than men, such as relying on a social network for emotional support (Weidner and Cain, 2006), leading to an assumption that men are unconcerned about their physical and psychological health. Indeed, this has led Courtenay (2000, p. 1386) to conclude that:

Being a woman may, in fact, be the strongest predictor of preventive and health-promoting behaviour . . .

In fact, there is some suggestion that health-promoting behaviours may be seen to be 'feminine', and may subsequently be seen to be incongruous with hegemonic masculinity. For example, Courtenay (2000) suggests that the most rapidly rising form of cancer in the United States, skin cancer, may be associated with a reluctance amongst some men to be seen to 'pamper' their bodies with sun screens and other lotions, which may be seen as a feminine activity, and a belief that a tan conveys 'rugged good looks'.

Interestingly, however, a recent study has found men with more socially constructed feminine qualities seem to have decreased mortality rates from coronary heart disease (Hunt *et al.*, 2007). Indeed, it seems that men tend to have poorer survival rates than women and are less psychologically adapted to cope with diagnosis of a physical illness, such as cancer (Nicholas, 2000). Furthermore, men may seek to deny or disregard pain and physical discomfort, and are less likely to seek help and may avoid medical care (Courtenay, 2000; Nicholas, 2000), although it has been suggested that men may have a poorer understanding of health and illness, and as such, may be less aware of symptoms requiring attention (Nicholas, 2000; Payne, 2004).

Men are also more at risk of accidents and have significantly higher rates of death and injury from road traffic accidents than women (Payne, 2004). This may stem not only from the fact that men are more likely to be employed in driving-related jobs, but also to patterns of high-risk behaviour whilst driving (WHO, 2002b), such as driving whilst intoxicated. Men thus are seemingly more cavalier regarding their physical health both in terms of risky lifestyle choices, and behaviours, which has led the World Health Organization to conclude that:

Gender role socialisation and the association of masculinity with risk taking behaviour, a greater acceptance of risk and disregard of pain and injury may be factors leading to hazardous actions on the part of men (WHO, 2002b, p. 3).

However, men who experience accidental deaths amongst peers seem less likely to engage in risk-taking behaviour, but this prudence can be overridden in some contexts, such as engaging in sport (Kippax *et al.*, 2002).

GENDERED MENTAL HEALTH

For Goldberg (1977), men 'in the harness' of hegemonic masculinity are at highest risk of mental health problems following stressful life events such as illness, divorce, job loss, retirement or other threats to the perceived masculine 'ideal'. Certainly, hegemonic masculine behaviour may lead to an inability to cultivate a supportive social network, such as intimate friendships with other men. As such, if support is sought it is usually from a spouse or partner, although as Goldberg (1977) indicates, in such a masculine world, there is often a reluctance to do so:

. . . the traditional male façade – cool, detached, controlled, guarded, and disengaged – is a protective mechanism that allows him to simply respond to external cues or inputs, like a programmed computer, rather than have to wrestle with constant conflict and ambiguity (Goldberg, 1977, p. 96).

The possible resultant bind and psychological conflicts between societal expectations and the hegemonic male psychological and emotional inner worlds, may lead to the possibility of developing anxiety and depression-related problems. As a consequence, this may increase the likelihood of adopting various maladaptive behaviours, such as the misuse of substances, as a means of managing such problems (Bennett and Jones, 2006).

However, rates of the clinical diagnosing of depression are commonly seen to be much higher for women than for men (Bennett and Jones, 2006). This would seem to indicate that femininity rather than masculinity is implicated in the development of depression. However, it seems that a diagnosis of depression is less likely to be made for men than women, despite the presentation of similar depressive symptoms (Potts *et al.*, 1991). Indeed, such differential rates of diagnosis, and subsequent care and treatment, may be further evidence of 'hegemonic masculinity', both in terms of assumptions made by those who are undertaking the diagnosing, and also as men are more likely than women to try to respond to depressive symptoms themselves rather than to seek help (Courtenay, 2000).

GENDERED SUICIDE

Suicide is a multi-factorial phenomenon with consistent findings from research implicating variables such as being male, living alone, unemployment, alcohol or drug misuse and mental health problems (DH, 2002b), particularly depression and the hearing of persecutory voices (Cutcliffe and Barker, 2004). An important factor in seeking to account for elevated rates of suicide is the perception of hopelessness (Collins and Cutcliffe, 2003) and loss of meaning to one's life, particularly in the face of chronic, terminal, debilitating or painful physical illnesses. Hence, the study of any one of these factors must be seen as part of the overall interactive backdrop with other variables.

According to the Office of National Statistics (ONS) (ONS, 2007), the overall male suicide rate since the 1990s has showed a downward trend. However, suicide is now one of the common causes of death of men aged under 35 in England. Suicide rates for men aged 15–24 are now more than twice as high as in 1971, and have almost doubled for men aged 25–44 (Men's Health Forum, 2002). In 2005, there were 5671 adult suicides in the United Kingdom. Almost three-quarters of these suicides were among men (ONS, 2007). A similar proportion of male to female suicides was reported in 'The Five Year Report Of The National Confidential Inquiry Into Suicide And Homicide By People With Mental Illness' (University of Manchester, 2006), where 74% were male. However, the ratio of males to females was highest in the 25–34 year age group, in whom 80% were male, and lowest in those over 75, where 61% were male.

Despite such obvious gender differences, there is little research undertaken on 'suicidal masculinity' (Scourfield, 2005). However, a repetitive theme in the literature associated with elevated rates of male suicides is an individual's perceived failure to live up to the 'ideals' of hegemonic masculinity, such as seeing oneself as a failure comparative to others (Kilmartin, 1994; Scourfield, 2005) and a possible internalized and negative perception of one's expression of masculinity as being subordinate to the 'ideal' (see Chapter 9: Homophobia in Mental Health Services). Indeed, Scourfield (2005) also implicates the limited emotional expressiveness (or 'emotional illiteracy') of hegemonic masculinity and the need for 'inner strength' to 'soldier' problems oneself (Men's Health Forum, 2002). As such, emotional expressive restraint may contribute to stress-related health problems (Möller-Leimkühler, 2003; Soulliere, 2005) compared with women, who often have a more extensive social support network than men to draw on in times of personal crises. Furthermore, women are more likely to recognize, acknowledge the need for, and ultimately seek professional psychological or psychiatric help (Möller-Leimkühler, 2003).

Indeed, this seems particularly true for younger men who tend to perceive emotional expressiveness and help-seeking behaviours as one of the significant differences between homosexual and heterosexual men (Men's Health Forum, 2002). Here, there may be a cultural dimension, for, in the Western world, a completed 'successful' suicide may be considered a more acceptable death for men than for women, with 'unsuccessful' attempts at suicide being perceived as emasculating or feminine (Canetto and Sakinofsky, 1998). There are also marked social class differences, with unskilled males being three-and-a-half times more likely to kill themselves than those in the professional social classes (Men's Health Forum, 2002).

GENDERED VIOLENCE AND CRIMINALITY

Newburn and Stanko claim (1994, p. 1) that the '. . . most significant fact about crime is that it is almost always committed by men'. Admittedly, 'crime' is a contested concept, and a social construction itself, but it is clear that males are over-represented as perpetrators of actions deemed 'criminal'. This disparity is even more marked when crimes are disaggregated and violent offences are considered separately. However, the fact that a minority of men overall engage in these activities – or, at least, only a small proportion are ever caught and appear in records/statistics – lends weight to the argument that *certain types* of masculinity are 'risky'. For example, men with strong perceptions of masculinity and few acceptable outlets in which to assert these are seemingly more prone to violence. This extends across all forms and levels of interpersonal violence. Unsurprisingly, then, this renders certain males both more likely to carry out violent, criminal acts and to be the victims of these.

Crichton (1995, p. 70) points out that the best demographic predictors of violence are shared between the mentally disordered and the non-mentally disordered, an example of the value of actuarial risk assessment frameworks to clinical risk assessment (however, see Chapter 16: A Systemic Approach to Violence Risk Assessment and Management). It has been recognized for some time that symbolic as well as pragmatic use of violence can be extremely important for the demonstration of masculinities amongst people of lower socio-economic status (Miller, 1958; Bruce *et al.*, 1998). Individuals who have been socialized within a framework of cultural capital that renders physical aggression central to concepts of ('real') manhood may use this to threaten, to cause harm and generally to avoid being seen to be 'disrespected' (Bruce *et al.*, 1998, p. 45; Hobbs *et al.*, 2003, p. 223). This is a matter which can of course extend to their behaviour in care settings and may well influence some to use aggression to resolve interpersonal difficulties.

At the extreme end of a violence continuum stands homicide. The deaths of adult females at the hands of their male partners or ex-partners are recognized as making up a startling proportion of homicides overall – 50% of all female homicide victims (Dorling, 2004, p. 181). In overall statistical terms males appear to be at greater risk of being the victims of homicide at all ages, and, on a very worrying note, homicides of young men appear to be increasing (Rooney and Devis, 1999; Dorling, 2004). Polk (1994, p. 166) points out that just over half of homicides are likely to involve males as both perpetrators and victims. The homicide rate of England and Wales is low overall, a merciful surprise given the high rates of interpersonal violence. (This is largely explained by relatively low levels of firearm and sharp weapon use, although availability of emergency medical facilities in towns and cities may save some victims (see Brookman, 2005).)

REDUCING THE RISK OF 'NEGATIVE' MASCULINITY

If hegemonic masculinity is such a bind (Goldberg, 1977), surely we should do away with it? Indeed, the impression is that acting according to masculine ideals places a great burden on men (Phillips, 2006; Thomas, 2006b), and as such masculinity is 'a gender in crisis' (Alt, 2001, p. 8). Not only is hegemonic masculinity implicated in a range of male health and risk behaviours, but there are clear implications for women (Payne, 2004) as reinforcement of male dominance is seen to support female subordination (Soulliere, 2005). Courtenay (2000) draws our attention to this bind situation:

By successfully using unhealthy beliefs and behaviours to demonstrate idealised forms of masculinity, men are able to assume positions of power – relative to women and less powerful men . . . By dismissing their health needs and taking risks, men legitimise themselves as the 'stronger' sex. In this way, men's use of unhealthy beliefs and behaviours helps to sustain and reproduce social inequality and the social structures that, in turn, reinforce and reward men's poor health habits (Courtney, 2000, p. 1397).

Indeed, some have argued for a new model of 'masculinity' to shed the 'armour' of social obligations where men can express and share their concerns with others and where there is greater patience and empathy with others and a concomitant ability to communicate meaningfully and demonstrate affection (Royo and Món-Catalunya, 2002). Others, however, point to signs that such hegemonic masculinity may be breaking down. Male mental health nurses are seen to have crossed the 'gender divide' by entering the profession (Bennett and Jones, 2006), but this, of course, assumes that such nurses have also shed any hegemonic loyalties and have openly embraced positive feminine qualities, such as emotional literacy, empathy and nurturance. Indeed, Phillips (2006) argues that the challenge to hegemonic masculinity in mental health practice can have positive and far-reaching implications:

. . . by encouraging clients and multidisciplinary colleagues to challenge, vocally and visibly, the pervasive cultural representations of a restrictive and governing 'normative' masculinity, we undermine the norm, expand identity possibilities, and positively impact physical and mental health at an individual and societal level (Phillips, 2006, p. 421).

However, while Connell (1995) similarly sees the problems associated with hegemonic masculinity, he also points out that there is a positive side. For example, legendary stories of heroes, sacrifice on behalf of others, strong and visionary leadership, sporting achievements and so forth are often associated with this form of masculinity. So we may question the value of 'overthrowing' this form of masculinity in its entirety, even if it were possible.

Perhaps an important strategy would be to support and encourage coping and help-seeking behaviours amongst 'at risk' men, for example, young men who have strong hegemonic orientation towards masculinity, and those at risk of suicide and mental health problems (such as young homosexual men, and those in young offender institutions). As such, courses and training programmes that seek to develop and broaden such men's coping strategies (for example, the ability to ask for help, recognizing emotions and the development of a range of supportive and meaningful social networks) may be a very useful foundation (Men's Health Forum, 2002).

Certainly, an awareness of 'hegemonic masculinity' amongst mental health nurses can afford insight into the potentially problematic interpersonal dynamics in clinical settings. Take, for example, what is termed the 'loss of face' – an issue that hinges on perceptions of one's appearance to others and the need to avoid humiliation and protect an individual's sense of honour. Indeed, a 'loss of face' is perhaps most prominent for those who see themselves through the eyes of others (Winlow *et al.*, 2001), so clients' experiences of nurses' actions and reactions become pivotal to their experiences of care. This is a relatively common experience among young men in penal custodial and other particularly masculine institutional settings. It is disappointing that there seems to be more attention to this in police studies (for example, Muir, 1977; Choongh, 1997; Westmarland, 2001) than in mental health care, and evidence, perhaps, of the inadequate attention that has been devoted to the social regulatory and controlling aspects of clinical nursing practice. However, an appreciation of this issue, and the development of an empathic understanding regarding why such behaviours arise and how one might respond personally and therapeutically to displays of hegemonic masculinity, could help to reduce the frequency of conflict, disharmony, marginalization and interpersonal violence.

Indeed, this may also be helpful to the reflections of nurses who lead the management of incidents involving disagreement or conflict. Some episodes become contests of wit or will, where 'weakness' cannot be shown (cf. Rhodes, 2004). Furthermore, self-awareness is crucial to ensure that wider social or cultural influences, such as hegemonic masculinity – with its emphasis on toughness and power struggles – do not become features of clinical practice (see Chapter 17: No Euphemisms: The Use of Force in Mental Health Care).

CONCLUSION

Men have higher rates of smoking, drinking and drug use and have poorer physical health, more accidents and higher rates of suicide and violence. Men are more likely to engage in risky behaviours, such as reckless driving, unprotected sex, unprotected exposure to sun and dangerous recreational activities. They have poorer social support networks and mechanisms, and are less likely to engage in health-promoting behaviours or to seek medical help (Alt, 2001). However, such issues are not a common focus within contemporary mental health nursing practice, which has implications for health promotion and the formation of therapeutic relationships. As such:

Even in studies that address health risks more common to men than women, the discussion of men's greater risks and of the influence of men's gender is often conspicuously absent. Instead, the 'gender' that is associated with greater risk remains unnamed . . . Left unquestioned, men's shorter life span is often presumed to be natural and inevitable (Courtenay, 2000, p. 1387).

All of this has enormous potential implications for the mental health nurse wishing to engage, support and care for the physical and mental health needs of male service users who may lack emotional literacy or the capacity to discuss issues that may indicate their 'vulnerability'. Indeed, nurses who similarly hold a hegemonic masculine ideal for themselves are likely to find the more positively feminine aspects of their practice (caring, compassion, empathy, nurturing and support) troublesome, and may prefer a more immediate, direct and tough approach to solving clinical problems (see Chapter 17: No Euphemisms: The Use of Force in Mental Health Care). This is likely to be incongruous with contemporary and professional understandings of mental health nursing practice, and the needs and wishes of service users navigating their journey to recovery (see Chapter 3: User Involvement and the Micro-Politics of Mental Health Care; Chapter 5: The Implications of Values-Based Practice in Mental Health Nursing; and Chapter 10: The Meaning of Recovery). The response to such situations here is likely to be complicated by wider societal and cultural expectations of masculine behaviour and the possibility of the unthinking adoption of such views and practices in health care scenarios. There may also be a concomitant reluctance to shed the 'armour' of social obligations, amongst staff and service users alike. Certainly, strategies which seek to address such issues will need to consider how such changes in behaviour may be facilitated without the exposure of an individual's vulnerability. For the nurse, considerations of hegemonic masculinity may be a springboard for personal and professional reflection, and a possible need to confront and challenge deeply felt beliefs and core values about gender identity and the cultural ascriptions of social roles which may impede care delivery. Indeed, it is here that we are reminded of the words of Oscar Wilde, who said in *The Importance of Being Earnest* (1895) – 'All women become like their mothers. That is their tragedy. No man does. That's his.'

CHAPTER 20
SOME CONSIDERATIONS FOR MENTAL HEALTH PRACTITIONERS WORKING WITH THOSE WHO SELF-NEGLECT

James Matthews and Steve Trenoweth

INTRODUCTION

Self-neglect is a relatively common problem in mental health care and individuals who neglect their own personal and household hygiene and health are familiar to mental health staff (Lauder, 1999a,b, 2005). As a result, the care and treatment of clients who self-neglect is a significant and contemporary issue for mental health services (Reed and Leonard, 1989) and a challenging, but nonetheless important, aspect of clinical risk assessment.

Self-neglect, as a concept, is also a poorly conceptualized and little researched phenomenon (Gibbons *et al.*, 2006; Lauder *et al.*, 2006) and in our current understanding of self-neglect, we appear to be in somewhat of a conceptual rut (Reed and Leonard, 1989). Furthermore, in mental health nursing textbooks it can be difficult to find reference made specifically to the issue of 'self-neglect', which has led some contemporary

Contemporary Issues in Mental Health Nursing, Edited by J. E. Lynch and S. Trenoweth
© 2008 John Wiley & Sons, Ltd

commentators to ponder the '. . . preparedness of nurses to deal with what is a relatively common problem' (Lauder *et al.*, 2006, p. 281) (see Chapter 2: Rebuilding Lives: A Critical Look at the Contemporary Role of the Mental Health Nurse). In this chapter, we offer some considerations for those who are working with clients who appear to neglect their health care needs.

POLICY FRAMEWORKS

In recent years, all mental health care providers have been required to provide comprehensive and structured plans of care for people who are under the supervision of specialist psychiatric services and have a severe mental health problem, via the Care Programme Approach (CPA) (DH, 1990, 1999c). Such clients may be in danger of losing contact with the mental health services or there may be a concern that the individual poses a significant risk to themselves or others. Risk may not be restricted to serious violence to others or to suicide/self-harm, but may also include concerns over severe self-neglect. In contemporary mental health practice, the employment of the CPA process not only acts as a significant guide to mental health workers in relation to identifying and addressing specific aspects of risk (Vick *et al.*, 2002; Lauder *et al.*, 2005), but its inclusive, comprehensive, multi-agency nature seeks to maximize chances of responding effectively to crises.

There are other legislative and policy frameworks which may be of assistance in the strategic management of clients who self-neglect. For example, the 'NHS Plan Implementation Programme' (DH, 2000b) and The Sainsbury's Centre for Mental Health (SCMH) Model on Crisis Resolution (SCMH, 2001b) offer guidance to community-based mental health teams in their approaches and responses to patient care, such as faster and easier access to health services, health promotion and better user involvement and feedback. It is also worth noting that other legislation, such as the National Assistance Acts of 1948/1951, can be enforced in cases of severe self-neglect (Gunstone, 2003), where there are specific fears to public health. The act covers specific issues relating to environmental hazards, such as hoarding, vermin and so forth, and can be utilized in conjunction with mental health legislation.

However, while the above policy frameworks and legislation can be useful for operationalizing and directing care, they will not provide answers or solutions as to *how* one addresses the specific needs of those who 'self-neglect' in a therapeutic, clinical or evidence-based way.

DEFINITIONS OF SELF-NEGLECT

A variety of definitions of self-neglect have been suggested, but overall a number of themes emerge from the literature. Severe self-neglect seems to reflect a constellation of behaviours (Lauder, 2001), and as such is a multi-dimensional problem (Lauder *et al.*, 2006) representing the disregard of, or inability to engage in, self-care activities despite available resources and knowledge (Reed and Leonard, 1989; Gibbons *et al.*, 2006). It is also '. . . a form of self care deficit in which those self-care activities that are thought to be necessary to maintain a socially accepted standard of personal and household hygiene are not undertaken' (Lauder, 2005, p. 46).

It is apparent that a subtle continuum exists in the field of self-neglect. Less serious deficits appear to lie on the lower end of the self-neglect scale, such as failure to look after diet, dental hygiene and not seeking medical attention when ill, whilst the more extreme *severe self-neglect* exists at the other. Such severe neglect may be: a significant deterioration in physical health; the hoarding of rubbish and animals, both alive and dead; the continual neglect of rotting food; poor personal hygiene resulting in parasitic infestations, and other infections; ignoring possible dangers from malfunctioning appliances; detachment from essential services; non-compliance with support and treatment; and leaving home with the doors unlocked and/or opened (Lauder, 2001; Arluke *et al.*, 2002; Gunstone, 2003; Gibbons *et al.*, 2006).

All of these highlight the intricate nature of this phenomenon, and the difficulties mental health practitioners may encounter in relation to the assessment and management of people that self-neglect. The concept of self-neglect is a multi-faceted one and is seemingly more complex than a 'mere' lack of attention to physical hygiene (Adams and Johnson, 1998; Lauder, 1999c, 2001; Gibbons *et al.*, 2006), and may also include a failure to manage finances, lack of social contacts, poor compliance with treatment and a client's failures to protect themselves from sexual, financial and property abuse (Gunstone, 2003).

PERSPECTIVES OF SELF-NEGLECT

Research on the subject of self-neglect has been to some extent sporadic (Adams and Johnson, 1998), which belies its prevalence, and the impact and implications for individual's health and well-being. Here we pause to consider various perspectives which have sought to account for self-neglect.

MENTAL ILLNESS

Self-neglect has long been associated with varying forms of mental illness or disturbances (Gibbons *et al.*, 2006), including obsessive–compulsive disorders (Maier, 2004), various forms of psychosis, depression, dementia (Halliday *et al.*, 2000; Abrams *et al.*, 2002), stress in later life (Clarke *et al.*, 1975) and personality disorder (Damecour and Charron, 1998; Abrams *et al.*, 2002). Self-neglect can also be found in those with frontal lobe atrophy, which can also be associated with aggression, hostility and paranoia (Orrell *et al.*, 1989). Higher rates of mental health problems have also been found amongst those who live in squalor, and self-neglect amongst this group seems to be exacerbated by a co-morbid alcohol abuse (Halliday *et al.*, 2000).

Mental illness, then, is often cited as a clinical precursor to self-neglect. However, approximately 50% of self-neglect cases in the over 60s have no clinically diagnosed mental disorder (Clarke *et al.*, 1975; MacMillan and Shaw, 1966). Thus, the links between a medical or nursing diagnosis and self-neglect is unclear (Lauder, 1999c). Whilst the experience of mental health problems and the use of psychiatric medication may go some way in explaining some clients' difficulties in coping with issues such as personal and household hygiene, finance, social interaction and concordance with treatment (see Chapter 11: Supporting Recovery: Medication Management in Mental Health Care), there is as yet no definitive evidence of a causal association between mental 'illness' and self-neglect (Vostanis and Dean, 1992).

AGE AND GENDER

Significant associations have also been suggested between the concept of self-neglect and cognitive decline in old age in particular, to the extent that in medical terms self-neglect in old age is often seen as a distinct syndrome (MacMillan and Shaw, 1966; Adams and Johnson, 1998; Rosenthal *et al.*, 1999; Abrams *et al.*, 2002). The term 'Diogenes Syndrome' is often used to describe self-neglect in the elderly, of which the most significant features are that of social withdrawal (Hettiaratchy and Manthorpe, 1989), malnutrition, the hoarding of rubbish and severe neglect of personal hygiene (Clark *et al.*, 1975). However, in recent years the term has provoked some discussion and may be inaccurate as the Greek philosopher *Diogenes* is recorded to have been a happy individual who sought out the company of others (Post, 1982; cited in Adams and Johnson, 1998). Indeed, some believe that *Diogenes* was making a political point against the hedonistic society he lived in by taking a vow of poverty (Vostanis and Dean, 1992).

The term 'Diogenes Syndrome' may also be clinically inappropriate and unhelpful. In their study on those living in squalor in their own homes in inner London, Halliday *et al.* (2000) found that both the younger and older people from their sample group were affected equally (age range: 18–94 years), and that those individuals who received assistance from specialist cleaning services appeared to have higher rates of mental health problems. They concluded that the definitions set out in Diogenes Syndrome may be a too narrow definition for people living in squalid conditions. Today, Diogenes Syndrome is seen to be of '. . . historical interest rather than of clinical utility' (Halliday *et al.*, 2000, p. 886).

There appears to be a dearth of research and discussion on the subject of self-neglect/ severe self-neglect in younger adults, specifically those under 60 (Cooney and Hamid, 1995). Often, it seems that younger adults who live in squalor do not come into contact with health services unless they have a co-existing mental health problem (Lauder, 2005) (see Chapter 14: Responding to the Needs of Younger People: The Bereaved

Adolescent). In a rare study in this area, Vostanis and Dean (1992) examined two cases of self-neglect in adults aged 35 and 38. Both subjects were women, unemployed and described as having an emotionally detached upbringing from their families and relatives. Although one client had been admitted to a psychiatric in-patient unit in the past, no evidence of a treatable psychiatric illness was diagnosed. The authors noted similarities in the personality traits of both subjects that correlated with previous findings on the social and interpersonal characteristics of those who self-neglect (MacMillan and Shaw, 1966), for example, few contacts with friends, rejection of help from outside agencies and both women described as being often suspicious and quarrelsome.

SOCIAL AND PSYCHOLOGICAL PERSPECTIVES

Social and psychological perspectives of self-neglect seek to understand and explain the phenomenon rather than classify it as a symptom of some underlying disorder (Lauder *et al.*, 2002). For example, Bristow *et al.* (2001) saw self-neglect as implicated in the (statistically significant) differences in the rates of admission to in-patient mental health facilities between inner and outer London. However, it is not clear if inner city life contributes to self-neglect or if people who are prone to self-neglect are somehow drawn to inner city areas.

Similarly, self-neglect may be indicative of a psychological need for an individual to seek approval or esteem from others. Fritz and Helgeson (1998), for example, described the phenomenon of 'unmitigated communion', where an individual becomes focused on, and perhaps over-involved with, the needs and welfare of others to the exclusion of his or her own personal needs. This may be especially valid when an individual comes to rely upon others to indicate self-worth.

The dominance of the medical model perspective of self-neglect over other professional constructed approaches is highlighted by Lauder (1999a) who points to the importance of the conceptualization of self-neglect, with a particular emphasis on how various members of a community may interpret or perceive self-neglect (see Chapter 8: Challenging Stigma and Promoting Social Justice). Social definitions and explanations of self-neglect centre on individual values, culturally acceptable norms and perceptions of citizenship (Lauder *et al.*, 2002, 2006; Gunstone, 2003). As such, self-neglect may be seen as a failure to engage in socially acceptable standards of personal and household hygiene as defined by culture (Lauder *et al.*, 2001) and, for example,

. . . *people who are 'dirty', 'unclean' and 'unhygienic' in Western Cultures are regarded as disordered, unhealthy and to be vanquished* (Lauder, 1999a, p. 60).

Self-neglect, it seems, can also be seen as a violation of social norms (Lauder, 2005). As such, notions of cleanliness and hygiene, like morality, vary enormously between cultures (and subcultures) (Lauder, 2001). Indeed, different groups of nurses have different constructions of self-neglect, and hence will make different social and clinical judgements, in part based on professional socialization and in part on their own cultural values (Lauder *et al.*, 2001) (see Chapter 5: The Implications of Values–Based Practice in Mental Health Nursing; Chapter 6: Truth, Uncertainty and the Mental Health Nurse; and Chapter 7: Where is your Evidence? Broadening the Scope of Professional Knowledge). Lauder also stresses the importance of considering issues such as how we as health professionals judge 'what are normal and abnormal levels of cleanliness and hygiene' (Lauder, 1999a, p. 61). In a broader sociological examination of the perception and construction of ideas relating to self-neglect, Lauder (2005) observes that the media may play a significant role in how society's (and inevitably health workers') views of self-neglect have been fashioned. Advertisements extolling the virtues of cleaning products for homes that eliminate germs in the 'war against dirt and bodily fluids' (Lauder, 2005, p. 47) do little to alleviate public anxiety in relation to matters of personal hygiene. Certainly, the phenomenon of 'animal hoarding', described by Arluke *et al.* (2002), indicates not so much a lack of mental competence or illness, but a lack of awareness of, and concern for, the risks to animals or humans. Why or how such individuals have a personal tolerance for such an extreme lack of sanitation and toxic atmospheres is unclear.

CHOICE AND SELF-DETERMINATION

Clinically, our decision to intervene (or indeed not to intervene) in cases of self-neglect can be seen as partly reflective of our perceptions of the phenomenon of self-neglect, including our personal perceptions of another's mental competence (Lauder *et al.*, 2006), and partly due to our own personal or cultural standards of hygiene.

However, not only does it seem that our clinical assessments and perceptions are influenced by our own personal and cultural factors, but whether or not to intervene likewise seems to be based, in part, on our beliefs regarding the extent to which we assume those who self-neglect choose to do so (Lauder, 2001) (see Chapter 16: A Systemic Approach to Violence Risk Assessment and Management). That is, our interventions may be based on whether we believe self-neglect is a deliberate decision – an intentional lifestyle choice on the part of the self-neglecting individual (Lauder, 1999b; Gibbons *et al.*, 2006) – or conversely whether we assume that self-neglect results from the unintentional consequences of circumstances beyond the person's control (Gibbons *et al.*, 2006), such as the experiencing of active symptoms of mental disorder. It is likely that such a decisional balance will inevitably influence the practitioner's clinical course of action (or inaction) (Longres, 1994; Lauder, 1999b, 2005).

Gunstone (2003) suggests a decisional equation by which to identify an individual clinician's subjective perception of the risk of self-neglect. Gunstone suggests that there exists a balance between, on the one hand, a practitioner's assessment of risk on the basis of safety and clinical duty of care, and on the other hand, personal concerns regarding social control and concerns over respecting the individual's right to self-determination. As such, consideration may be given in this decisional balance to the rights of people to neglect themselves or to engage in behaviours which might be detrimental to their health, such as smoking (Lawn, 2004), the practitioner's own personal tolerance of self-neglect, and the local or national policy or legislative frameworks, such as the Nursing and Midwifery Code of Professional Conduct (NMC, 2004b) (see Chapter 16: A Systemic Approach to Violence Risk Assessment and Management). Indeed, the latter point was identified by Symonds (1995), who argued that the socio–political climate may legitimize professional inaction with regards to self-neglect under a banner of user empowerment and that most disabled:

. . . in the present climate, appear to be suffering from the ideology of right wing libertarianism, whereby neglect passes as self-determination in an increasingly self-care society (Symonds, 1995, p. 100).

That is, by not helping the person to address issues of self-neglect, and in particular self-care or hygiene needs, there is a danger that such individuals become stigmatized and shunned by communities, or avoided by members of the general public, which may serve merely to reinforce their isolation and exclusion from wider society (see Chapter 8: Challenging Stigma and Promoting Social Justice). Indeed, as Woods *et al.* (1999, p. 79) argued:

. . . an individual is required to alter or modify his/her behaviour in order to function effectively, to be accepted by society

Risk, it seems, is '. . . always culturally constituted and as such is always imbued with culturally determined values' (Crowe and Carlyle, 2002, p. 23). Therefore, one might argue that one role for the mental health nurse is to assist people to 'conform' to society's expectations regarding appropriate standards of conduct, and in particular, hygiene. This is likely to be uncomfortable for those who are concerned about the role of the mental health nurse as an agent of social control (Glenister, 1997; Morrall, 1998) (see Chapter 2: Rebuilding Lives: A Critical Look at the Contemporary Role of the Mental Health Nurse and Chapter 3: User Involvement and the Micro–Politics of Mental Health Care).

There is a clear issue here regarding whether we perceive that a respect for human dignity arises from our intervening, or by our not intervening. Some argue that we need to expand on our understanding of human dignity within our own ethical framework. For example, Gallagher (2004, p. 593) suggests that there is an endless potential for us to 'degrade, devalue, and humiliate and also to be degraded, devalued, and humiliated'. Gallagher suggests that for us as practitioners to improve our ethical practice in relation to dignity, we should look towards an ethic of aspiration, in that we aspire to be better while acknowledging our shortcomings and weaknesses and our potential to violate others' dignity (see Chapter 4: Compassion and Chapter 5: The

Implications of Values-Based Practice in Mental Health Nursing). In contrast, Macklin (2003) suggests that dignity may be a useless and vague concept that has spilled over from religious sources into the realm of medical ethics, and implies that the word should be avoided, to be replaced by its predecessor and more appropriate term, *respect for the individual*. Although Gallagher and Macklin disagree on the terms used to describe how we treat, care or show empathy for others, they do agree on the importance of this issue and the ethics associated with it.

Achieving a balance between what is perceived to be in a client's best interest and one's own obligation to duty of care, while considering significant issues relating to health, dignity, personal autonomy and freedom can be difficult (Crowe and Carlyle, 2003; Lawn, 2005; Gibbons *et al.*, 2006) (see Chapter 16: A Systemic Approach to Violence Risk Assessment and Management). For instance, one has to consider the disparity that seemingly exists between how one will interpret, apply and balance mental health legislation requirements, and one's own professional obligations and one's personal commitment to caring for the client. Of course, an important issue here is how one might clinically and practically respond to clients who self-neglect.

RESPONDING TO SELF-NEGLECT

It seems that not only is a 'universal' theory or perspective of self-neglect unobtainable (Lauder, 1999a), but there can be no objective or universal measures about what is the 'best' standard of hygiene or self-care or when someone is 'self-neglecting'. This has implications not only for the choice of clinical interventions, but also for evaluation of success of care interventions.

The response, if any, to self-neglect is based in part on an ethical decision about whether or not one has the moral or legal right or duty to paternalistically intervene in the lives of another. Another compelling issue is how to *effectively* respond. Assuming that one has made the decision to intervene, there is a lack of research and practical guidance for mental health practitioners relating to how to assess and therapeutically work with clients that have been identified as being at risk of self-neglect (Lauder, 1999b; Gunstone, 2003). Here, we review some of the work that is available, and make some recommendations based on research and literature from other areas which may assist us in our clinical nursing response to self-neglect.

ASSESSMENT

As with all risk events, self-neglect '. . . can go undetected until either a pattern of behaviour is observed by health care personnel or the individual is acutely hospitalised in a state of severe neglect' (Gibbons *et al.*, 2006, p. 11). Hence, risk assessments of self-neglect can often only be made a posteriori and often then only following a crisis. However, there is a clear need for the early identification of self-neglect, not only so that early preventative action may be taken (if, of course, this is perceived to be necessary) (Lauder, 1999b), but also because self-neglect may be part of a 'relapse signature' which might be indicative of a client's deteriorating mental state (Gunstone, 2003). Therefore, the regular monitoring of those at risk for nutrition and dietary intake, physical health status, self-care and hygiene, along with treatment concordance, is essential (Tierney *et al.*, 2004) (see Chapter 12: Physical Co-Morbidity in Mental Health).

Gunstone (2003), however, found that although mental health workers who worked with people who self-neglect did not resist the use of formal assessment tools, most used a number of other approaches to underpin their assessments that included direct personal observation, information from the client and carers, social networks and previous medical histories. Gunstone also highlighted the significant problem that exists for clinical staff in the application of actuarial risk assessment tools, in that most have been developed for research, and do little to meet the everyday needs that emerge in individual cases (see Chapter 16: A Systemic Approach to Violence Risk Assessment and Management). For mental health clinicians working with people who self-neglect, this highlights a significant weakness associated with interpretations and outcomes of clinical risk assessments. Such assessments – for example, The Camberwell Assessment of Need (Slade *et al.*, 1999) or the Expanded Brief Psychiatric Rating Scale (Lukoff *et al.*, 1986) (Figure 20.1) – may indicate or describe a health care need in a global sense but there exist few comprehensive tools to assess the risk of self-neglect in day-to-day clinical practice, which offer practitioners clarification of, and clinical insight into, the complex and multi-faceted nature of self-neglect.

The lack of a universal and standardized benchmark by which to identify 'deficits' in hygiene and the neglect of other needs, means that assessing and monitoring requires clinicians to be aware as to how the phenomenon appears to different groups and to different people, and

. . . to explore both the similarities between cases and to recognise the essentially unique and personal experience of every single case of self neglect (Lauder, 1999a, p. 62).

Hence, in our assessment of self-neglect we perhaps need to develop a unique profile of an individual, including an awareness of their personal beliefs surrounding the importance of hygiene and other factors; their ability to respond to their own perceived need; a clear baseline for their 'usual' standards of hygiene and variations from this baseline; and factors which might underpin a movement away from this baseline.

One tool that may be useful in addressing the complexity of 'social' risk, whilst capturing the 'personal and social realities' of self-neglect (Woods *et al.*, 1999, p. 84) as experienced from the client's perspective, is that of the Behavioural Status Index (BSI) (Woods *et al.*, 1999). The BSI aims to generate data that facilitates risk assessment by three subscales: those risks most commonly associated with a forensic context;

Score	Rating	Criteria
2	Very mild	Hygiene/appearance somewhat below usual standards, e.g. shirt out of pants buttons, unbuttoned
3	Mild	Hygiene/appearance much below usual standards, e.g. clothing dishevelled and stained, hair uncombed
4	Moderate	Hygiene/appearance below socially acceptable standards, e.g. large holes in clothing, bad breath, hair uncombed and oily, eating irregular and poor
5	Moderately severe	Hygiene highly erratic and poor, e.g. extreme body odour, eating very irregular and poor, e.g. eating only potato chips
6	Severe	Hygiene and eating potentially life threatening, e.g. eats and/or bathes only when prompted
7	Extremely severe	Hygiene and eating life threatening, e.g. does not eat or engage in hygiene

Figure 20.1

Self-Neglect Symptom Construct (Expanded BPRS – Lukoff *et al.*, 1986)
Hygiene, appearance, or eating behaviour below usual expectations, below socially acceptable standards, or life threatening within the past 2 weeks.

the degree of insight or awareness; and the skills associated with effective social interaction and communication. The aim is to assist the person to achieve an optimum
level of functioning that is meaningful to the client rather than a clinically derived,
theoretical optimum. As such, items are rated ordinally (degree to which the item is
present or absent) rather than categorically (presence/absence of an item).

While there is always a danger of using such tools beyond their original intended
application (there are implications for the validity and reliability of the findings), it is
the BSI subscales of 'insight' and 'communication and social skills' which may be of

potential use in assessing self-neglect. The 'insight' subscale, for example, affords the analysis of meanings that are attributed to personal experiences and seeks to identify personal interpretations and intentions behind behaviours. Here, items relating to an awareness of personal relationships, the perceived awareness of the need for care/treatment and self-appraisal may be particularly pertinent. Similarly, the 'communication and social skills' subscale offers items which seek to assess a wide range of social behaviours, including non-verbal communication, the ability to engage in social activities and conversation and, perhaps most importantly for self-neglect, the physical presentation of self.

The BSI suggests that the various subscales will interact:

Suppose . . . it could be consistently demonstrated that the social 'risk' presented by a patient tends to vary inversely with his/her degree of personal insight and capacity to perform well in key communicative skills (Woods *et al.*, 1999, p. 88).

As such, it may be that there is less assessed risk of self-neglect if one has more insight/ awareness into the nature and extent of one's self-neglect, and the social or communicative factors which underpin same. However, the BSI is not an 'off the shelf' risk assessment tool for self-neglect, and we are required to be mindful of its intended use with a forensic client group. Our suggestion here is that the BSI possesses several features which may be of value in the assessment of self-neglect.

Finally, when we are undertaking risk assessments of self-neglect, there is a need to consider how we might help the person who has a tendency to pose a risk to themselves or others to become integrated into communities (Woods *et al.*, 1999). While there is a recognition that there are considerable individual differences in standards of personal care, there will still be the rather uncomfortable notion of assessing the individual against the yardstick of socially mandated standards of personal conduct.

INTERVENTIONS

In recent years, the development of National Occupational Standards has been developed to provide details of a standardized approach to describing and assessing the competence for the mental health workforce. Of particular relevance to those who are working with clients who self-neglect are competencies which assist practitioners to 'enable individuals to obtain and maintain household and personal goods' (Skills for Health, 2005a) and to 'enable individuals to maintain their personal hygiene and appearance' (Skills for Health, 2005b). However, while such competencies are useful in that they provide an overall detailed framework for practical care and support, the heterogeneous nature of the phenomena of self-neglect often seems to require an individualized rather than a generalized approach in clinical interventions (Lauder, 1999b). Similarly, the competencies appear to assume that the client is willing to accept such assistance, or is aware of the need for such support from practitioners. As Lauder (2005) pointed out, there is often a reluctance of those who are prone to self-neglect to actively engage with treatment, and that self-neglect '. . . is often accompanied by a strong sense of independence and a reluctance to accept professional interference' (Lauder *et al.*, 2006, p. 280). In fact, disengagement and non-concordance may be important characteristics of self-neglect (Lauder, 1999c). Whatever specific interventions are offered, an issue to be addressed will have to be how to actively engage, work in partnership (Lauder *et al.*, 2006) and maintain contact with clients who self-neglect (see Chapter 2: Rebuilding Lives: A Critical Look at the Contemporary Role of the Mental Health Nurse and Chapter 3: User Involvement and the Micro-Politics of Mental Health Care).

Therefore, therapeutic interventions, psychological support and practical measures may also be required. Thus far, some authors have offered suggestions regarding the types of therapeutic interventions which may be helpful to some clients, such as behaviour therapy (Klosterkotter and Peters, 1985) and psychopharmacology (Ungvari and Hantz, 1991), especially if there are co-existing mental health problems (Lauder, 1999b; Gibbons *et al.*, 2006) (see Chapter 10: The Meaning of Recovery and Chapter 11: Supporting Recovery: Medication Management in Mental Health Care). Similarly, a number of practical measures have been suggested. Vostanis and Dean (1992) found that clients' self-care improved by moving to more protected accommodation, while structured day activities may be of benefit to others (Reyes-Ortiz, 2001).

Indeed, a nurse may choose *not* to intervene in cases of perceived self-neglect. This may be an intentional strategy reflective of the perception that an individual has made an active, intentional decision to neglect their self-care needs. That is, in pursuance of a belief of the importance of respecting the user's voice, we may choose to do nothing (see Chapter 5: The Implications of Values-Based Practice in Mental Health Nursing and Chapter 6: Truth, Uncertainty and the Mental Health Nurse). Unfortunately, this may also be seen as neglect of a clinical duty, or collusion with the person's neglect of their self-care or health care-related needs (Lawn, 2005). However, due to the overall lack of research in this area (with some commendable exceptions, such as the pioneering work of Lauder and his colleagues), more research needs to be undertaken to discover effective, evidence-based or helpful interventions that will assist the self-neglecting client (see Chapter 7: Where is your Evidence? Broadening the Scope of Professional Knowledge).

What is clear, however, is that an effective and co-ordinated multi-agency response is needed (Lauder *et al.*, 2005; Gibbons *et al.*, 2006) due to the complexity of responding to those who self-neglect (Kerzner *et al.*, 2003), and this may include health and social care staff as well as environmental health officers (Lauder, 1999b) and sometimes even animal welfare organizations.

THE WAY FORWARD?

Mental health practitioners are obligated to explore and examine the deeper and more intricate factors that will affect the personal autonomy, freedom and dignity of the individual by any interventions from mental health professionals. For example, issues such as self-governance, lifestyle choice, conformity, cultural and individual differences have to be given significant consideration, irrespective of the individual's legal status. Within the rights-based approach in mental health, self-governance and autonomy are seen to be part of one's humanity, but construing someone to be incompetent (in this case in terms of one's ability to meet self-care needs) or lacking of mental capacity, may also have a dehumanizing effect (Crowe and Carlyle, 2002; Olsen, 2003). This is why the extent of input in any interventions of self-neglect will have to be carefully considered, particularly in relation to how it will be perceived and appreciated by the client.

Some argue for changes in the way we conceptualize mental health problems, to the extent that mental heath professionals need to look more closely at the intertwined relationship between power, knowledge, esteem and personal governance (Godin, 2000; Kuokkanen and Katajisto, 2003; Davidson, 2005). Lauder (1999b) argues for better training and support to deal with pressures and ethical dilemmas and an under-standing of notions of hygiene as socially constructed, which allows us to consider and reflect upon our own values and beliefs (Lauder, 2001) (see Chapter 5: The Implica-tions of Values-Based Practice in Mental Health Nursing).

It is notable that there is a significant lack of research on the subject of self-neglect, particularly in relation to adults under age 60. This appears to have a direct effect on the application of knowledge and guidelines available in relation to the subject. As such, there is a tendency to refer to, and infer from, related or associated work (such as that which relates to an elderly client group), which might explain the propensity to opt for a medical explanation for self-neglect. Indeed, there is a danger here of overlooking the possibility that these may be 'symptoms' emanating from another 'condition' entirely (Damecour and Charron, 1998; Lauder, 2001), such as the inten-tional and strategic use of behaviour that might be considered self-neglecting for per-sonal protests or to draw attention to political issues (Hall, 1997). Here, the individual may also be seeking to demonstrate or assert their own personal freedom to a perceived 'oppressor' when they believe that their autonomy has been threatened. As a result of this, mental health nurses may find themselves drawing on models that would normally be allied to general nursing or the criminal justice system; hence in many cases the primary focus becomes the physical, rather than psychological or even psychiatric, aspect of a client's condition (Lauder, 2001).

CONCLUSIONS

There are many considerations for mental health practitioners who work with individu-als who self-neglect. First, there is a need to review and update one's knowledge of available research, other literature and legislation that can be utilized when assessing and intervening in cases of self-neglect. Second, there is a need to look at the wider aspects of each case, particularly in relation to how the client sees themselves, and one's own views and the views of carers and other clinicians regarding personal perceptions of an individual's lifestyle.

Most importantly, a number of professional, clinical and ethical issues should be given consideration when responding to cases of self-neglect. These include a duty of care to the individual, the roles and responsibilities of health care professionals to assist the client to improve their health and well-being, and considerations of autonomy, personal choice, coercion and freedom. One must also be mindful of the potential dangers of pathologizing self-neglect as an irrational life choice, which subsequently affords '. . . a negation of that person as a fully affiliated citizen and justifying their subjugation' (Crowe and Carlyle, 2002, p. 24) (see Chapter 8: Challenging Stigma and Promoting Social Justice). In responding to self-neglect, and health improvement in general, there often seems to be a stark and unsatisfactory choice between those who support '. . . a heavy handed nanny state on one hand, and those supporting inactivity bordering on neglect in the name of individual freedom on the other' (DH, 2004c, p. 1). There is an urgent need to review our practice and knowledge base so as to effectively respond to the needs of clients who are prone to self-neglect, to assist them to become included within society, but without compromising their capacity for self-determination and their human dignity (see Chapter 4: Compassion).

CHAPTER 21
THE FUTURE OF MENTAL HEALTH NURSING

Steve Trenoweth, Jonathon E. Lynch and Peter Nolan

The scope and practice of the mental health nurse in the future are likely to be very different from what we see around us today. The impacts of modernization, restructuring and reform of mental health services, the Chief Nursing Officer's (CNO) Review of Mental Health Nursing (DH, 2005a, 2006a) and the 'Ten Essential Shared Capabilities' (DH, 2004a) will be significant and undoubtedly have far-reaching influences. Further developments, such as changes to the Mental Health Act 1983 (which are proposed but unconfirmed at the time of writing) and nurse prescribing are also likely to alter the focus and future role of the mental health nurse. The imperative for the mental health nursing profession, then, is to be able to rise to the challenge of delivering care that meaningfully and therapeutically responds to the holistic needs of service users, and in a positive, evidential and supportive way. This is a time, therefore, of great challenges and opportunities to develop innovative approaches to overcome the various systemic barriers that may undermine the quality of mental health nursing care. In this final chapter we review some of the contemporary issues and themes raised in this book and point to future challenges which await the profession.

MEETING NEEDS OF SERVICE USERS

The changing socio-political context has increased expectations from service users for the delivery of care, which values and empowers them as individuals (see in particular

Contemporary Issues in Mental Health Nursing, Edited by J. E. Lynch and S. Trenoweth
© 2008 John Wiley & Sons, Ltd

Chapter 3: User Involvement and the Micro-Politics of Mental Health Care). Nurses will need to consider their professional response to such expectations, and how they may subsequently support service users, with complex and diverse needs, on their own personal journey to recovery (see Chapter 2: Rebuilding Lives: A Critical Look at the Contemporary Role of the Mental Health Nurse and Chapter 10: The Meaning of Recovery). This will require not only an extensive evidence base but also an ethical appreciation and (re-)consideration of the values which underpin their practice. In particular, explicit appreciation will need to be given to the subjectivity of the user's voice and the individual's lived experience of mental distress (see Chapter 5: The Implications of Values–Based Practice in Mental Health Nursing and Chapter 6: Truth, Uncertainty and the Mental Health Nurse). However, to ensure that the needs of service users are met, the profession must deliver a consistently high standard of care, regardless of the context. As such, nurses will need to develop therapeutic alliances based explicitly on the foundation of partnership and a desire and willingness to work alongside service users without prejudice or bias (see Chapter 3: User Involvement and the Micro-Politics of Mental Health Care).

All service users have the right to receive care based on what is known to work, but it is important that the value of treatment options and nursing interventions is not seen simply in terms of what has been shown to improve clinical 'outcomes' under research conditions. More importantly, nurses need to assist the individual service user to identify and choose interventions that are most helpful to the individual's recovery, are reflective of their own needs, hopes and aspirations (see Chapter 10: The Meaning of Recovery and Chapter 11: Supporting Recovery: Medication Management in Mental Health Care). Arguably, in mental health care the highest form of evidence is that provided by the experience of service users themselves. Ultimately it is what works best for them that matters. The mental health nurse in the contemporary context, therefore, needs to be much more than a technician who blindly applies research findings (which may, in any case, not help to respond effectively to clinical needs). To this extent, nurses will need to manage their own personal and professional anxieties surrounding resultant clinical complexity, ambiguity and uncertainty, and must be able to draw upon a variety of different sources of knowledge to offer suggestions regarding recovery pathways and treatment options (Chapter 6: Truth, Uncertainty and the Mental Health Nurse and Chapter 7: Where is your Evidence? Broadening the Scope of Professional Knowledge).

The care offered to service users, of course, needs to be not only informed but compassionate (see Chapter 4: Compassion). In a contemporary context, there is a requirement for a clear and explicit focus on recovery and improving overall health and well-being in a holistic sense. The broader aim of mental health nursing care will, therefore, need to be that of improving quality of life by instilling hope and optimism and rebuilding lives which have been blighted by mental distress (see Chapter 2: Rebuilding Lives: A Critical Look at the Contemporary Role of the Mental Health Nurse and Chapter 14: Responding to the Needs of Younger People: The Bereaved

Adolescent). The contemporary goal is to assist individuals on their journeies to recovery, in coming to terms with their difficulties and/or disabilities, and in living lives that are as happy and fulfilled as possible. Nurses need to be aware that people have different ways of living and consequently they experience mental health problems differently, and choose different solutions to their problems. Here, there is also a need for mental health nurses to address the very real fears and worries experienced by service users about their care, and to consider how they might overcome possible barriers to the development of, and engagement in, supportive and therapeutic relationships.

PROVIDING HOLISTIC CARE AND IMPROVING PHYSICAL CARE

In recent years, the poor quality of physical health of mental health service users has become a particularly significant issue (see Chapter 12: Physical Co-Morbidity in Mental Health). There is a contemporary recognition of the higher morbidity and mortality rates from chronic diseases within this group compared with the general population. There are important opportunities for mental health nurses to play a significant role in improving both the physical and mental health of people with serious mental illness (Robson and Gray, 2007) (see Chapter 13: Physical Illness: Promoting Effective Coping in Clients with Co-Morbidity). Future mental health nurses will therefore be required to develop their clinical and research practice to improve the mental and physical well-being of service users. To this end, an awareness of aetiological and risk factors associated with the development of physical ill health is essential to improve skills in the screening and early detection of a wide range of medical illnesses. There will also be a need for effective responses to the identified needs and concerns of service users regarding their physical and mental health, including ensuring timely referrals to specialist medical services. In turn, this has significant implications for pre- and post-registration education.

Assisting service users to take responsibility for their own physical health is a powerful means of engaging them in the skills of self-monitoring, self-reflection and self-management and in supporting attempts at autonomous living. Service users and nurses alike will need to recognize that biological well-being is a precondition for a productive and meaningful life. Here, mental health nurses will need to consider their roles as health educators and health promoters, possibly through measures such as: developing smoking cessation programmes; undertaking comprehensive annual health checks; ensuring appropriate and equal access to medical care; advising on diet and ensuring adequate nutrition to support recovery; bespoke exercise programmes; monitoring effects and side-effects of medication, including weight gain and reduced glucose intolerance; and advice on maintenance of sexual health. Nurses will also need to assist service users to recognize and accept the consequences of ill health; to recognize the complex interplay between stress and health; and appreciate the many ways in which disabilities can be overcome.

A crucial aspect of work here is helping to identify and clarify personal and meaningful health-related goals and supporting each individual to work towards them (see Chapter 10: The Meaning of Recovery; Chapter 11: Supporting Recovery: Medication Management in Mental Health Care; and Chapter 14: Responding to the Needs of Younger People: The Bereaved Adolescent). This may well have implications for knowledge and skills development in the provision of holistic care amongst mental health nurses who report being unprepared for this role (Brimblecombe et al., 2007).

IMPROVING IN-PATIENT CARE

In 1999, the Standing Nursing and Midwifery Advisory Council (SNMAC) felt that '. . . the picture of mental health nursing in acute settings is often a demoralised group, with ineffective clinical leadership, inadequately prepared in terms of education and training, with patently inadequate support from other professional groups and administrative staff' (SNMAC, 1999, p. 21). There have, of course, been some improvements since this time, but it is clear that the service user's experience of acute in-patient care remains negative and broadly speaking, the overall conclusions of SNMAC remain highly relevant (SCMH, 2005) (see Chapter 2: Rebuilding Lives: A Critical Look at the Contemporary Role of the Mental Health Nurse). Indeed, reports of inadequate staffing, a general custodial atmosphere, overcrowding and high levels of boredom continue to emerge. For the mental health nurse, acute in-patient environments remain areas of great tension and stress and as such, 'The poor quality of work life contributes to the problems of recruiting and retaining highly qualified and motivated mental health nurses' (SNMAC, 1999, p. 6). However, despite difficulties such as these – which are largely rooted in decades of structural neglect – nurses have demonstrated that if given support they can transform even the most dire conditions (Holmes, 2006).

There remains a need for quality clinical leadership and management support for mental health nurses who work in such environments. Certainly, many of the training needs of staff in acute care environments identified by SNMAC (1999) seem to have remained unmet, such as evidence-based cognitive, family and behavioural interventions and medication management. Perhaps, though, we must come to accept that the current model of generic acute in-patient care is not capable of responding to the needs and wishes of service users, and that we are asking too much of mental health nurses to provide therapeutic care in such environments. Perhaps it is time to consider alternatives to acute in-patient care and escalate the provision of primary and secondary mental health community services – both in terms of their responsiveness to service user needs, and a broader health promotion/prevention focus. Perhaps a future focus for mental health nursing practice might be on the early engagement with people who may be experiencing mental distress and improving the availability of psychological treatments in primary care settings to offset the need for in-patient admission? Dare we think the unthinkable and consider what the future would look like without psychiatric in-patient facilities (Rethink, 2005b)?

TAKING A POSITIVE APPROACH TO RISK

A positive approach to risk requires multi-factorial, systemic, context-specific and comprehensive assessments and an awareness of the ways in which individuals and organizations seek to contain and defend themselves against the anxieties generated by uncertainty (see Chapter 6: Truth, Uncertainty and the Mental Health Nurse and Chapter 16: A Systemic Approach to Violence Risk Assessment and Management). This requires health care practitioners to rise to the challenge of supporting those who do not wish to engage with care and the subsequent ethical dilemmas this poses (in terms of achieving a balance between respecting human dignity, the capacity for self-determination and personal freedoms, and acting in the perceived best interests of the individual, obligations of duty of care and role of protecting the public). There is also a need for mental health nurses to develop awareness as to how their own personal values and subjectivity (see Chapter 5: The Implications of Values-Based Practice in Mental Health Nursing) (influenced by such factors as availability and provision of personal support and team work (see Chapter 15: Enhancing Effective Multidisciplinary Team-Working: A Psychoeducational Approach)) can shape perceptions of risk (see Chapter 16: A Systemic Approach to Violence Risk Assessment and Management).

Furthermore, it is crucial for mental health nurses to appreciate that there are many risks to which the service users themselves are exposed, such as those associated with masculinity (see Chapter 19: Masculinity as a Risk Variable in Physical and Mental Ill Health), self neglect (see Chapter 20: Some Considerations for Mental Health Practitioners Working with Patients who Self-Neglect), lack of equal access to medical health care (see Chapter 12: Physical Co-Morbidity in Mental Health), stigma and social exclusion (see Chapter 8: Challenging Stigma and Promoting Social Justice and Chapter 9: Homophobia in Mental Health Services), lack of involvement and partnership working (see Chapter 3: User Involvement and the Micro-Politics of Mental Health Care), experiences of restrictive and custodial care (see Chapter 17: No Euphemisms: The Use of Force in Mental Health Care) and restraint (Chapter 18: The Psychological Impact of Restraint: Examining the Aftermath for Staff and Patients). With restraint, there is a clear need to develop strategies of being able to respond effectively to the challenges of managing violence and aggression whilst also considering the aftermath and the possible psychological impact of physical interventions for both staff and patients. It is not only ourselves that we should strive to satisfy on these matters. Service users' de facto experiences must be crucial to ongoing efforts to identify and research good practice (see Chapter 7: Where is your Evidence? Broadening the Scope of Professional Knowledge). Nor should the perceptions of those who seek to speak for and protect the interests of service users be seen as hostile to clinical practice. Rather, practice should be informed by the views and influences and, crucially, efforts should be made to ensure that practices are transparent, professionally acceptable and positive about those who receive them (see Chapter 3: User Involvement and the Micro-Politics of Mental Health Care).

BECOMING VISIBLE

An important contemporary and recurrent theme which has emerged from the previous chapters is the need for the development of a positive modern mental health nursing profession that is alert and responsive to the needs of service users and able to make significant contributions to their recovery (see Chapter 2: Rebuilding Lives: A Critical Look at the Contemporary Role of the Mental Health Nurse). As such, there is a subsequent need to *demonstrate* clearly what the mental health nursing profession has to offer service users and society in general. At present, many have argued that much of the work of mental health nurses goes unrecognized and is seemingly invisible or not obvious (Barker and Buchanan–Barker, 2005). A future challenge, therefore, will be to make visible the real work of mental health and that should also be the aim of those who deliver, manage, research, commission and receive mental health nursing services. This will inevitably require developing a subject-specific knowledge base and undertaking research into the wealth of knowledge embedded in its own practice, whilst being critically analytical about its contribution to health care practice (see Chapter 7: Where is your Evidence? Broadening the Scope of Professional Knowledge). That is, the profession needs to celebrate and publicize achievements, whilst simultaneously acknowledging its areas for development and demonstrating a commitment to continuous quality assurance. This may require new ways of working and new settings for practice. For example, increasing the visibility of mental health nursing in primary care can support responses to the psychological needs of people in distress outside specialist secondary services, whilst ensuring that service users in secondary care settings receive appropriate and equitable primary health care.

DEVELOPING A PROFESSIONAL PARADIGM

To become visible, it is necessary to review historical links and, in particular, to consider breaking free from the paternalistic influence of medicine and finding a distinctive professional voice. Furthermore, whilst we must acknowledge that the slavish adherence to a unifying paradigm can hinder and constrain the generation of new knowledge (Kuhn, 1970), many authors see the current ideological fragmentation and heterogeneity as being problematic for the profession and service users. That is, there have been calls for an explicitness and clarity regarding the work of mental health nurses, in terms of fundamental or core roles and responsibilities (see Chapter 2: Rebuilding Lives: A Critical Look at the Contemporary Role of the Mental Health Nurse).

Central to the development of core roles and responsibilities is an appreciation of the use of evidence that underpins clinical practice and, more broadly, what is considered to be valuable professional knowledge (see Chapter 7: Where is your Evidence? Broadening the Scope of Professional Knowledge). That is, which sources of information help mental health nurses to make sense of, and understand, the personal experience of service users? If this extends to undertaking 'research', then consideration needs to be given to methodologies and approaches that will help us to investigate clinical concerns meaningfully and generate knowledge that is applicable to real-life contexts. The application of such knowledge, however, is likely to encompass the need for an appreciation of the professional values which must underpin ethical decision making.

There is also an imperative to capitalize upon, and utilize, knowledge which is alive in the practitioner's consciousness. Perhaps, then, a unifying mental health nursing framework emphasizes not so much the hoarding of 'facts' to be indiscriminately applied, but the wisdom of interpretation, and the recognition that people search for their own personal truths and are active interpreters of experiences in their own lives (see Chapter 6: Truth, Uncertainty and the Mental Health Nurse). This affords the opportunity of valuing lived experiences and of stressing the importance of subjectivity, and the negotiation and sharing of meanings between individuals. Above all, this approach recognizes the ephemeral nature of knowledge and of 'knowing', and a willingness and openness to embrace change and new ideas.

There are many '. . . oases [of] high quality care and innovation . . .' (Holmes, 2006, p. 404) in contemporary mental health nursing. Indeed, there is evidence that mental health nurses are capable of effective and successful therapeutic interventions, such as cognitive behavioural interventions, and medication management (Curran and Brooker, 2007). However, much work remains to be done. There is a clear need to address the 'identity crisis' that is currently bedevilling mental health nurses, and urgent clarification is needed regarding the profession's primary function. Without this, practitioners can feel isolated, adrift on a sea of incessant policies and guidelines, caught up in internecine conflicts brought about by power struggles and 'turf wars' where lines of professional demarcation may be increasingly blurred. Thus, in order to give the best possible service, nurses should endeavour to be free from the demands of over-expanding bureaucracy, endless form-filling, desk-hopping and the myriad quasi-clerical tasks that conceal scarcity of resources (Klein *et al.*, 1996). Moreover, this is not a time for complacency or inertia. To avoid the possible 'slow death of psychiatric nursing' (Holmes, 2006), the profession must ensure its future by proactively and positively embracing contemporary challenges and opportunities. This may mean ensuring its representation and involvement in policy development, both locally and nationally.

The ever-increasing pool of educated, informed and motivated nurses make the time right for consolidation and progress in our professional aims of improving the care we seek to offer service users. We must be prepared to acknowledge and celebrate robust examples of good clinical practice amongst our nursing colleagues, which should be held as beacons to guide the development of all mental health nursing care. This is the springboard from which good practice can spread, and service users' experiences of care can be improved. However, we must nurse in the present with one eye to the future. Indeed, the current pace of change in contemporary mental health care is truly astonishing. As Giuseppe di Lampedusa wrote in *The Leopard* (1958), even 'if we want things to stay as they are, things will have to change'. We must, therefore, be prepared to invest our time and energy in the next generation of mental health nurses – our student nurses – whose enthusiasm, ideals and commitment will be the driving force to shape future mental health nursing care.

References

Abbott, P and Wallace, C (eds) (1990) *The Sociology of the Caring Professions*. Basingstoke: Falmer.

Abrams, RC, Lachs, M, McAvay, G, Keohane, DJ and Bruce, ML (2002) 'Predictors of self-neglect in community-dwelling elders' *The American Journal of Psychiatry* **159**(10): 1724–1730.

Adams, J and Johnson, J (1998) 'Nurses' perceptions of gross self-neglect amongst older people living in the community' *Journal of Clinical Nursing* **7**: 547–552.

Adams, R (1994) *Prison Riots in Britain and the USA*, 2nd edn. Basingstoke: Macmillan.

Agan, RD (1987) 'Intuitive knowing as a dimension of nursing' *Advances in Nursing Science* **10**(1): 63–70.

Aiken, F and Tarbuck, P (1995) 'Practical ethical and legal aspects of caring for the assaultive patient' in Stark, C and Kidd, B (eds) *Management of Violence and Aggression*. London: Gaskell.

Alazewski, A, Manthorpe, J and Walsh, M (1995) 'Risk: the sociological view of perception and management' *Nursing Times* **9**(47): 34–35.

Allebeck, P (1989) 'Schizophrenia: a life shortening disease' *Schizophrenia Bulletin* **15**: 81–89.

Allen, J (1997) 'Assessing and managing risk of violence in the mentally disordered' *Journal of Psychiatric and Mental Health Nursing* **4**: 369–378.

Allison, D and Casey, D (1999) 'Antipsychotic induced weight gain: a comprehensive research synthesis' *The American Journal of Psychiatry* **156**(11): 1686–1696.

Allison, DB, Mackell, JA and Mcdonnell, DD (2003) 'The impact of weight gain on quality of life among persons with schizophrenia' *Psychiatric Services* **54**(4): 565–567.

Almost, J (2006) 'Conflict within nursing work environments: concept analysis' *Journal of Advanced Nursing* **53**(4): 444–453.

Almvik, R and Woods, P (2003) 'Short-term risk prediction: the Bröset violence checklist' *Journal of Psychiatric and Mental Health Nursing* **10**: 231–238.

Alpert, GP and Dunham, RG (2004) *Understanding Police Use of Force: Officers, Suspects and Reciprocity*. New York: Cambridge University Press.

Alt, R (2001) 'A gender in crisis' *WMJ* **100**(3): 8–12, 78.

American Diabetes Association/American Psychiatric Association/American Association of Endocrinologists/North American Association for the Study of Obesity (2004) 'Consensus development conference on antipsychotic drugs and obesity and diabetes' *Diabetes Care* **27**: 596–601.

American Psychiatric Association (APA) (2000) *Diagnostic and Statistical Manual of Mental Disorders*, 4th edn. Washington, DC: APA Publications.

Anderson, IM (2000) 'Selective serotonin reuptake inhibitors versus tricyclic antidepressants: a meta-analysis of efficacy and tolerability' *Journal of Affective Disorders* **58**: 19–36.

Contemporary Issues in Mental Health Nursing, Edited by J. E. Lynch and S. Trenoweth
© 2008 John Wiley & Sons, Ltd

Anderson, M (1983) 'Nursing interventions: what did you do that helped?' *Perspectives in Psychiatric Care* **XXI**: 4–8.

Anderson, R, Funnell, M, Carlson, A, Saleh Statin, N, Cradock, S and Skinner, C (2000) 'Facilitating self care through empowerment' in Snoeck, J and Skinner, TC (eds) *Psychology in Diabetes Care*. London: John Wiley & Sons.

Andresen, R, Oades, L and Caputi, P (2003) 'The experience of recovery from schizophrenia: towards an empirical validated stage model' *Australian and New Zealand Journal of Psychiatry* **37**: 586–594.

Andrews, A and Harlen, W (2006) 'Issues in synthesising research in education' *Educational Research* **48**(3): 287–299.

Anonymous (2006) 'Serious mental illness: a view from within' in Gamble, C and Brennan, G (eds) *Working with Serious Mental Illness: A Manual for Clinical Practice*, 2nd edn. Edinburgh: Elsevier.

Anthony, WA (1993) 'Recovery from mental illness: the guiding vision of the mental health service system in the 1990s' *Psychiatric Rehabilitation Journal* **16**: 11–24.

Appels, A, Bar, FW, Bruggeman, C and De Baets, M (2000) 'Inflammation, depressive symptomatology, and coronary artery disease' *Psychosomatic Medicine* **61**: 378–386.

Arluke, A, Frost, R, Luke, C, Messner, E, Nathanson, J, Patronek, G, Papazian, M and Steketee, G (2002) 'Health implications of animal hoarding' *Health and Social Work* **27**(2): 125–132.

Arthur, D (2007) 'A view of the English Mental Health Nursing Review from the South East Asian Pacific Rim *International Journal of Nursing Studies* **44**: 331–333.

Auciello, P and Foy, D (1998b) 'Trauma and posttraumatic stress disorder in severe mental illness' *Journal of Consulting and Clinical Psychology* **66**: 439–499.

Audit Commission (2001) *A Spoonful of Sugar: Medicines Management in NHS Hospitals*. London: Audit Commission.

Aursnes, I, Tvete, IF, Gaasemyr, J and Natvig, B (2005) 'Suicide attempts in clinical trials with paroxetine randomised against placebo' *BMC Medicine* **3**: 14.

Awad, AG (1992) 'Quality of life of schizophrenic patients on medications and implications for new drug trials' *Hospital and Community Psychiatry* **43**(3): 262–265.

Badger, F and Nolan, P (2007) 'Attributing recovery from depression: perceptions of people cared for in primary care' *Journal of Nursing and Healthcare of Chronic Illness* **16**(3a): 25–34.

Baily, KR (1987) Inter-study differences: how should they influence the interpretation and analysis of results? *Statistics in Medicine* **6**: 351–360.

Baker, C, Beglinger, J, King, S, Salyards, M and Thompson, A (2000) 'Transforming negative work cultures: a practical strategy' *JONA* **30**(7/8): 357–363.

Baldessarini, RJ, Cohen, BM and Teicher, M (1990) 'Pharmacologic treatment' in Levy, ST and Ninan, PT (eds) *Schizophrenia: Treatment of Acute Psychotic Episodes*. Washington, DC: American Psychiatric Press.

Balk, DE (1983) 'Effects of sibling death on teenagers' *Journal of School Health* **53**: 14–18.

Balk, DE (1996) 'Psychological development during four years of bereavement: a longitudinal case study' *Death Studies* **22**(1): 23–42.

Balk, DE and Corr, CA (2001) 'Bereavement during adolescence: a review of research' in Stroebe, MS, Hansson, RO, Stroebe, W and Schut, H (eds) (2001) *Handbook of Bereavement Research, Consequences, Coping and Care*. Washington, DC: American Psychological Association.

Bandura, A (1996) *Social Foundations of Thought and Action: A Social Cognitive Theory*. Englewood Cliffs, NJ: Prentice-Hall.

Bandura, A (1997) 'Toward a unifying theory of behaviour change' *Psychological Review* **84**: 191–215.

Bandura, A (1998) 'Health promotion from the perspective of social cognitive theory' *Psychology and Health* **13**: 623–649.

Banerjee, S, Bingley, W and Murphy, E (1995) *Deaths of Detained Patients: A Review of Reports to the Mental Health Act Commission*. London: Mental Health Foundation.

Banks, S (2001) *Ethics and Values in Social Work*, 2nd edn. Basingstoke: Palgrave (Practical Social Work).

Bannister, D (1983) 'Self in personal construct theory' in Adams-Webber, J and Mancuso, JC (eds) *Applications of Personal Construct Theory*. Ontario: Academic Press.

Bannister, D (2005) 'The logic of passion' in Fransella, F (ed.) *The Essential Practitioner's Handbook of Personal Construct Psychology*. Chichester, John Wiley & Sons.

Bannister, D and Fransella, F (1986) *Inquiring Man: The Psychology of Personal Constructs*, 3rd edn. London: Routledge.

Barker, P (1998) 'Editorial' *Journal of Psychiatric and Mental Health Nursing* **5**: 227.

Barker, P (2001) 'The Tidal Model: developing an empowering, person-centred approach to recovery within psychiatric and mental health nursing' *Journal of Psychiatric and Mental Health Nursing* **8**: 233–240.

Barker, P (2003) 'The Tidal Model: psychiatric colonisation, recovery and the paradigm shift in mental health care' *Journal of Psychiatric and Mental Health Nursing* **12**: 96–102.

Barker, P (2004) *Assessment in Psychiatric and Mental Health Nursing: In Search of the Whole Person*. Cheltenham: Nelson Thornes.

Barker, P and Buchanan-Barker, P (2004) 'Caring as a craft' *Nursing Standard* **19**(9): 17–18.

Barker, P and Buchanan-Barker, P (2005) 'Still invisible after all these years: mental health nursing on the margins' *Journal of Psychiatric and Mental Health Nursing* **12**: 252–256.

Barker, P and Stevenson, C (2000) *The Construction of Power and Authority in Psychiatry*. Oxford: Butterworth-Heinemann.

Barker, P, Jackson, S and Stevenson, C (1998) 'The need for psychiatric nursing: towards a multidimensional theory of caring' *Nursing Inquiry* **6**: 103–111.

Barker, P, Jackson, S and Stevenson, C (1999) 'What are psychiatric nurses needed for? Developing a theory of essential nursing practice' *Journal of Psychiatric and Mental Health Nursing* **6**: 273–282.

Barker, P, Reynolds, W and Stevenson, C (1997) 'The human science basis of psychiatric nursing: theory and practice' *Journal of Advanced Nursing* **25**(4): 660–667.

Barlow, JH, Ellard, DR, Hainsworth, JM, Jones, FR and Fisher, A (2005) 'A review of self-management interventions for panic disorders, phobias and obsessive-compulsive disorders' *Acta Psychiatrica Scandinavica* **111**: 272–285.

Baron, RA and Richardson, DR (1994) *Human Aggression*, 2nd edn. New York: Plenum Press.

Barratt, E (1994) 'Impulsiveness and aggression' in Monahan, J and Steadman, H (eds) *Violence and Mental Disorder: Developments in Risk Assessment*. Chicago: University of Chicago Press.

Bartels, SJ, Drake, RE and Wallace, MA (1995) 'Long-term course of substance use disorders among patients with severe mental illness' *Psychiatric Services* **46**: 248–251.

Bartlett, P and Sandland, R (2003) *Mental Health Law: Policy and Practice*, 2nd edn. Oxford: Oxford University Press.

Barton, R (1976) *Institutional Neurosis*. Bristol: John Wright and Sons.

Basky, G (2000) 'Does religion speed recovery in mental illness?' *Canadian Medical Association Journal* **163**: 1497.

Bassman, R (2000) 'Agents, not objects: our fights to be' *Journal of Clinical Psychology/In Session* **56**: 1395–1411.

Bateman, AW and Tyrer, P (2004) 'Services for personality disorder: organisation for inclusion' *Advances in Psychiatric Treatment* **10**: 425–433.

Battersby, MW (2004) 'Community models of mental care warrant governmental support' *British Medical Journal* **329**(7475): 1140–1141.

Baumeister, RF (1999) *Evil: Inside Human Violence and Cruelty*. New York: WH Freeman & Co.

BBC (2004) Health toll of anti-gay prejudice [on-line]. Available at: http://news.bbc.co.uk/1/hi/health/4055801.stm

Beck, A (1976) *Cognitive Therapy and the Emotional Disorders*. New York: International University Press.

Beck, A, Freeman, A & Associates (1990) *Cognitive Therapy of Personality Disorders*. New York: Guilford.

Beck, U (1992; first published in German, 1986) *Risk Society: Towards a New Modernity* (translated by Mark Ritter). London: SAGE.

Beech, I (1998) 'What future for research in mental health nursing – rediscovering the Yin' *Journal of Psychiatric and Mental Health Nursing* **5**: 234–235.

Beech, P and Norman, I (1995) 'Patients' perceptions of the quality of psychiatric nursing care: findings from a small-scale descriptive study' *Journal of Clinical Nursing* **4**(2): 117–123.

Benner, P (1984) *From Novice to Expert: Excellence and Power in Clinical Nursing Practice*. Menlo Park, CA: Addison-Wesley.

Benner, P and Tanner, C (1987) 'How expert nurses use intuition' *American Journal of Nursing* **Jan**: 23–31.

Bennett, G and Jones, R (2006) 'Men, masculinity and mental health' *Issues in Mental Health Nursing* **27**: 333–336.

Bennett, J, Done, J and Hunt, B (1995a) 'Assessing the side effects of antipsychotic drugs: a survey of CPN practice' *Journal of Psychiatric and Mental Health Nursing* **2**: 177–182.

Bennett, J, Done, J, Harrison-Read, P and Hunt, B (1995b) 'Development of a rating scale/checklist to assess the side effects of antipsychotics by community psychiatric nurses' in Brooker, C and White, E (eds) *Community Psychiatric Nursing: A Research Perspective*, Vol. 3. London: Chapman and Hall.

Bentall, R (2003) *Madness Explained: Psychosis and Human Nature*. London: Penguin.

Benton, D and Donohoe, RT (1999) 'The effects of nutrients on mood' *Public Health Nutrition* **2**: 403–409.

Beresford, P (2005) 'A new day' *Openmind* **May/Jun**: 133.

Beresford, P and Beales, A (2005) 'We did it our way' *Openmind* **Nov/Dec**: 136.

Berren, MR, Santiago, JM, Zent, MR and Carbone, CP (1999) 'Health care utilization by persons with severe and persistent mental illness' *Psychiatric Services* **50**(4): 559–561.

Bertalanffy, IV (1973) *General Systems Theory*. Harmondsworth: Penguin.

Bertram, G and Stickley, T (2005) 'Mental health nurses: promoters of inclusion or perpetrators of exclusion?' *Journal of Psychiatric and Mental Health Nursing* **12**: 387–395.

Bertram, M (2005) 'Reforms, rights or wrongs? A Foucauldian exploration of the new Mental Health Bill in the United Kingdom' *International Journal of Sociology and Social Policy* **25**(12): 1–21.

Bevan, M (1998) 'Nursing in the dialysis unit: technological enframing and a declining art, or an imperative for caring?' *Journal of Advanced Nursing* **27**: 730–736.

Bhui, K, Stansfeld, S, Hull, S, Priebe, S, Mole, F and Feder, G (2003) 'Ethnic variations in the pathways to and use of specialist services in the UK: systematic review' *British Journal of Psychiatry* **182**: 105–116.

Black, D (1996) 'Childhood bereavement' *British Medical Journal* **312**(7045): 1496.

Black, DW, Goldstein, RB, Nasrallah, A and Winokur, G (1991) 'The prediction of recovery using a multivariate model in 1471 depressed inpatients' *European Archives of Psychiatry and Clinical Neuroscience* **241**: 41–45.

Blofeld, J (Chair) (2004) *Independent Inquiry into the Death of David Bennett*. Cambridge: Norfolk, Suffolk and Cambridgeshire Strategic Health Authority.

Blom-Cooper, L, Hally, H and Murphy, E (1995) *The Falling Shadow: One's Patient's Mental Health Care 1978–1993*. London, Duckworth.

Bodenheimer, T, Lorig, K, Holman, HR and Grumbach, K (2002) 'Patient self management of chronic disease in primary care' *Journal of the American Medical Association* **288**: 2469–2475.

Boettcher, EG (1983) 'Preventing violent behaviour: an integrated theoretical model for nursing' *Perspectives in Psychiatric Care* **XXI**: 54–58.

Bonner, G (2007) *Examination of the Aftermath of Restraint in UK Mental Health Settings*. Unpublished PhD thesis. London: Thames Valley University.

Bonner, G and Wellman, N (2007) Examining the Aftermath of Restraint in UK Acute Mental Health Settings – Evaluation of the Thames Valley University (TVU) Post Incident Review Framework: The Experience of Hospital Staff.

Bonner, G, Lowe, T, Rawcliffe, D and Wellman, N (2002) 'Trauma for all: a pilot study of the subjective experience of physical restraint for mental health inpatients and staff in the UK' *Journal of Psychiatric and Mental Health Nursing* **9**(4): 465–473.

Boseley, S (1999) 'Risk of helping children to grieve' *The Guardian* 10th May, p. 8.

Bott, E (1976) 'Hospital and society' *British Journal of Medical Psychology* **49**: 97–140.

Bott-Spillius, E (1990) 'Asylum and society' in Trist, E and Murray, H (eds) *The Social Engagement of Social Science*, Vol. 1. London: Free Association Books.

Bourner, T (1996) 'The research process: four steps to success' in Greenfield, T (ed) *Research Methods: Guidance for Postgraduates*. London: Arnold.

Bowers, L (2005) 'Reasons for admission and their implications for the nature of acute inpatient psychiatric nursing' *Journal of Psychiatric and Mental Health Nursing* **12**(2): 231–236.

Bowers, L, Alexander, J, Simpson, A, Ryan, C and Carr-Walker, P (2007a) 'Student psychiatric nurses' approval of containment measures: relationship to perception of aggression and attitudes to personality disorder' *International Journal of Nursing Studies* **44**: 349–356.

Bowers, L, Allan, T, Simpson, A, Nijman, H and Warren, J (2007c) 'Adverse incidents, patient flow, and nursing workforce variables on acute psychiatric wards: the Topkins Acute Ward Study' *International Journal of Social Psychiatry* **53**(1): 75–84.

Bowers, L, van der Werf, B, Vokkolainen, A, Muir-Cochrane, E, Allan, T and Alexander, J (2007b) 'International variation in containment measures for disturbed psychiatric inpatients: a comparative questionnaire survey' *International Journal of Nursing Studies* **44**: 357–364.

Bowles, N and Jones, A (2005) 'Whole systems working and acute inpatient psychiatry: an exploratory study' *Journal of Psychiatric and Mental Health Nursing* **12**: 283–289.

Bowling, B and Phillips, C (2002) *Racism, Crime and Justice*. Harlow: Pearson/Longman.

Box, S (1989) *Power, Crime and Mystification*, 2nd edn. London: Routledge.

Box, S and Russell, K (1975) 'The politics of discredibility: disarming complaints against the police' *Sociological Review* **23**: 325–349.

Bracken, P and Thomas, P (2005) *Postpsychiatry: Mental Health in a Postmodern World*. Oxford: Oxford University Press.

Bradley, EH, Bogardus, ST, Tinetti, ME and Inouye, SK (1999) 'Goal setting in clinical medicine' *Social Science and Medicine* **49**: 267–278.

Brase-Smith, S (1995) 'Restraints: retraumatization for rape victims?' *Journal of Psychosocial Nursing* **3**(7).

Bray, J (1999) 'An ethnographic study of psychiatric nursing' *Journal of Psychiatric and Mental Health Nursing* **6**: 297–305.

Brennan, G (2006) 'Stress vulnerability model of serious mental illness' in Gamble, C and Brennan, G (eds) *Working with Serious Mental Illness: A Manual for Clinical Practice*, 2nd edn. London: Elsevier.

Brewin, C, Rose, S, Andrews, B, Green, J, Tata, P, McEvedy, C, Turner, S and Foa, E (2002) 'Brief screening instrument for post-traumatic stress disorder' *British Journal of Psychiatry* **181**: 158–162.

Brimblecombe, N (2005) 'The changing relationship between mental health nurses and pychiatrists in the United Kingdom' *Journal of Advanced Nursing* **49**(4): 344–353.

Brimblecombe, N, Tingle, A, Tunmore, R and Murrell, T (2007) 'Implementing holistic practices in mental health nursing: a national consultation' *International Journal of Nursing Studies* **44**: 339–348.

Bristow, M, Kohen, D and O'Mahony, G (2001) 'Effects of social and behavioural factors in acute psychiatric admissions: a comparison between inner and outer London' *Journal of Mental Health* **10**(1): 109–113.

British Medical Association (BMA) (2003) *Adolescent Health*. London: British Medical Association. Available at: http://www.bma.org.uk/ap.nsf/AttachmentsByTitle/PDFAdolescentHealth/$FILE/Adhealth.pdf

British Medical Association (BMA) (2006) *Child and Adolescent Mental Health, A Guide for Healthcare Professionals*. London: British Medical Association. Available at: http://www.bma.org.uk/ap.nsf/AttachmentsByTitle/PDFChildAdolescentMentalHealth/$FILE/ChildAdolescentMentalHealth.pdf

Brooker, C (2007) 'The Chief Nursing Officer's Review of Mental Health Nursing in England: an ode to "Motherhood and Apple Pie"?' *International Journal of Nursing Studies* **44**: 327–330.

Brookes (1988) *Control and restraint techniques: A study into effectiveness at HMP Gartree*. DPS Report, Series II, No. 156. London: Home Office.

Brookman, F (2005) *Understanding Homicide*. London: SAGE.

Brown, J (2006) 'Young people and bereavement counselling: what influences the decision to access professional help?' *Bereavement Care* **25**(1): 3–6.

Brown, J, Kitson, A and McKnight, T (1992) 'Caring and being cared for' in Brown, J, Kitson, A and McKnight, T (eds) *Challenges in Caring – Exploration in Nursing and Ethics*. London: Chapman and Hall.

Brown, RI (1986) *Management and Administration in Rehabilitation Programmes*. San Diego: College-Hill.

Brown, S, Birtwistle, J, Roe, L and Thompson, C (1999) 'The unhealthy lifestyle of people with schizophrenia' *Psychological Medicine* **29**(3): 697–701.

Brownlee, S, Leventhal, H and Leventhal, EA (2000) 'Regulation, self regulation and construction of the self in the maintenance of physical health' in Boekartz, M, Pintrich, PR and Zeidner, M (eds) *Handbook of Self Regulation*. San Diego: Academic Press.

Bruce, MA, Roscigno, VJ and McCall, PL (1998) 'Structure, context, and agency in the reproduction of black-on-black violence' *Theoretical Criminology* **2**(1): 29–55.

Buber, M (1923/2004) *I and Thou*. New York: Continuum Publishing.

Buchanan-Barker, P (2004) 'The Tidal Model: uncommon sense' *Mental Health Nursing* **24**: 6–10.

Buchanan-Barker, P and Barker, P (2005) 'Observation: the original sin of mental health nursing? *Journal of Psychiatric and Mental Health Nursing* **12**: 541–549.

Buckenham, M (1998) 'Socialisation and personal change: a personal construct psychology approach' *Journal of Advanced Nursing* **28**(4): 874–881.

Bulman, C and Schutz, S (eds) (2004) *Reflective Practice in Nursing*, 3rd edn. Oxford: Blackwell.

Burke, D, Herman, H, Evans, M, Cockram, A and Trauer, T (2000) 'Educational aims and objectives for working in multidisciplinary teams' *Australasian Psychiatry* **8**(4): 336.

Burke, L (2003) 'Integration into higher education: key implementers' views on why nurse education moved into higher education' *Journal of Advanced Nursing* **42**(4): 382–389.

Burnard, P (1989) 'The "sixth" sense' *Nursing Times* **85**(50): 52–53.

Burnard, P and Hannigan, B (2000) 'Qualitative and quantitative approaches in mental health nursing: moving the debate forward' *Journal of Psychiatric and Mental Health Nursing* **7**: 1–6.

Burr, J and Chapman, T (1998) 'Some reflections on cultural and social considerations in mental health nursing' *Journal of Psychiatric and Mental Health Nursing* **5**: 431–437.

Burr, V and Butt, T (1992) *Invitation to Personal Construct Psychology*. London: Whurr.

Bury, M (1998) 'Postmodernity and health' in Scambler, G and Higgs, P (eds) *Modernity, Medicine and Health: Medical Sociology Towards 2000*. London: Routledge.

Butler, M and Drake, DH (2007) 'Reconsidering respect: its role in Her Majesty's Prison Service' *The Howard Journal* **46**(2): 115–127.

Butterworth, T (1994) 'Working in partnership: a collaborative approach to care: the review of mental health nursing' *Journal of Psychiatric and Mental Health Nursing* **1**: 41–44.

Butterworth, T, Studdy, S, Martin, E, Glen, S and James, V (1999) 'Higher education broadens nursing opportunities' *Nursing Standard* **13**(19): 10.

Byrne, P. (2001) 'Psychiatric stigma' *British Journal of Psychiatry* **178**: 281–284.

Caldwell, M (1992) 'Incidence of PTSD among staff victims of patient violence' *Hospital and Community Psychiatry* **43**: 838–839.

Callaghan, P and Owen, S (2005) 'Editorial – Psychiatric and mental health nursing: past, present and future' *Journal of Psychiatric and Mental Health Nursing* **12**: 639–641.

Cameron, D, Kapur, R and Campbell, P (2005) 'Releasing the therapeutic potential of the psychiatric nurse: a human relations perspective of the nurse–patient relationship' *Journal of Psychiatric and Mental Health Nursing* **12**: 64–74.

Campbell, K, Twenge, J, Clementz, B, McDowell, J, Krusemark, E, Dyckman, K and Brunnell, A (2006) 'Social exclusion and poor decision making' *Social Neuroscience* [on-line journal]. Available at: http://www.mentalhealth.org.uk

Campbell, P (1996a) 'The history of the user movement in the UK' in Heller, T *et al.* (eds) *Mental Health Matters: A Reader*. Basingstoke: Macmillan.

Campbell, P (1996b) 'Working with service users' in Sandford, T and Gournay, K (eds) *Perspectives in Mental Health Nursing*. London: Bailliere Tindall.

Campbell, P (1999) 'The service user/survivor movement' in Newnes, C, Holmes, G and Dunn, C (eds) *This is Madness: A Critical Look at the Future of Mental Health Services*. Ross-on-Wye: PCCS Books.

Campbell, P (2005) 'From little acorns – the mental health service user movement' in Bell, A and Lindley, P (eds) *Beyond the Water Towers: The unfinished revolution in mental health services 1985–2005*. London: Sainsbury Centre for Mental Health.

Canetto, S and Sakinofsky, I (1998) 'The gender paradox in suicide' *Suicide and Life-Threatening Behaviour* **28**(1): 1–23.

Card, R (2006) *Card, Cross and Jones Criminal Law*, 17th edn. Oxford: Oxford University Press.

Care Services Improvement Partnership/National Institute for Mental Health in England (CSIP/NIMHE) (2006) *Our Choices in Mental Health: A Framework for Improving Choice for*

People Who Use Mental Health Services and Their Carers. Available at: http://www.csip-plus. org.uk/CPT/Our%20Choices%20Doc%20-%20Final.pdf

Carper, B (1978) 'Fundamental patterns of knowing in nursing' *Advances in Nursing Science* **1**(1): 1–23.

Carr, A (ed.) (2000) *What Works with Children and Adolescents? A Critical Review of Psychological Interventions with Children, Adolescents and their Families.* London: Routledge.

Carter, S, Garside, P and Black, A (2003) 'Multidisciplinary team working, clinical networks and chambers: opportunities to work differently in the NHS' *Quality and Safety in Health Care* **12**: 25–28.

Cascardi, M, Mueser, K, DeGiralomo, J and Murring, M (1996) 'Physical aggression against psychiatric inpatients by family members and partners' *Psychiatric Services* **47**(5): 531–533.

Casey, DE, Haupt, DW, Newcomer, JW, Henderson, DC, Sernyak, MJ, Davidson, M, Lindenmayer, JP, Manoukian, SV, Banerji, MA, Lebovitz, HE and Hennekens, CH (2004) 'Anti-psychotic induced weight gain and metabolic abnormalities: implications for increased mortality in patients with schizophrenia' *Journal of Clinical Psychiatry* **65**(Suppl 7): 257–269.

CASP (2006) *Critical Appraisal Tools.* Public Oxford: Health Resource Unit. Available at: http://www.phru.nhs.uk/casp/critical_appraisal_tools.htm

Cater, S and Coleman, J (2006) *Adolescent Health Provision: Factors Facilitating the Provision of Young People's Health Services.* A Report for the Department of Health, Brighton, Trust for the Study of Adolescence. Available at: http://www.studyofadolescence.org.uk/_assets/doc/ Report.doc

Cavadino, M and Dignan, J (2002) *The Penal System: An Introduction*, 3rd edn. London: SAGE.

Chamberlin, J (1998) 'Citizenship, rights and psychiatric disability' *Psychiatric Rehabilitation Journal* **21**: 405–408.

Chamberlin, J (2001) 'Equal rights, not public relations' *World Psychiatric Association Conference 'Together Against Stigma'*, Leipzig, September 2001.

Chambers, M (1998) 'Interpersonal mental health nursing: research issues and challenges' *Journal of Psychiatric and Mental Health Nursing* **5**: 203–211.

Chan, A, Graves, V and Shea, TB (2006) 'Apple juice concentrate maintains acetylcholine levels following dietary compromise' *Journal of Alzheimer's Disease* **9**: 287–291.

Chan, P and Rudman, M (1998) 'Paradigms for mental health nursing: fragmentation or integration?' *Journal of Psychiatric and Mental Health Nursing* **5**: 143–146.

Chen, J (1999) '"Medication concordance" is best helped by improving consultation skills' *British Medical Journal* **March**(318): 670.

Children's Society (2006) *The Good Childhood, A National Inquiry.* Launch Report. London: The Children's Society. Available at: http://www.childrenssociety.org.uk/NR/rdonlyres/ 7A2AF2ED-B8BE-40C1-9FA2-DB88C28ACC81/0/TGCILaunchReportSeptember 2006NEW.pdf

Chin, C (1998) 'Dangerousness: myth or reality?' *Psychiatric Care* **5**(2): 66–71.

Choongh, S (1997) *Policing as Social Discipline.* Oxford: Clarendon Press.

Citrome, L and Yeomans, D (2005) 'Do guidelines for severe mental illness promote physical health and well-being?' *Journal of Psychopharmacology* **19**(6): 102–109.

Clarke, ANG, Manikar, GO and Gray, I (1975) 'Diogenes syndrome: a clinical study of gross neglect in old age' *The Lancet* **1**: 338–366.

Clarke, L (1999a) *Challenging Ideas in Psychiatric Nursing.* London: Routledge.

Clarke, L (1999b) 'Darkness visible' *Nursing Times* **95**(36): 36–37.

Clay, J (1996) *R.D. Laing: A Divided Self.* London: Hodder and Stoughton.

Clay, T (1987) *Nurses – Power and Politics.* London: Heinemann Nursing.

Cleary, M (2004) 'The realities of mental health nursing in acute inpatient environments' *International Journal of Mental Health Nursing* **13**: 53–60.

Cleary, M and Edwards, C (1999) 'Something always comes up: nurse–patient interaction in an acute psychiatric setting' *Journal of Psychiatric and Mental Health Nursing* **6**: 469–477.

Clulow, C (1994) 'Balancing care and control: the supervisory relationship as a focus for promoting organisational health' in Obholzer, A and Roberts, V (eds) *The Unconscious at Work: Individual and Organisational Stress in the Human Services.* London: Routledge.

Cobb, A (1993) *Safe and Effective? MIND's Views on Psychiatric Drugs, ECT and Psychosurgery.* London: MIND.

Cohen, A and Hove, M (2001) *Physical Health of the Severe and Enduring Mentally Ill: A Training Pack for GP Educators.* Available at: http://www.scmh.org.uk/80256FBD004F6342/vWeb/wpKHAL6G7K9Z

Cohen, A and Phelan, M (2001) 'The physical health of patients with mental illness: a neglected area' *Mental Health Promotion Update* **2**: 15–16.

Cohen, D and Prusak, L (2001) *In Good Company: How Social Capital Makes Organisations Work.* Boston: Harvard Business School Press.

Cohen, O (2005) 'How do we recover? An analysis of psychiatric survivor oral histories' *Journal of Humanistic Psychology* **45**: 333–354.

Cohen, S (2001) *States of Denial: Knowing About Atrocities and Suffering.* Cambridge: Polity.

Cohen, S and Rodriguez, MS (1995) 'Pathways linking affective disturbances and physical disorders' *Health Psychology* **14**(5): 374–380.

Coid, J, Petruckevitch, A, Wai-Shan, C, Richardson, J, Moorey, S and Feder, G (2003) 'Abusive experiences and psychiatric morbidity in women primary care attenders' *British Journal of Psychiatry* **183**: 332–339.

Coleman, JC and Hendry, LB (1999) *The Nature of Adolescence*, 3rd edn. London: Routledge.

Coleman, M and Jenkins, E (1998) 'Developments in mental health nursing: a critical voice' *Journal of Psychiatric and Mental Health Nursing* **5**: 355–359.

Collins, S and Cutcliffe, J (2003) 'Addressing hopelessness in people with suicidal ideation: building upon the therapeutic relationship utilizing a cognitive behavioural approach' *Journal of Psychiatric and Mental Health Nursing* **10**: 175–185.

Collins, S and Long, A (2003) 'Too tired to care? The psychological effects of working with trauma' *Journal of Psychiatric and Mental Health Nursing* **10**: 17–27.

Commission for Healthcare Audit and Inspection (2006) *A Review of Healthcare in the Community for Young People who Offend.* London: Commission for Healthcare Audit and Inspection.

Connell, RW (1995) *Masculinities.* Berkeley, CA: University of California Press.

Connolly, M and Kelly, C (2005) 'Lifestyle and physical health in schizophrenia' *Advances in Psychiatric Treatment* **11**: 125–132.

Connor, SL and Wilson, R (2006) 'It's important that they learn from us for mental health to progress' *Journal of Mental Health* **15**(4): 461–474.

Conroy, J (2001) *Unspeakable Acts, Ordinary People: The Dynamics of Torture.* London: Vision.

Coodin-Schiff, A (2004) 'Recovery and mental illness: analysis and personal reflections' *Psychiatric Rehabilitation Journal* **27**: 212–218.

Cook, AS (1995) 'Ethical issues in bereavement research' *Death Studies* **19**: 103–122.

Cook, AS (2001) 'The dynamics of ethical decision making in bereavement research' in Stroebe, MS, Hansson, RO, Stroebe, W and Schut, H (eds) *Handbook of Bereavement Research, Consequences, Coping and Care.* Washington, DC: American Psychological Association.

Cooney, C and Hamid, W (1995) 'Review: Diogenes syndrome' *Age and Aging* **24**(5): 451–453.

Cordess, C (2000) 'A forensic psychiatry perspective' in Robinson, D and Kettle, A (eds) *Forensic Nursing and Multidisciplinary Care of the Mentally Disordered Offender*. London: Jessica Kingsley.

Cordwell, JS and Farr, C (2007) *The Psychoeducational Approach: An Evaluation of Intervention Efficacy with Severe Personality Disorder*. West London Mental Health NHS Trust. DSPD Service Evaluation Report. Unpublished.

Cordwell, JS, Farr, C and Bradley, L (2004) *Psychoeducation Programme for Personality Disorders: DSPD Programme Manual*. West London Mental Health NHS Trust. Unpublished.

Cormack, I, Martin, D and Ferriter, M (2004) 'Improving the physical health of long stay psychiatric in-patients' *Advances in Psychiatric Treatment* **10**: 107–115.

Corr, CA and Balk, DE (eds) (1996) *Handbook of Adolescent Death and Bereavement*. New York: Springer Publishing Company.

Corr, CA and McNeil, JN (eds) (1986) *Adolescence and Death*. New York: Springer Publishing Company.

Corrigan, PW (2000) 'Mental health stigma as social attribution: implications for research methods and attitude change' *Clinical Psychology: Science and Practice* **7**: 48–67.

Corrigan, PW (2005) *On the Stigma of Mental Illness: Practical Strategies for Research and Social Change*. Washington, DC: American Psychological Association.

Corrigan, PW and Lundin, KR (2001) *Don't Call Me Nuts. Coping with the Stigma of Mental Illness*. University of Chicago: Recovery Press.

Corrigan, PW and Phelan, SM (2004) 'Social support and recovery in people with serious mental illnesses' *Community Mental Health Journal* **40**: 513–523.

Coulter, A (1997) 'Partnerships with patients: the pros and cons of shared clinical decision-making' *Journal of Health Services Research Policy* **2**(2): 112–121.

Courtenay, W (2000) 'Constructions of masculinity and their influence on men's well-being: a theory of gender and health' *Social Science & Medicine* **50**: 1385–1401.

Cowman, S, Farelly, M and Gilheany, P (2001) 'An examination of the role and function of psychiatric nurses in clinical practice in Ireland' *Journal of Advanced Nursing* **34**(6): 745–753.

Crabtree, BF and Miller, WL (1999) *Doing Qualitative Research*. Thousand Oaks: Sage.

Craine, L, Henson, C and MacLean, D (1988) 'Prevalence of a history of sexual abuse among female psychiatric patients in a state hospital system' *Hospital and Community Psychiatry* **39**(3): 300–304.

Crichton, J (1995) 'The response to psychiatric inpatient violence' in Crichton, J (ed.) *Psychiatric Patient Violence: Risk and Response*. London: Duckworth.

Crisp, H, Rix, M, Meltzer, I and Rowlands, J (2000) 'Stigmatisation of people with mental illness' *British Journal of Psychiatry* **177**: 4–7.

Cross, S (2002) *'I Can't Stop Feeling Sad': Calls to Childline about Bereavement*. London: Childline.

Crossley, N (1999) 'Fish, field, habitus and madness: the first wave mental health users movement in Great Britain' *British Journal of Sociology* **50**(4): 647–670.

Crowe, M and Carlyle, D (2003) 'Deconstructing risk assessment and management in mental health nursing' *Journal of Advanced Nursing* **43**(1): 19–27.

Cruse Bereavement Care (2004) *After Someone Dies: A Leaflet about Death, Bereavement and Grief for Young People*. Richmond: Cruse Bereavement Care.

Cunningham, K, Wolbert, R, Graziano, A and Slocum, J (2005) 'Acceptance and change: the dialectic of recovery' *Psychiatric Rehabilitation Journal* **29**: 146–148.

Curran, C, Grimshaw, C and Deery, A (2006) 'Government proposals to close the Bourne-wood gap' *Open Mind* **142**: 24–25.

Curran, J and Brooker, C (2007) 'Systematic review of interventions delivered by UK mental health nurses' *International Journal of Nursing Studies* **44**: 479–509.

Cutcheon, H and Pincombe, J (2001) 'Intuition: an important tool in the practice of nursing' *Journal of Advanced Nursing* **35**(5): 342–348.

Cutcliffe, J (2003) 'Assessing risk of suicide and self-harm' in Barker, P (ed.) *Psychiatric and Mental Health Nursing: The Craft of Caring.* London: Arnold.

Cutcliffe, J and Barker, P (2004) 'The nurses' global assessment of suicide risk (NGASR): developing a tool for clinical practice' *Journal of Psychiatric and Mental Health Nursing* **11**: 393–400.

Cutcliffe, JR and Hannigan, B (2001) 'Mass media monsters and mental health clients: the need for increased lobbying' *Journal of Psychiatric and Mental Health Nursing* **8**: 315–321.

Cutcliffe, JR and Koehn, CV (2007) 'Hope and interpersonal psychiatric/mental health nursing: a systematic review of the literature – Part two' *Journal of Psychiatric and Mental Health Nursing* **14**: 141–147.

D'Silva, K and Duggan, C (2002) 'Service innovations: development of a psychoeducational programme for patients with personality disorder' *Psychiatric Bulletin* **26**: 268–271.

D'Zurilla, T and Goldfried, M (1971) 'Problem solving and behaviour modification' *Journal of Abnormal Psychology* 107–126.

Daisy's Dream (2002) *The Bereaved Child in School: Information to Help Schools Support a Child or Young Person who has Experienced the Death of Someone Significant to them.* Reading: Daisy's Dream.

Dale, C, O'Hare, G and Rae, M (2006) *A Report on the NIMHE/NPSA Project on the Prevention and Management of Aggression and Violence in Mental-Health Services.* Final Report. Available at: http://www.nimhe.csip.org.uk/silo/files/project-report-with-contents1pdf.pdf

Daley, AJ (2002) 'Exercise therapy and mental health in clinical populations: is exercise therapy a worthwhile intervention?' *Advances in Psychiatric Treatment* **8**: 262–270.

Damecour, C and Charron, M (1998) 'Hoarding: a symptom, not a syndrome' *Journal of Clinical Psychiatry* **59**: 267–272.

Daniel, B and Wassell, S (2002) *Adolescence, Assessing and Promoting Resilience in Vulnerable.* London: Jessica Kingsley.

Davidson, K (2000) *Cognitive Therapy for Personality Disorders: A Guide for Clinicians.* Oxford: Butterworth-Heinemann.

Davidson, L (2005) 'Recovery, self management and the expert patient – changing the culture of mental health from a UK perspective' *Journal of Mental Health* **14**(1): 25–35.

Davis, H (2003) *Human Rights and Civil Liberties.* Cullompton, Devon: Willan.

Davis, JM, Barter, JT and Kane, JM (1989) 'Antipsychotic drugs' in Kaplan, HI and Sadock, BJ (eds) *Comprehensive Textbook of Psychiatry Vol. 5.* Baltimore, MD: Williams and Wilkms.

Davison, S (1997) 'Risk assessment and management – a busy practitioner's perspective' *International Review of Psychiatry* **9**: 201–206.

Day, JC, Wood, G, Dewey, M and Bentall, RP (1995) 'A self-rating scale or measuring neuroleptic side-effects: validation in a group of schizophrenic patients' *British Journal of Psychiatry* **166**: 650–653.

De Groot, L, Lloyd, C and King, R (2003) 'An evaluation of a family psychoeducation programme in community mental health' *Psychiatric Rehabilitation Journal* **27**(1): 18–23.

Dean, J, Todd, G, Morrow, H and Sheldon, K (2001) '"Mum, I used to be good looking . . . look at me now": the physical health needs of adults with mental health problems: the perspectives of users, carers and front-line staff' *International Journal of Mental Health Promotion* **3**(4): 16–24.

Deegan, P (1993) 'Recovering our sense of value after being labelled mentally ill' *Journal of Psychosocial Nursing and Mental Health Services* **31**: 7–11.

Deegan, P (2001) 'Recovery as a self-directed process of healing and transformation' *Occupational Therapy in Mental Health: A Journal of Psychosocial Practice and Research* **17**: 5–21.

Department for Constitutional Affairs (2007) *Mental Capacity Act 2005. Code of Practice (2007 Final Edition)*. London: The Stationery Office.

Department of Health (DH) (1990) *Caring for People. The Care Programme Approach for People with a Mental Illness Referred to Specialist Mental Health Service*. London: HMSO.

Department of Health (DH) (1994a) *Working in Partnership: A Collaborative Approach to Care (Report of the Mental Health Nursing Review Team)*. London: HMSO.

Department of Health (DH) (1994b) *Nutritional Aspects of Cardiovascular Disease*. London: HMSO.

Department of Health (DH) (1997a) *The New NHS – Modern, Dependable*. London: HMSO.

Department of Health (DH) (1997b) *Health Committee Third Report, Health Services for Children and Young People in the Community; Home and School*. London: HMSO.

Department of Health (DH) (1998a) *A First Class Service: Quality in the New NHS*. Available at: www.dh.gov.uk/en/Publicationsandstatistics/Publications/PublicationsPolicyAndGuidance/DH_4006902

Department of Health (DH) (1998b) *Modernising Mental Health Services: Safe, Sound and Supportive*. Available at: http://www.dh.gov.uk/en/Publicationsandstatistics/Publications/PublicationsPolicyAndGuidance/DH_4003105

Department of Health (DH) (1998c) *Smoking Kills: Executive Summary* [on-line]. Available at: http://www.dh.gov.uk/en/Publicationsandstatistics/Publications/PublicationsPolicyAndGuidance/DH_4008708

Department of Health (DH) (1999a) *National Service Framework for Mental Health: Modern Standards and Service Models*. Available at: http://www.dh.gov.uk/en/Publicationsandstatistics/Publications/PublicationsPolicyAndGuidance/DH_4009598

Department of Health (DH) (1999b) *Making a Difference: Strengthening the Nursing, Midwifery and Health Visiting Contribution to Health and Healthcare*. Available at: http://www.dh.gov.uk/en/Publicationsandstatistics/Publications/PublicationsPolicyAndGuidance/DH_4007977

Department of Health (DH) (1999c) *Effective Care Co-ordination in Mental Health Services: A Policy Booklet Modernising the Care Programme Approach*. Available at: http://www.dh.gov.uk/en/Publicationsandstatistics/Publications/PublicationsPolicyAndGuidance/DH_4009221

Department of Health (DH) (1999d) *Independent Inquiry into Inequalities in Health (Chair: Sir Donald Acheson)*. London: HMSO.

Department of Health (DH) (1999e) *Clinical Governance: Quality in the New NHS*. HSC 1999/065. London: HMSO.

Department of Health (DH) (2000a) *The NHS Plan: A Plan for Investment, a Plan for Reform*. Available at: http://www.dh.gov.uk/en/Publicationsandstatistics/Publications/PublicationsPolicyAndGuidance/DH_4002960

Department of Health (DH) (2000b) *NHS Plan Implementation Programme* [on-line]. Available at: http://www.dh.gov.uk/en/Publicationsandstatistics/Publications/PublicationsPolicyAndGuidance/DH_4002690

Department of Health (DH) (2001a) *The Journey to Recovery: The Government's Vision for Mental Health Care*. Available at: http://www.dh.gov.uk/en/Publicationsandstatistics/Publications/PublicationsPolicyAndGuidance/DH_4002700

Department of Health (DH) (2001b) *The Expert Patient: A New Approach to Chronic Disease Management for the 21st Century*. Available at: http://www.dh.gov.uk/en/Publicationsandstatistics/Publications/PublicationsPolicyAndGuidance/DH_4006801

Department of Health (DH) (2001c) *Safety First: Five Year Report of the National Confidential Inquiry into Suicides and Homicides by People with Mental Illness.* London: HMSO.

Department of Health (DH) (2001d) *Making it Happen: A Guide to Delivering Mental Health Promotion* [on-line]. Available at: http://www.dh.gov.uk/en/Publicationsandstatistics/ Publications/PublicationsPolicyAndGuidance/DH_4007907

Department of Health (DH) (2002a) *Mental Health Policy Implementation Guide: Dual Diagnosis Good Practice Guide* [on-line]. Available at: http://www.dh.gov.uk/en/Publicationsandstatistics/ Publications/PublicationsPolicyAndGuidance/DH_4009058

Department of Health (DH) (2002b) *National Suicide Prevention Strategy for England.* Available at: http://www.dh.gov.uk/en/Publicationsandstatistics/Publications/PublicationsPolicyAnd Guidance/DH_4009474

Department of Health (DH) (2003) *Mainstreaming Gender and Women's Mental Health: Implementation Guidance.* London: HMSO.

Department of Health (DH) (2004a) *The Ten Essential Shared Capabilities: A Framework for the Whole of the Mental Health Workforce.* Available at: http://www.dh.gov.uk/en/Publicationsandstatistics/ Publications/PublicationsPolicyAndGuidance/DH_4087169

Department of Health (DH) (2004b) *The National Service Framework for Mental Health – Five Years On.* London: HMSO.

Department of Health (DH) (2004c) *Choosing Health: Making Health Choices Easier* [on-line]. Available at: http://www.dh.gov.uk/en/Publicationsandstatistics/Publications/Publications PolicyAndGuidance/DH_4094550

Department of Health (DH) (2004d) *Scientific Committee on Tobacco and Health. Secondhand Smoke. Review of Evidence Since 1998* [on-line]. Available at: http://www.dh.gov.uk/en/ Publicationsandstatistics/Publications/PublicationsPolicyAndGuidance/DH_4101474

Department of Health (DH) (2004e) *National Service Framework for Children, Young People and Maternity Services: The Mental Health and Psychological Well-being of Children and Young People.* Available at: http://www.dh.gov.uk/en/Publicationsandstatistics/Publications/ PublicationsPolicyAndGuidance/DH_4089114

Department of Health (DH) (2005a) *Chief Nursing Officer's Review of Mental Health Nursing: Consultation Document.* Available at: http://www.dh.gov.uk/en/Consultations/ Closedconsultations/DH_4121787

Department of Health (DH) (2005b) *Creating a Patient-Led NHS: Delivering the NHS Improvement Plan.* Available at: http://www.dh.gov.uk/en/Publicationsandstatistics/Publications/ PublicationsPolicyAndGuidance/DH_4106506

Department of Health (DH) (2005c) *A Workforce Response to Local Delivery Plans: A Challenge for NHS Boards.* London: HMSO.

Department of Health (DH) (2005d) *Mental Health and Deafness – Towards Equity and Access: Best Practice Guidance.* London: HMSO.

Department of Health (DH) (2005e) *Valuing People: A New Strategy for Learning Disability for the 21st Century.* London: HMSO.

Department of Health (DH) (2005f) *Delivering Race Equality in Mental Health Care: An Action Plan for Reform Inside and Outside Services and the Government's Response to the Independent Inquiry into the Death of David Bennett.* London: HMSO.

Department of Health (DH) (2005g) *You're Welcome Quality Criteria, Making Health Services Young People Friendly.* London: HMSO.

Department of Health (DH) (2006a) *From Values to Action: The Chief Nursing Officer's Review of Mental Health Nursing.* Available at: http://www.dh.gov.uk/en/Publicationsandstatistics/ Publications/PublicationsPolicyAndGuidance/DH_4133839

Department of Health (DH) (2006b) *Our Health, Our Care, Our Say: A New Direction for Community Services*. London: HMSO.

Department of Health (DH) (2006c) *Dual Diagnosis in Mental Health Inpatient and Day Hospital Settings* [on-line]. Available at: http://www.dh.gov.uk/en/Publicationsandstatistics/Publications/PublicationsPolicyAndGuidance/DH_062649

Department of Health (DH) (2006d) *Choosing Health: Supporting the Physical Needs of People with Severe Mental Illness – Commissioning Framework* [on-line]. Available at: http://www.dh.gov.uk/en/Publicationsandstatistics/Publications/PublicationsPolicyAndGuidance/DH_4138212

Department of Health (DH) (2006e) *Promoting the Mental Health and Psychological Well-being of Children and Young People and Maternity Services: Report on the Implementation of Standard 9 of the National Service Framework for Children, Young People and Maternity Services*. Available at: http://www.dh.gov.uk/en/Publicationsandstatistics/Publications/PublicationsPolicyAndGuidance/DH_062778

Department of Health and Welsh Office (1999) *Code of Practice. Mental Health Act 1983* [3rd version]. London: The Stationery Office. Available at: http://www.dh.gov.uk/assetRoot/04/07/049/61/04074961.pdf

Dickersin, K (1990) 'The existence of publication bias and risk factors for its occurrence' *Journal of the American Medical Association* **263**: 1385–1389.

Dickersin, K and Min, YI (1993) 'NIH clinical trials and publication bias' *Online Journal of Current Clinical Trials* **50**: 4967.

Dickersin, K, Min, YL and Meinert, CL (1992) 'Factors influencing publication of research results: follow-up of applications submitted to two institutional boards' *Journal of the American Medical Association* **267**(3): 374–378.

DiClemente, R and Ponton, L (1993) 'HIV related risk behaviours among psychiatrically hospitalised adolescents and school based adolescents' *American Journal of Psychiatry* **150**: 324–325.

Dingwall, R and Allen, D (2001) 'The implications of healthcare reforms for the profession of Nursing' *Nursing Inquiry* **8**: 64–74.

Disability Rights Commission (DRC) (2005) *Equal Treatment: Closing the Gap*. Interim Report of a Formal Investigation into Health Inequalities. Available at: www.drc.org.uk

Disability Rights Commission (DRC) (2006) *Equal Treatment: Closing the Gap*. Available at: http://www.drc.org.uk/library/health_investigation.aspx

Dixon, L, Weiden, P and Delahanty, J et al. (2000) 'Prevalence and correlates of diabetes in national schizophrenia samples' *Schizophrenia Bulletin* **26**: 903–912.

Dixon, LB, Kreyenbuhl, JA, Dickerson, FB, Donner, TW, Brown, CH, Wolheiter, K, Postrado, L, Goldberg, RW, Fang, L, Marano, C and Messias, E (2004) 'A comparison of type 2 diabetes outcomes among persons with and without severe mental illnesses' *Psychiatric Services* **55**(8): 892–900.

Dixon, WA (2000) 'Problem-solving appraisal and depression: evidence for a recovery model' *Journal of Counselling and Development* **78**: 87–91.

Dobash, RE and Dobash, RP (1984) 'The nature and antecedents of violent events' *British Journal of Criminology* **24**: 269–288.

Dobos, C (1992) 'Defining risk from the perspective of nurses in clinical roles' *Journal of Advanced Nursing* **17**: 1303–1309.

Donovan, C and Suckling, HC (2004) *Difficult Consultations with Adolescents*. Oxford: Radcliffe Medical Press.

Dorais, M (with Lajeunesse, SL; translated by Pierre Trembley) (2004) *Dead Boys Can't Dance: Sexual Orientation, Masculinity and Suicide*. Montreal: McGill-Queens' University Press.

Dorling, D (2004) 'Prime suspect: murder in Britain' in Hillyard, P, Pantazis, C, Tombs, S and Gordon, D (eds) *Beyond Criminology: Taking Harm Seriously*. London: Pluto.

Dorrer, N (2006) *Evidence of Recovery: The 'Ups' and 'Downs' of Longitudinal Outcome Studies*. SRN Discussion Paper Series. Report No. 4. Glasgow: Scottish Recovery Network.

Dowdney, L, Wilson, R, Maughan, B, Allerton, M, Schofield, P and Skuse, D (1999) 'Psychological disturbance and service provision in parentally bereaved children: prospective case-control study' *British Medical Journal* **319**: 354–357.

Dowson, CA, Kuijer, RG and Mulder, RT (2004) 'Anxiety and self-management behaviour in chronic obstructive pulmonary disease: what has been learned? *Chronic Respiratory Disease* **1**(4): 213–220.

Doyle, M (1996) 'Assessing risk of violence from clients' *Mental Health Nursing* **16**: 20–23.

Doyle, M and Dolan, M (2002) 'Violence risk assessment: combining actuarial and clinical information to structure clinical judgements for the formulation and management of risk' *Journal of Psychiatric and Mental Health Nursing* **9**: 649–657.

Drake, RE, Mueser, KT, Clarke, RE and Wallace, MA (1996) 'The course, treatment, and outcome of substance disorder in persons with severe mental illness' *American Journal of Orthopsychiatry* **66**: 42–51.

Drury, J (2006) 'Compassion for the mentally ill' *American Journal of Nursing* **106**(5): 15.

Duxbury, J (2002) 'An evaluation of staff and patients' views of and strategies employed to manage patient aggression and violence on one mental health unit' *Journal of Psychiatric and Mental Health Nursing* **9**: 325–337.

Duxbury, J and Paterson, B (2005) 'The use of physical restraint in mental health nursing: an examination of principles, practice and implications for training' *The Journal of Adult Protection* **7**(4): 13–24.

Duxbury, J and Whittington, R (2005) 'Causes and management of patient aggression and violence: staff and patient perspectives' *Journal of Advanced Nursing* **50**(5): 469–478.

Easen, P and Wilcockson, J (1996) 'Intuition and rational decision-making: a false dichotomy?' *Journal of Advanced Nursing* **24**: 667–673.

Easterbrook, PJ, Berlin, J, Gopalan, R and Matthews, DR (1991) 'Publication bias in clinical research' *Lancet* **337**: 867–872.

Ebrahim, S and Smith, GD (1997) 'Systematic review of randomised controlled trials of multiple risk factor interventions for preventing coronary heart disease' *British Medical Journal* **314**: 1666–1674.

Edney, D (2004) *Mass Media and Mental Illness: A Literature Review*. Available at: http://www.ontario.cmha.ca/docs/about/mass_media.pdf

Edwards, J and Weary, G (1998) 'Antecedents of causal uncertainty and perceived control: a prospective study' *European Journal of Personality* **12**: 135–148.

Egger, M, Smith, D and Altman, I (eds) (2001) *Systematic Reviews in Health Care: Meta-analysis in Context*. London: BMJ Books.

Ellinson, M, Thomas, J and Patterson, A (2004) 'A critical evaluation of the relationship between serum vitamin B12 folate and total homocysteine with cognitive impairment in the elderly' *Journal of Human Nutrition and Dietetics* **17**: 371–383.

English, J and Card, R (2005) *Police Law*, 9th edn. Oxford: Oxford University Press.

Eustace, B (1990) *The Police Self-defence Handbook*. London: A&C Black.

Evans, M (2006) 'Making room for madness in mental health: the importance of analytically informed supervision of nurses and other mental health professionals' *Psychoanalytical Psychotherapy* **20**(1): 16–29.

Evans, P (1980) *Prison Crisis*. London: George Allen and Unwin.

Fagen, L and Garelick, A (2004) 'The doctor–nurse relationship' *Advances in Psychiatric Treatment* **10**: 277–286.

Faulkner, A (2004) 'Strategies for surviving acute care' in Harrison, M, Howard, D and Mitchell, D (eds) *Acute Mental Health Nursing: From Acute Concerns to the Capable Practitioner*. London: Sage.

Faulkner, A and Layzell, S (2000) *Strategies for Living: The Research Report*. London: Mental Health Foundation.

Fernando, S (2003) *Cultural Diversity, Mental Health and Psychiatry: The Struggle Against Racism*. London: Routledge.

Ferner, R (2003) 'Should medical students be taught rational prescribing?' *Student BMJ* **11**(Apr): 89–90.

Finlay, IG and Jones, NK (2000) 'Unresolved grief in young offenders in prison' *British Journal of General Practice* **50**(456): 569–570.

Finzen, A and Hoffmann-Richter, U (1999) 'Mental illness as metaphor' in Guimon, J, Fischer, W and Sartorius, N (eds) *The Image of Madness*. Basel: Karger.

Firth-Cozens, J (2001a) 'Cultures for effective learning' in Vincent, C (ed.) *Clinical Risk Management*. London: BMJ Books.

Firth-Cozens, J (2001b) 'Multidisciplinary teamwork: the good, bad, and everything in between' *Quality in Health Care* **10**: 65–69.

Fishbein, M and Ajzen, I (1975) *Belief, Attitude, Intention and Behaviour: An Introduction to Theory and Research*. Reading, MA: Addison-Wesley.

Fisher, D (2003) 'People are more important than pills in recovery from mental disorder' *Journal of Humanistic Psychology* **43**: 65–68.

Fitzgerald, M and Sim, J (1982) *British Prisons*, 2nd edn. Oxford: Blackwell.

Fleming, S and Balmer, L (1996) 'Bereavement in adolescence' in Corr, CA and Balk, DE (eds) *Handbook of Adolescent Death and Bereavement*. New York: Springer Publishing Company.

Fleming, SF and Adolph, R (1986) 'Helping bereaved adolescents: needs and responses' in Corr, CA and McNeill, JN (eds) *Adolescence and Death*. New York: Springer Publishing Company.

Fletcher, J (1997a) 'Do nurses really care? Some unwelcome findings from recent research and inquiry' *Journal of Nursing Management* **5**(1): 43–50.

Fletcher, J (1997b) 'Do nurses really care? An agenda for higher education following recent mergers' *Journal of Nursing Management* **5**(2): 97–104.

Food Standards Agency (FSA) (2001) *The Balance of Good Health*. Available at: http://www.food.gov.uk/multimedia/pdfs/bghbooklet.pdf

Forchuk, C (2001) 'Evidence-based psychiatric/mental nursing' *Evidence Based Mental Health* **4**: 39–40.

Forchuk, C, Jewell, J, Tweedell, D and Steinnagel, L (2003) 'Role changes experienced by clinical staff in relation to clients' recovery from psychosis' *Journal of Psychiatric and Mental Health Nursing* **10**: 269–276.

Ford, R (2004) 'The policy and service context for mental health nursing' in Norman, I and Ryrie, I (eds) *The Art and Science of Mental Health Nursing: A Textbook of Principles and Practice*. Maidenhead: Open University Press.

Ford, R, Durcan, G, Warner, L, Hardy, P and Muijen, M (1998) 'One day survey by the Mental Health Act Commission of acute adult psychiatric inpatient wards in England and Wales' *BMJ* **317**: 1279–1283.

Foucault, M (1971) *Madness and Civilization*. London: Tavistock.

Foucault, M (1977) *Discipline and Punish: The Birth of the Prison*. London: Penguin.

Fox, L (1999) 'Personal accounts: missing out on motherhood' *Psychiatric Services* **50**: 193–194.

Frackiewicz, EJ, Sramek, JJ, Herrera, JM, Kurtz, NM and Cutler, NR (1997) 'Ethnicity and antipsychotic response' *The Annals of Pharmacotherapy* **31**(11): 1360–1369.

France, A (2004) 'Young people' in Fraser, S, Lewis, V, Ding, S, Kellett, M and Robinson, C (eds) (2004) *Doing Research with Children and Young People*. London: SAGE/Open University.

Franks, V (2004) 'Evidence-based uncertainty in mental health nursing' *Journal of Psychiatric and Mental Health Nursing* **11**: 99–105.

Fransella, F (1972) *Personal Change and Reconstruction: Research on the Treatment of Stuttering*. London: Academic Press.

Fransella, F and Neimeyer, R (2005) 'George Alexander Kelly: the man and his theory' in Fransella, F (ed.) *The Essential Practitioner's Handbook of Personal Construct Psychology*. Chichester: John Wiley & Sons.

Friedli, L and Dardis, C (2002) 'Smoke gets in their eyes' Mental Health Today **Jan**: 18–21.

Fritz, H and Helgeson, V (1998) 'A theory of unmitigated communion' *Personality and Social Psychology Review* **2**(3): 173–183.

Fulford, KWM and Williams, R (2003) 'Values-based child and adolescent mental health services?' *Current Opinion in Psychiatry* **16**: 369–376.

Fultz, NH, Ofstedal, MB, Herzog, AR and Wallace, RB (2003) 'Additive and interactive effects of comorbid physical and mental conditions on functional health' *Journal of Aging and Health* **15**(3): 465–481.

Gadsby, A (2006) Opinion: if service users felt listened to they'd be happier to compromise' *Nursing Times* **102**(47): 10.

Gafoor, M and Hussein-Rassool, G (1998) 'The co-existence of psychiatric disorders and substance misuse: working with dual diagnosis patients' *Journal of Advanced Nursing* **27**: 497–502.

Gallagher, A (2004) 'Dignity and respect for dignity – two key health professional values: implications for nursing practice' *Nursing Ethics* **11**(6): 587–599.

Gallant, MP (2003) 'The influence of social support on chronic illness self-management: a review and directions for research' *Health Education and Behavior* **30**(2): 170–195.

Galletly, CA and Watson, DP (2006) 'Substance misuse in patients with acute mental illness' *Medical Journal of Australia* **184**: 645.

Gallop, R and Reynolds, W (2004) 'Putting it all together: dealing with complexity in the understanding of the human condition' *Journal of Psychiatric and Mental Health Nursing* **11**: 357–364.

Gallop, R, McCay, E and Guah, M (1999) 'The experience of hospitalization and restraint of women who have a history of childhood sexual abuse' *Health Care for Women International* **10**: 401–416.

Gamble, C (2006) 'Building relationships: lessons to be learnt' in Gamble, C and Brennan, G (eds) *Working with Serious Mental Illness: A Manual for Clinical Practice*, 2nd edn. London: Elsevier.

Garcia, I (2006) *A Report on the Administrative Workload for Mental Health Workers*. London: Sainsbury Centre for Mental Health.

Garland, D (2001) *The Culture of Control: Crime and Social Order in Contemporary Society*. Oxford: Oxford University Press.

Gibbons, S, Lauder, W and Ludwick, R (2006) Self-neglect: a proposed new NANDA diagnosis' *International Journal of Nursing Terminologies and Classifications* **17**(1): 10–18.

Giddens, A (2002) *Runaway World: How Globalisation is Shaping Our Lives*. London: Profile Books.

Gijbels, H (1995) 'Mental health nursing skills in an acute admission environment: perceptions of mental health nurses and other mental health professionals' *Journal of Advanced Nursing* **21**: 460–465.

Gijbels, H and Burnard, P (1995) *Exploring the Skills of Mental Health Nurses.* Aldershot: Ashgate.

Gilbody, SM, Song, F, Eastwood, AJ and Sutton, A (2000) 'The causes, consequences and detection of publication bias in psychiatry' *Acta Psychiatrica Scandinavica* **102**: 241–249.

Gilland, R (1871) *Annual Report for Moulsford Asylum.* Unpublished archive material. Fair Mile Hospital, Oxford.

Glazer, S (2002) 'Response to critique of "therapeutic touch and postmodernism in nursing"' *Nursing Philosophy* **3**: 63–65.

Glenister, D (1997) 'Coercion, control and mental health nursing' in *The Mental Health Nurse: Views of Practice and Education.* Oxford: Blackwell Science.

Gochman, DS (1997) *Handbook of Health Behaviour Research.* New York: Plenum.

Godin, P (2000) 'A dirty business: caring for people who are a nuisance or a danger' *Journal of Advanced Nursing* **32**(6): 1396–1402.

Goffman, E (1961) *Asylums: Essays on the Social Situation of Mental Patients and Other Inmates.* London: Penguin.

Goffman, E (1963) *Stigma: Notes on the Management of Spoiled Identity.* New York: Simon and Schuster, Inc.

Goldberg, H (1977) *The Hazards of Being Male: Surviving the Myth of Masculine Privilege.* New York: Signet Books.

Goldman, LS (1999) 'Medical illness in patients with schizophrenia' *Journal of Clinical Psychiatry* **60**: 10–15.

Goldson, B and Coles, D (2005) *In the Care of the State? Child Deaths in Penal Custody in England and Wales.* London: INQUEST.

Gomm, R, Hammersley, M and Foster, P (2002) *Case Study Method.* Thousand Oaks: Sage.

Gostin, L (1986) *Institutions Observed: Towards a New Concept of Secure Provision in Mental Health.* London: King's Fund.

Gournay, K (1994) Redirecting the emphasis to severe mental illness. *Nursing Times* **90**(25): 40–41.

Gournay, K (1996) 'Schizophrenia: a review of the contemporary literature and implications for mental health nursing theory, practice and education' *Journal of Psychiatric and Mental Health Nursing* **3**: 7–12.

Gournay, K (2001) 'Mental health nursing in 2001: what happens next?' *Journal of Psychiatric and Mental Health Nursing* **8**: 473–476.

Gournay, K (2005) 'The changing face of psychiatric nursing' *Advances in Psychiatric Treatment* **11**: 6–11.

Gournay, K and Ritter, S (1998) 'What future for research in mental health nursing: rejoinder to Parsons, Bech and Rolfe' *Journal of Psychiatric and Mental Health Nursing* **5**: 227–230.

Gournay, K, Sandford, T, Johnson, S and Thornicroft, G (1997) 'Dual diagnosis of severe mental health problems and substance misuse/dependence: a major priority for mental health nursing' *Journal of Psychiatric and Mental Health Nursing* **4**: 89–95.

Gournay, K, Ward, M and Thornicroft, G *et al.* (1998) 'Crisis in the capital: in-patient care in inner London' *Mental Health Practice* **1**: 10–18.

Graham, HL, Maslin, J, Copello, A, Birchwood, M, Mueser, K, McGovern, D and Georgiou, G (2001) 'Drug and alcohol problems amongst individuals with severe mental health problems in an inner city area of the UK' *Social Psychiatry and Psychiatric Epidemiology* **36**: 448–455.

Granat-Goldstein, J (2001) 'Personal accounts: color within the lines . . . Think outside the box' *Psychiatric Services* **52**: 769–770.

Gray, R (2000) 'Does patient education enhance compliance with clozapine? A preliminary investigation' *Journal of Psychiatric and Mental Health Nursing* **7**: 285–286.

Gray, R, Leese, M, Bindman, J, Becker, T, Burti, L, David, A, Gournay, K, Kikkert, M, Koeter, M, Puschner, B, Schene, A, Thornicroft, G and Tansella, M (2006) 'Adherence therapy for people with schizophrenia: European multicentre randomised controlled trial' *British Journal of Psychiatry* **189**: 508–514.

Green, P and Ward, T (2004) *State Crime: Governments, Violence and Corruption*. London: Pluto.

Griffin, N (1989) 'Multi professional care in forensic psychiatry' *Psychiatric Bulletin* **13**: 613–615.

Griffiths, M. (2003) 'Terms of engagement – reaching hard to reach adolescents' *Young Minds Magazine* **62**(Jan/Feb). Available at: http://www.youngminds.org.uk/magazine/62/griffiths. php

Griffiths, R (1983) *Report of the NHS Management Inquiry*. London: DHSS.

Griffiths, S (2002) *Addressing the Health Needs of Rough Sleepers*. London: ODPM/HMSO. Available at: http://www.communities.gov.uk/pub/122/Addressingthehealthneedso froughsleepersPDF135Kb_id1150122.pdf

Guarnaccia, PJ and Parra, P (1996) 'Ethnicity, social status, and families' experiences of caring for a mentally ill family member' *Community Mental Health Journal* **32**: 243–260.

Guimon, J (2001) 'Mass media and psychiatry' *Current Opinion in Psychiatry* **14**(6): 533–534.

Guimon, J, Fischer, W and Sartorious, N (1999) *The Image of Madness*. Basel: Karger.

Gunstone, S (2003) 'Risk assessment and management of patients who self-neglect: a 'grey area' for mental health workers' *Journal of Psychiatric and Mental Health Nursing* **10**: 287–296.

Guy, W (1976) *ECDEU Assessment Manual for Psychopharmacology*. Washington, DC: US Department of Health, Education and Welfare.

Hadfield, P (2006) *Bar Wars: Contesting the Night in Contemporary British Cities*. Oxford: Oxford University Press.

Hagerty, B, Bissonnette, T, Bostrom, A, Lovell, B and Sieloff, C (1995) 'The status of psychiatric nursing: characteristics and perceptions of nurses in the State of Michigan' *Issues in Mental Health Nursing* **16**: 419–432.

Hagger, M and Orbell, S (2003) 'A meta-analytic review of the common sense model of illness representations' *Psychology and Health* **18**: 141–184.

Haglund, K, Von Knorring, L and Von Essen, L (2003) 'Forced medication in psychiatric care: patient experiences and nurse perceptions' *Journal of Psychiatric and Mental Health Nursing* **10**: 65–72.

Halbreich, U and Palter, S (1996) 'Accelerated osteoporosis in psychiatric patients: possible pathophysiological processes' *Schizophrenia Bulletin* **22**: 447–454.

Halbreich, U, Shen, J and Panaro, V (1996) 'Are chronic psychiatric patients at increased risk for developing breast cancer?' *American Journal of Psychiatry* **153**: 559–560.

Hall, J (1997) 'Dirty protests: a phenomenological assessment' *Medicine, Science and the Law* **37**(1): 35–36.

Hall, S (1997) 'The spectacle of the "other"' in Hall, S (ed.) *Representation: Cultural Representations and Signifying Practices*. London: SAGE/Open University.

Halliday, G, Banerjee, S, Philpot, M and Macdonald, A (2000) 'Community study of people who live in squalor' *The Lancet* **355**: 882–886.

Hamblett, C (2000) 'Obstacles to defining the role of the mental health nurse' *Nursing Standard* **14**(51): 34–37.

Harding, M and Zahniser, H (1994) 'Empirical correction of seven myths about schizophrenia with implications for treatment' *Acta Psychiatrica Scandinavica* **90**(Suppl. 384): 140–146.

Harlen, W and Schlapp, U (2005) *Literature Reviews*. The Scottish Centre for Research in Education. Available at: http://www.scre.ac.uk/spotlight/spotlight71.html

Harrington, R (1996) 'Childhood bereavement: bereavement is painful but does not necessarily make children ill' *British Medical Journal* **313**(7060): 822.

Harrington, R and Harrison, L (1999) 'Unproven assumptions about the impact of bereavement on children' *Journal of the Royal Society of Medicine* **92**(5): 230–233.

Harris, EC and Barraclough, B (1998) 'Excess mortality of mental disorder' *British Journal of Psychiatry* **173**: 11–53.

Harris, G, Rice, M and Quinsey, V (1993) 'Violent recidivism of mentally disordered offenders: the development of a statistical prediction instrument' *Criminal Justice Behaviour* **20**: 315–335.

Harrison, L and Harrington, R (2001) 'Adolescents' bereavement experiences, prevalence, association with depressive symptoms, and use of services' *Journal of Adolescence* **24**: 159–169.

Harrison, S (2005) 'Where next for mental health?' *Nursing Standard* **19**(23): 12.

Harrow, M, Grossman, L, Jobe, T and Herbener, E (2005) 'Do patients with schizophrenia ever show signs of recovery? A 15-year multi-follow-up study' *Schizophrenia Bulletin* **31**: 723–724.

Hayward, P and Bright, J (1997) 'Stigma and mental illness: a review and critique' *Journal of Mental Health* **6**: 345–354.

Health Education Authority (1997) *Speech for Mr Tim O'Malley T.D., Minister of State at the Department of Health and Children at the Conference of Partners for Health in Education*. Available at: http://www.dohc.ie/press/speeches/2006/20060311.html

Healthcare Commission (2005) *Count Me In. Results of a National Census of Inpatients in Mental Health Hospitals and Facilities in England and Wales*. London: Department of Health.

Healthcare Commission (2006a) *Survey of Users of Services 2006: Community Mental Health Services*. Available at: http://www.healthcarecommission.org.uk/_db/_documents/Community_MH_survey_report.pdf

Healthcare Commission (2006b) *State of Healthcare 2006*. London: Commission for Healthcare, Audit and Inspection.

Healthcare Commission (2007) *Talking About Medicines: The Management of Medicines in Trusts Providing Mental Health Services*. London: Commission for Healthcare Audit and Inspection. Available at: http://www.healthcarecommission.org.uk/_db/_documents/Talking_about_medicines_mental_health_trust_report.pdf

Healy, D (2005) *Psychiatric Drugs Explained*, 4th edn. Edinburgh: Churchill Livingstone.

Heidegger, H (1977) *The Question Concerning Technology and Other Essays* (trans. William Lovitt). New York: Harper and Row.

Heidi, F and Helgeson, V (1998) 'Distinctions between unmitigated communion from communion: self neglect and over-involvement with others' *Journal of Personality and Social Psychology* **75**(1): 121–140.

Hem, M and Heggen, K (2003) 'Being professional and being human: one nurse's relationship with a psychiatric patient' *Journal of Advanced Nursing* **43**(1): 101–108.

Hemingway, H and Marmot, M (1999) 'Evidence based cardiology: psychosocial factors in the aetiology and prognosis of coronary heart disease. Systematic review of prospective cohort studies' *British Medical Journal* **318**: 1460–1467.

Herbert, J (1997) 'Fortnightly review: stress, the brain, and mental illness' *British Medical Journal* **315**(7107): 530–535.

Herbig, B, Büssing, A and Ewert, T (2001) 'The role of tacit knowledge in the work context of nursing' *Journal of Advanced Nursing* **34**(5): 687–695.

Herdman, E (2004) 'Nursing in a postemotional society' *Nursing Philosophy* **5**: 95–103.

Herman, H (2001) 'The need for mental health promotion' *Australian and New Zealand Journal of Psychiatry* **39**: 709–715.

Herman, J (1992) *Trauma and Recovery: From Domestic Abuse to Political Terror.* London: Pandora.

Hettiaratchy, P and Manthorpe, J (1989) 'The "hidden" nature of self-neglect' *Care of the Elderly* **1**(1): 14–15.

Hewitt, J and Coffey, M (2005) 'Therapeutic working relationships with people with schizophrenia: literature review' *Journal of Advanced Nursing* **52**(5): 561–570.

Hewitt, P (2005) *Speech at the 'Britain Speaks – Effective Public Engagement and Better Decision Making' Conference*, London, 23 June. Available at: http://www.dh.gov.uk/NewsHome/Speeches

Higgins, R, Hurst, K and Wisyow, G (1999) *Psychiatric Nursing Revisited: The Care Provided for Acute Psychiatric Patients.* London: Whurr.

Himelhoch, S, Lehman, A, Kreyenbuhl, J, Daumit, G, Brown, C and Dixon, L (2004) 'Prevalence of chronic obstructive pulmonary disease among those with serious mental illness' *American Journal of Psychiatry* **161**: 2317–2319.

Hinshelwood, RD and Skogstad, W (2000) 'The dynamics of health care institutions' in Hinshelwood, RD and Skogstad W (eds) *Observing Organisations Anxiety, Defence and Culture in Health Care.* London: Routledge.

Hipwell, AE, Singh, K and Clark, A (2000) 'Substance misuse among clients with severe and enduring mental illness: service utilisation and implications for clinical management' *Journal of Mental Health* **9**: 37–50.

Hitchon, G, Westra, A, Beales, A and Beresford, P (2006) 'Putting users in control' *Mental Health Today* **June**.

Hobbs, D, Hadfield, P, Lister, S and Winlow, S (2003) *Bouncers: Violence and Governance in the Night-time Economy.* Oxford: Oxford University Press.

Hoggett, B (1996) *Mental Health Law*, 4th edn. London: Sweet and Maxwell.

Holland, J (2001) *Understanding Children's Experiences of Parental Bereavement.* London: Jessica Kingsley.

Holmbeck, GN (2002) 'A developmental perspective on adolescent health and illness: an introduction to the special issues' *Journal of Pediatric Psychology* **27**(5): 409–416.

Holmes, C (2006) 'The slow death of psychiatric nursing: what next?' *Journal of Psychiatric and Mental Health Nursing* **13**: 401–415.

Holmes, CL, Simmons, H and Pilowsky, LS (2001) 'Rapid tranquilisation' in Beer, MD, Pereira, SM and Paton, C (eds) *Psychiatric Intensive Care.* London: Greenwich Medical Media Ltd.

Holmes, D, Murray, SJ, Perron, A and Rail, G (2006) 'Deconstructing the evidence-based discourse in health sciences: truth power and fascism' *International Journal of Evidence Based Healthcare* **4**(3): 180–186.

Holmes-Eber, P and Riger, S (1990) 'Hospitalisation and the composition of patients' social networks' *Schizophrenia Bulletin* **16**: 157–164.

Holzer, CE, Shea, BM, Swanson, JW, Leaf, PJ, Myers, JK, George, L, Weissman, MM and Bednarske, P (1986) 'The increased risk for specific psychiatric disorders among persons of low socioeconomic status' *American Journal of Social Psychiatry* **6**: 259–271.

Home Office (2003) *World Prison Population List.* Findings 234. London: Home Office.

Honkasalo, M (2006) 'Fragilities in life and death: engaging in uncertainty in modern society' *Health, Risk and Society* **8**(1): 27–41.

Hospers, J (1997) *An Introduction to Philosophical Analysis*, 4th edn. London: Routledge.

House of Commons (2005) *Joint Committee on the Draft Mental Health Bill – First Report*. London: House of Commons.

House of Lords/House of Commons Joint Committee on Human Rights (2004) *Deaths in Custody: Third Report of Session 2004–05 Volume 1. Report, Together with Formal Minutes*. HL Paper 15-1 HC137-1. London: The Stationery Office.

House of Lords/House of Commons Joint Committee on Human Rights (2007) *Deaths in Custody: Further Developments. Seventh Report of Session 2006–07*. HL Paper 59 HC 364. London: The Stationery Office.

Howard League for Penal Reform (2002) *Children in Prison: Barred Rights*. London: HLPR.

Howard, GS (1991) 'Culture tales: a narrative approach to thinking, cross-cultural psychology and psychotherapy' *American Psychologist* **46**(3): 187–197.

Howard, LM, Kumar, C and Thornicroft, G (2002) 'The general fertility rate in women with psychotic disorders' *American Journal of Psychiatry* **159**(6): 991–997.

Hugman, R (2005) *New Approaches in Ethics for the Caring Professions*. Basingstoke: Palgrave.

Humphries, M (2005) 'The multidisciplinary team and clinical team meetings' in Wix, S and Humphries, M (eds) *Multidisciplinary Working in Forensic Mental Health Care*. London: Churchill Livingstone.

Hunot, VM, Horne, RM, Leese, MN and Churchill, RC (2007) 'A cohort study of adherence to antidepressants in primary care: the influence of antidepressant concerns and treatment preferences' *The Primary Care Companion to the Journal of Clinical Psychiatry* **9**(2): 91–99.

Hunt, K, Lewars, H, Emslie, C and Batty, G (2007) 'Decreased risk of death from coronary heart disease amongst men with higher "femininity" scores: a general population cohort study' *International Journal of Epidemiology* [on-line]. Published April 2007, 10.1093/ije/dym022, 1–9

Hurd, RC (1999) 'Adults view their childhood bereavement experiences' *Death Studies* **23**: 17–41.

INQUEST (2004) *Inquest Briefing: The Restraint Related Death of David 'Rocky' Bennett*. London: INQUEST.

Institute of Race Relations (1991) *Deadly Silence: Black Deaths in Custody*. London: Institute for Race Relations.

Inventor, B, Henricks, J, Rodman, L, Imel, J, Holermon, L and Hernandez, F (2005) 'The impact of medical issues in inpatient geriatric psychiatry' *Issues in Mental Health Nursing* **26**(1): 23–46.

Irala-Estevez, JD, Groth, M and Johansson, L *et al.* (2000) 'A systematic review of socio-economic differences in food habits in Europe: consumption of fruit and vegetables' *European Journal of Clinical Nutrition* **54**: 706–714.

Ireland, L (2006) Evidence-based practice' in Brown, J and Libberton, P (eds) *Principles of Professional Studies in Nursing*. Basingstoke: Palgrave Macmillan.

Ito, H, Koyama, A and Higuchi, T (2005) 'Polypharmacy and excessive dosing: psychiatrists' perceptions of anti-psychotic drug prescriptions' *British Journal of Psychiatry* **187**: 243–247.

Jackson, L, Leclerc, J, Erskine, Y and Linden, W (2005) 'Getting the most out of cardiac rehabilitation: a review of referral and adherence predictors' *Heart* **91**(1): 10–14.

Jackson, S and Stevenson, C (1998) 'The gift of time from the friendly professional' *Nursing Standard* **12**(51): 31–33.

Jackson-Koku, G (2001) 'Mental illness and substance misuse: a nursing challenge' *British Journal of Nursing* **10**: 242–246.

Jacobson, N and Greenley, D (2001) 'What is recovery? A conceptual model and explication' *Psychiatric Services* **52**(4): 482–485.

Jameson, N and Allison, E (1995) *Strangeways 1990: A Serious Disturbance.* London: Larkin.

Jankowicz, D (2001) 'Why does subjectivity make us nervous?' *Journal of Intellectual Capital* **2**(1): 61–73.

Janssen, I, Hanssem, M, Bak, M, Bijl, R, DeGraaf, R, Vollebergh, W, McKenzie, K and Van Os, J (2003) 'Discrimination and delusional ideation' *British Journal of Psychiatry* **182**: 71–76.

Jaques, E (1955) 'Social systems as a defence against persecutory and depressive anxiety' in Klein, M, Heimann, P and Money-Kyrle, R (eds) *New Directions in Psychoanalysis.* London: Tavistock.

Jessop, J and Ribbens McCarthy, J (2005) 'The social contexts of bereavement experiences and interventions' in Ribbens McCarthy, J with Jessop, J *Young People, Bereavement and Loss, Disruptive Transitions.* York: Joseph Rowntree Foundation/National Children's Bureau.

Jeste, D, Gladsjo, J, Lindamer, L and Lacro, J (1996) 'Medical co-morbidity in schizophrenia' *Schizophrenia Bulletin* **22**: 413–430.

Jewitt, C (1997) 'Images of men: male sexuality in sexual health leaflets and posters for young people' *Sociological Research Online* **2**(2). Available at: http://www.socresonline.org.uk/2/2/6.html

Jindal, R, Mackenzie, EM, Baker, GB and Yeragani, VK (2005) 'Cardiac risk and schizophrenia' *Journal of Psychiatry Neuroscience* **30**(6): 393–395.

Jobe, T and Harrow, M (2005) 'Long-term outcome of patients with schizophrenia: a review' *Canadian Journal of Psychiatry* **50**: 892–900.

Johns, A (1997) 'Substance misuse: a primary risk and a major problem of comorbidity' *International Review of Psychiatry* **9**: 233–241.

Johnson, A, Mercer, C, Erens, B, Copas, A, McManus, S, Wellings, K, Fenton, K, Korovessis, C, Macdowall, W, Nanchahal, K, Purdon, S and Field, J (2001) 'Sexual behaviour in Britain: partnerships, practices and HIV risk behaviours' *The Lancet* **358**: 1835–1842.

Johnson, M and Webb, C (1995) 'Rediscovering unpopular patients: the concept of social judgement' *Journal of Advanced Nursing* **21**: 466–475.

Johnson, S (1997) 'Dual diagnosis of severe mental illness and substance misuse: a case for specialist services?' *British Journal of Psychiatry* **171**: 205–208.

Jolobe, O (2002) 'Clinical decision-making: coping with uncertainty' *Postgraduate Medical Journal* **78**: 764.

Jones, DR, Macias, C and Barreira, PJ *et al.* (2004) 'Prevalence, severity, and co-occurrence of chronic physical health problems of persons with serious mental illness' *Psychiatric Services* **55**(11): 1250–1257.

Jones, G (2005) *Young Adults and the Extension of Economic Dependence.* London: National Family and Parenting Institute.

Jones, K (1972) *A History of the Mental Health Services.* London: Routledge and Kegan Paul.

Jones, K (1993) *Asylums and After.* London: Althorne Press.

Jones, K (2004) 'Mission drift in qualitative research, or moving toward a systematic review of qualitative studies, moving back to a more systematic narrative review' *The Qualitative Report* **9**(1): 95–112.

Jones, M (1968) *Social Psychiatry in Practice.* Harmondsworth: Pelican.

Jordan, J, Ellis, S and Chambers, R (2002) 'Defining shared decision making and concordance: are they one and the same?' *Postgraduate Medical Journal* **78**: 383–384.

Jordan, S, Knight, J and Pointon, D (2004) 'Monitoring adverse drug reactions: scales, profiles, and checklists' *International Nursing Review* **51**(4): 208.

Jorm, AF, Christensen, H, Griffiths, KM and Rodgers, B (2002) 'Effectiveness of complimentary and self-help treatments for depression' *Medical Journal of Australia* **176**(10): S84–S95.

Jung, W and Irwin, M (1999) 'Reduction of natural killer cytotoxic activity in major depression: interaction between depression and cigarette smoking' *Psychosomatic Medicine* **61**: 263–270.

Kane, B (1979) 'Children's concepts of death' *The Journal of Genetic Psychology* **134**: 141–153.

Kane, JM and Marder, SR (1993) 'Psychopharmacologic treatment of schizophrenia' *Schizophrenia Bulletin* **19**(2): 287–302.

Karoly, P and Ruehlman, LS (1996) 'Motivational implications of pain: chronicity, psychological distress and work goal construal in a national sample of adults' *Health Psychology* **15**: 383–390.

Kelly, C and McCreadie, RG (1999) 'Smoking habits, current symptoms and premorbid characteristics of schizophrenia patients in Nithsdale, Scotland' *American Journal of Psychiatry* **156**: 1751–1757.

Kelly, GA (1955/1991) *The Psychology of Personal Constructs: Volume One. A Theory of Personality.* London: Routledge.

Kelly, GA (1969) 'The threat of aggression' in Maher, B (ed.) *Clinical Psychology and Personality: The Selected Papers of George Kelly.* New York: John Wiley & Sons.

Kelly, GA (1970) 'A brief introduction to personal construct psychology' in Bannister, D (ed.) *Perspectives in Personal Construct Psychology.* London: Academic Press.

Kelly, GA (1977) 'The psychology of the unknown' in Bannister, D (ed.) *New Perspectives in Personal Construct Theory.* London: Academic Press.

Kelly, M and Gamble, C (2005) 'Exploring the concept of recovery in schizophrenia' *Journal of Psychiatric and Mental Health Nursing* **12**: 245–251.

Kemp, R, Kirov, G, Everitt, B, Hayward, P and David, A (1998) 'Randomised controlled trial of compliance therapy: 18-month follow-up' *British Journal of Psychiatry* **172**: 413–419.

Kendall, D (2004) *Social Problems in a Diverse Society*, 3rd edn. Boston, MA: Pearson/Allyn and Bacon.

Kendall, RE (2001) 'The distinction between mental and physical illness' *British Journal of Psychiatry* **178**: 490–493.

Kendrick, T (1996) 'Cardiovascular and respiratory risk factors and symptoms among general practice patients with long term mental illness' *British Journal of Psychiatry* **169**: 733–739.

Kennedy, A, Gately, C and Rogers, A (2004) *Assessing the Process of Embedding EPP in the NHS: Preliminary Survey of PCT Pilot Sites.* National Primary Care Research and Development Centre. Universities of Manchester and York.

Kerzner, L, Dobmeyer, T, Murphy, C, Rowan, F and Hagen, R (2003) 'Benefits associated with interdisciplinary homes visits to self-neglecting vulnerable adults' *JAGS* **51**(4): S71.

Kessler, R, Berglund, P, Foster, C, Saunders, W, Stang, PE and Walters, EE (1997) 'Social consequences, psychiatric disorders, 11: Teenage parenthood' *American Journal of Psychiatry* **154**: 1405–1411.

Kiechl, S, Egger, G and Mayr, M *et al.* (2001) 'Chronic infections and the risk of carotid atherosclerosis: prospective results from a large population study' *Circulation* **103**(8): 1064–1070.

Kiecolt-Glaser, JK, Preacher, KJ and Maccallum, RC *et al.* (2003) 'Chronic stress and age-related increases in the proinflammatory cytokine IL-6' *Proceedings of the National Academy of Sciences USA* **100**(15): 9090–9095.

Kilmartin, CT (1994) *The Masculine Self.* New York: Macmillan.

King, L and Appleton, J (1997) 'Intuition: a critical review of the research and rhetoric' *Journal of Advanced Nursing* **26**: 194–202.

King, M and McKeown, E (2003) *Mental Health and Social Wellbeing of Gay Men, Lesbians and Bisexuals in England and Wales.* London: Mind.

Kippax, S, Crawford, J, Abelson, J and Lambevski, S (2002) 'Masculinity, mortality and risk' *International Conference on AIDS*, July 7–12, Abstract No. ThPeE7798.

Klass, D, Silverman, PR and Nickman, PA (eds) (1996) *Continuing Bonds: New Understandings of Grief.* London: Taylor & Francis.

Klein, M (1946) 'Notes on some schizoid mechanisms' in Klein, M (ed.) *Envy and Gratitude and Other Works 1946–1963.* London: Virago; 1–24.

Klein, M (1959) 'Our adult world and its roots in infancy' in Klein, M (ed.) *Envy and Gratitude and Other Works 1946–1963.* London: Virago.

Klein, R, Day, P and Redmayne, S (1996) *Managing Scarcity.* Buckingham: Open University Press.

Klosterkotter, J and Peters, U (1985) 'Diogenes syndrome' *Forschr Neurological Psychiatry* **53**: 427–434.

Koehn, D (1994) *The Ground of Professional Ethics.* London: Routledge.

Koivisto, K, Janhonen, S and Väisänen, L (2004) 'Patients' experiences of being helped in an inpatient setting' *Journal of Psychiatric and Mental Health Nursing* **11**: 268–275.

Korff, M, Gruman, J and Schaefer, JEA (1997) 'Collaborative management of chronic illness' *Annals of Internal Medicine* **127**: 1097–1102.

Koro, CE, Fedder, DO and L'italien, GJ *et al.* (2002) 'An assessment of the independent effects of olanzapine and risperidone exposure on the risk of hyperlipidaemia in schizophrenic patients' *Archive of General Psychiatry* **59**: 1021–1026.

Koss, M, Bailey, J, Yuan, N, Herrera, V and Lichter, E (2003) 'Depression and PTSD in survivors of male violence: research and training initiatives to facilitate recovery' *Psychology of Women Quarterly* **27**(2): 130–142.

Krumberger, J (2002) 'A priceless resource' *RN* **65**(5): 36ac18, 38ac20.

Kubler-Ross, E (1970) *On Death and Dying.* London: Tavistock.

Kuh, D and Ben-Shlomo, Y (2004) *A Life Course Approach to Chronic Disease Epidemiology.* Oxford: Oxford University Press.

Kuhn, T (1970) *The Structure of Scientific Revolutions*, 2nd edn. Chicago: University of Chicago Press.

Kulis, S and Nieri, T (2007) *Gender, Gender Identity and Risk Behaviours of Youth from Mexican Immigrant Communities.* Conference Proceedings: Bridging Disciplinary Boundaries (Jan 11–14). Available at: http://sswr.confex.com/sswr/2007/techprogram/P6258.HTM

Kumar, S, Guite, H and Thornicroft, G (2001) 'Service-users' experience of violence within a mental health system: a study using a grounded theory approach' *Journal of Mental Health* **10**(6): 597–611.

Kuokkanen, L and Katajisto, J (2003) 'Promoting or impeding empowerment?' *Journal of Nursing Administration* **33**(4): 209–215.

Laing, RD and Esterson, A (1964) *Sanity, Madness and the Family.* London: Penguin.

Lake, V and Hall, B (2005) *Young Offenders and Mental Health.* Available at: http://www.rcn.org.uk/mhz/good_practice/young_offenders_and_mental_health

Lakeman, R (2003) 'Ethical issues in psychiatric and mental health nursing' in Barker, P (ed.) *Psychiatric and Mental Health Nursing: The Craft of Caring.* London: Arnold.

Lakeman, R (2004) 'Standardised routine outcome measurement: pot holes in the road to recovery' *International Journal of Mental Health Nursing* **13**: 210–215.

Lalani, N and London, C (2006) 'The media: agents of social exclusion for people with a mental illness?' Politics of Health Group. Available at: http://www.pohg.org.uk/support/publications.html

Lalani, N, Scriven, A and London, C (2006) 'Mental health and media: why stigma should be old news' *Healthmatters* **64**: 16.

Lambert, TJR, Velakoulis, D and Pantelis, C (2003) 'Medical co-morbidity in schizophrenia' *Medical Journal of Australia* **178**: S67–70.

Lambo, T (1970) 'The importance of cultural factors in psychiatric treatments' in Al-Issa, I and Dennis, W (eds) *Cross Cultural Studies of Behaviour*. New York: Holt, Rinehart and Winston.

Lansdown, R and Benjamin, G (1985) 'The development of the concept of death in children aged 5–9 years' *Child Care, Health and Development* **11**: 13–20.

Lanza, ML (1983) 'The reactions of nursing staff to physical assault by a patient' *Hospital and Community Psychiatry* **34**: 44–47.

Lauder, W (1999a) 'The medical model and other constructions of self-neglect' *International Journal of Nursing Practice* **5**: 58–63.

Lauder, W (1999b) 'A survey of self-neglect in patients living in the community' *Journal of Clinical Nursing* **8**: 95–102.

Lauder, W (1999c) 'Constructions of self-neglect: a multiple case study design' *Nursing Inquiry* **6**(1): 48–57.

Lauder, W (2001) 'The utility of self-care theory as a theoretical basis for self-neglect' *Journal of Advanced Nursing* **34**(4): 545–551.

Lauder, W (2005) 'Self-neglect: the role of judgement and applied ethics' *Nursing Standard* **19**(18): 45–51.

Lauder, W, Anderson, I and Barclay, A (2002) 'Sociological and psychological theories of self-neglect' *Journal of Advanced Nursing* **40**(3): 331–338.

Lauder, W, Anderson, I and Barclay, A (2005) 'A framework for good practice in interagency interventions with cases of self-neglect' *Journal of Psychiatric and Mental Health Nursing* **12**: 192–198.

Lauder, W, Ludwick, R, Zeller, R and Winchell, J (2006) 'Factors influencing nurses' judgements about self-neglect cases' *Journal of Psychiatric and Mental Health Nursing* **13**: 279–287.

Lauder, W, Meehan, T and Moxham, L (2004) 'Changing face of mental health nursing' *Journal of Psychiatric and Mental Health Nursing* **11**: 1–2.

Lauder, W, Scott, P and Whyte, A (2001) 'Nurses' judgements of self-neglect: a factorial survey' *International Journal of Nursing Studies* **38**(5): 601–608.

Launer, J (2002) *Narrative-Based Primary Care: A Practical Guide*. Abingdon: Radcliffe Medical Press.

Laurance, J (2003) *Pure Madness: How Fear Drives the Mental Health System*. London: Routledge.

Lawn, S (2004) 'Cigarette smoking in psychiatric settings: occupational health, safety, welfare and legal concerns' *Australian and New Zealand Journal of Psychiatry* **39**: 886–891.

Lazarus, R and Folkman, S (1984) *Psychological Stress and the Coping Process*. New York: Springer.

Leathard, A (1994) *Going Interprofessional: Working Together for Health and Welfare*. London: Routledge.

Lee, S, Gray, R, Gournay, K, Wright, S, Parr, A and Sayer, J (2003) 'Views of nursing staff on the use of physical restraint' *Journal of Psychiatric and Mental Health Nursing* **10**(4): 425–430.

Lee, S, Wright, S, Sayer, J, Parr, A, Gray, R and Gournay, K (2001) 'Physical restraint training for nurses in English and Welsh psychiatric intensive care and regional secure units' *Journal of Mental Health* **10**(2): 151–162.

Leff, J (2001) 'Why is care in the community perceived as a failure?' *British Journal of Psychiatry* **179**: 381–383.

Lehane, M (1996) 'What the papers say' *Nursing Standard* **10**(28): 22–23.

Lelliott, P, Paton, C, Harrington, M, Konsolaki, M, Sensky, T and Okocha, C (2002) 'The influence of patient variables on polypharmacy and combined high dose of antipsychotic drugs prescribed for in-patients' Psychiatric Bulletin 26: 411–414.

Lett, HS, Blumenthal, JA and Babyak, MA (2004) 'Depression as a risk factor for coronary artery disease; evidence, mechanisms and treatment' Psychosomatic Medicine 66: 305–315.

Leung, J and Arthur, DG (2004) 'Clients and facilitators' experiences of participating in Hong Kong self-help group for people recovering from mental illness' International Journal of Mental Health Nursing 13: 232–241.

Leventhal, H and Nerenz, DR (1983) 'A model for stress research with implications for the control of stress disorders' in Meichenbaum, D and Jaremko, M (eds) Stress Reduction and Prevention. New York: Plenum.

Lewis, A and Webster, C (2004) 'General instruments for risk assessment' Current Opinion in Psychiatry 17: 401–405.

Liberman, RP, Hilty, MD, Drake, RE and Tsang, HWH (2001) 'Requirements for multi-disciplinary teamwork in psychiatric rehabilitation' Psychiatric Services 52(10): 1331–1342.

Liberman, RP, Kopelowicz, A, Ventura, J and Gutkind, D (2002) 'Recovery from schizophrenia: a challenge for the 21st century' International Review of Psychiatry 14(4): 256–272.

Lieberman, JA, Stroup, TS, McEvoy, JP, Swartz, MS, Rosenheck, RA, Perkins, DO, Keefe, RSE, Davis, SM, Davis, CE, Lebowitz, BD, Severe, J and Hsiao, JK (2005) 'Effectiveness of antipsychotic drugs in patients with chronic schizophrenia' New England Journal of Medicine 353: 1209–1223.

Link, B and Phelan, J (1999) 'Labelling and stigma' in Aneshensel, C and Phelan, J (eds) Handbook of Sociology and Social Research. New York: Kluwer Academic/Plenum.

Link, BG and Phelan, JC (2001) 'Conceptualizing stigma' Annual Review of Sociology 27: 363–385.

Link, BG, Stuening, EL, Neese-Todd, S, Asmussen, S and Phelan, JC (2001) 'The consequences of stigma for the self-esteem of people with mental illnesses' Psychiatric Services 52: 1621–1626.

Lipscomb, JA and Love, CC (1992) 'Violence towards health care workers; an emerging occupational hazard' AAOHN Journal 40: 219–228.

Lipsky, M (1980) Street-Level Bureaucracy: Dilemmas of the Individual in Public Services. New York: Russel-Sage Foundation.

Lister, R (2001) 'New Labour: a study in ambiguity from a position of ambivalence' Critical Social Policy 21(4): 425–447.

Little, L (1999) 'Risk factors for assaults on nursing staff: childhood abuse and education level' Journal of Nursing Administration 29(12): 22–29.

Littlejohn, C (2003) 'Critical realism and psychiatric nursing: a philosophical inquiry' Journal of Advanced Nursing 43(5): 449–456.

Littlewood, R and Lipsedge, M (1997) Aliens and Alienists: Ethnic Minorities and Psychiatry, 3rd edn. London: Routledge.

Livesely, J (2001) Handbook of Personality Disorders: Theory, Research, and Treatment. New York: Guilford Press.

Lloyd-Williams, M, Wilkinson, C and Lloyd-Williams, FF (1998) 'Do bereaved children consult the primary health care team more frequently?' European Journal of Cancer Care 7: 12–124.

Lockwood, S (2004) '"Evidence of me" in evidence based medicine?' British Medical Journal 329: 1033–1035.

London South Bank University (LSBU) (2007) Inventing Adulthoods, A Qualitative Longitudinal Dataset on Young People Growing Up in England and Northern Ireland between 1996–2006. Available at: http://www.lsbu.ac.uk/inventingadulthoods.

London, C, Scriven, A and Lalani, N (2006) 'Sir Winston Churchill: Greatest Briton used as an anti-stigma icon' *Journal of The Royal Society for the Promotion of Health* **126**(4): 163–164.

Longres, J (1994) 'Self neglect and social control: a modest test of an issue' *Journal of Gerontological Social Work* **22**(3/4): 3–20.

Lord Carlile of Berriew (Chair) (2006) *An Independent Inquiry into the Use of Physical Restraint, Solitary Confinement and Forcible Strip Searching of Children in Prisons, Secure Training Centres and Local Authority Secure Children's Homes.* London: Howard League for Penal Reform.

Lorig, K, Kraines, R and Holman, H (1981) 'A randomised, prospective controlled study of the effects of health education' *Arthritis and Rheumatology* **24**: S90.

Lowe, F and O'Hara, S (2000) 'Multidisciplinary team working in practice: managing the transition' *Journal of Interprofessional Care* **14**(3): 269–279.

Lowe, T (1992) 'Characteristics of effective nursing interventions in the management of challenging behaviour' *Journal of Advanced Nursing* **17**: 1226–1232.

Lowe, T, Wellman, N and Taylor, R (2003) 'Limit-setting and decision-making in the management of aggression' *Journal of Advanced Nursing* **41**(2): 154–161.

Luban, D (2006) 'Liberalism, torture and the ticking bomb' in Greenberg, KJ (ed.) *The Torture Debate in America.* New York: Cambridge University Press.

Luborsky, L, Diguer, L, Seligman, DA, Rosenthal, R, Krause, ED, Johnson, S, Halperin, G, Bishop, M, Berman, JS and Schweizer, E (1999) 'The researcher's own therapy allegiances: a "wild card" in comparisons of treatment efficacy' *Clinical Psychology: Science and Practice* **6**: 95–106.

Lukoff, D, Nuechterlein, KH and Ventura, J (1986) 'Brief psychiatric rating scale (expanded – 1986)' *Schizophrenia Bulletin* **12**: 594–602.

Lunt, A (2001) 'Risk and uncertainty: the unknown and psychiatric rehabilitation' *Psychiatric Rehabilitation Journal* **25**: 89–92.

Lunt, A (2004) 'The implications for the clinician of adopting a recovery model: the role of choice in assertive treatment' *Psychiatric Rehabilitation Journal* **28**: 93–97.

Lützén, K and Schreiber, R (1998) 'Moral survival in a nontherapeutic environment' *Issues in Mental Health Nursing* **19**: 303–315.

Lynch, JE and Kemp, P (2005) 'Social problems as political resource' *Talking Politics* **18**(1): 47–50.

Lyon, C and Pimar, A (2004) *Physical Interventions and the Law.* London: BILD.

Lyons, D and McLoughlin, MD (2001) 'Clinical review: recent advances' *British Medical Journal* **323**: 1228–1231.

MacGillivary, H, Nefson, G and Pilleltensky, I (1998) *Partnerships for solidarity with disadvantaged people: Values, stakeholders, context, processes, and outcomes.* Unpublished manuscript, Wilfrid Laurier University.

Machin, T and Stevenson, C (1999) 'Review: towards a framework for clarifying psychiatric nursing roles' *Journal of Psychiatric and Mental Health Nursing* **4**: 81–87.

Macintyre Undercover (1999) BBC1 TV, 16 November.

Macklin, R (2003) 'Dignity is a useless concept' *British Medical Journal* **327**: 1419–1420.

MacMillan, D and Shaw, P (1966) 'Senile breakdown in standards of personal and environmental cleanliness' *British Medical Journal* **2**: 1032–1037.

Maes, S and Karoly, P (2005) 'Self regulation assessment and intervention in physical health and illness: a review' *Applied Psychology: An International Review* **54**(2): 267–299.

Mahon, MM, Goldberg, EZ and Washington, SK (1999) 'Concept of death in a sample of Israeli kibbutz children' *Death Studies* **23**: 43–59.

Maier, T (2004) 'On phenomenology and classification of hoarding: a review' *Acta Psychiatrica Scandinavica* **110**: 323–337.

Main, TF (1990) 'Knowledge, learning and freedom from thought' *Psychoanalytic Pschotherapy* **5**(1): 59–74.

Mann, JI (2002) 'Diet and risk of coronary heart disease and type 2 diabetes' *Lancet* **360**: 783–789.

Mann, S and Cowburn, J (2005) 'Emotional labour and stress within mental health nursing' *Journal of Psychiatric and Mental Health Nursing* **12**: 154–162.

Marangos-Frost, S and Wells, D (2000) 'Psychiatric nurses' thoughts and feelings about restraint use: a decision dilemma' *Journal of Advanced Nursing* **32**(2): 362–369.

Marengo, J (1994) 'Classifying the courses of schizophrenia' *Schizophrenia Bulletin* **20**: 519–536.

Markowitz, FE (2001) 'Modelling processes in recovery from mental illness: relationships between symptoms, life satisfaction, and self-concept' *Journal of Health and Social Behaviour* **42**: 64–79.

Marmot, M and Wilkinson, R (1999) *Social Determinants of Health.* Oxford: Oxford University Press.

Marshall, TH (1950) *Citizenship and Social Class.* Cambridge: University of Cambridge Press.

Marshall, TH and Bottomore, T (1992) *Citizenship and Social Class.* London: Pluto Press.

Martin, DV (1962) *Adventure in Psychiatry.* Oxford: Bruno Cassirer.

Martin, JP (1984) *Hospitals in Trouble.* London: Basil Blackwell.

Marwaha, S and Johnson, S (2005) 'Views and experiences of employment among people with psychosis: a qualitative descriptive study' *International Journal of Social Psychiatry* **51**: 302–316.

Marx, K (1964) *Early Writings* (trans. TB Bottomore). New York: McGraw-Hill.

Mason, D (2000) *Race and Ethnicity in Modern Britain*, 2nd edn. Oxford: Oxford University Press.

Mason, T (1998) 'Models of risk assessment in mental health practice: a critical examination' *Mental Health Care* **1**: 405–407.

Mason, T and Chandley, M (1999) *Managing Violence and Aggression: A Manual for Nurses and Health Care Workers.* Edinburgh: Churchill Livingstone.

Mavundla, T (2000) 'Professional nurses' perception of nursing mentally ill people in a general hospital setting' *Journal of Advanced Nursing* **32**(6): 1569–1578.

McAllister, M and Walsh, K (2004) 'Different voices: reviewing and revising the politics of working with consumers in mental health' *International Journal of Mental Health Nursing* **13**: 22–32.

McCloughen, A (2003) 'The association between schizophrenia and cigarette smoking: a review of the literature and implications for mental health nursing practice' *International Journal of Mental Health Nursing* **12**: 119–129.

McCormick, J, Rodney, P and Varcoe, C (2003) 'Reinterpretations across studies: an approach to meta-analysis' *Qualitative Health Research* **13**(7): 933–944.

McCormick, K (2002) 'A concept analysis of uncertainty in illness' *Journal of Nursing Scholarship* **34**(2): 127–131.

McCreadie, R (2003) 'Diet, smoking and cardiovascular risk in people with schizophrenia' *British Journal of Psychiatry* **183**: 534–539.

McFarlane, A, Bookless, C and Air, T (2001) 'Life events and psychiatric disorder: the role of a natural disaster' *British Journal of Psychiatry* **151**: 362–367.

McFarlane, L (1998) *Diagnosis: Homophobic. The experiences of lesbians, gay men and bisexuals in mental health services.* Available at: http://www.pacehealth.org.uk/NR/rdonlyres/FA99EE96-BE60-45AF-B45B-A6859C740E24/0/diagnosis_homophobic.pdf.

McGorry, P, Curry, C and Elkins, K (1997) 'Psychosocial interventions in mental disorders: developing evidenced-based practice' *Current Opinion in Psychiatry* **10**: 173–177.

McManus, P, Mant, A, Mitchell, PB, Montgomery, WS, Marley, J and Auland, ME (2000) 'Recent trends in the use of antidepressants in Australia, 1990–1998' *Medical Journal of Australia* **173**(9): 458–461.

McMillan, M (2004) *The Person-Centred Approach to Therapeutic Change*. London: Sage.

McNeil, JN, Silliman, B and Swihart, JJ (1991) 'Helping adolescents cope with the death of a peer' *Journal of Adolescent Research* **6**: 132–145.

Meddings, S and Perkins, R (2002) 'What "getting better" means to staff and users of a rehabilitation service: an exploratory study' *Journal of Mental Health* **11**(3): 319–325.

Medical Research Council (MRC) (2000) *A Framework for Development and Evaluation of RCTs for Complex Interventions to Improve Health*. London: Medical Research Council Health Services and Public Health Research Board.

Meek, I (1998) 'Evaluation of the role of the health care assistant within a community mental health intensive care team' *Journal of Nursing Management* **6**: 11–19.

Megargee, E (1976) 'The prediction of dangerous behaviour' *Criminal Justice and Behaviour* **3**: 3–21.

Mellor, JE, Laugharne, JDE and Peet, M (1996) 'Omega-3 fatty acid supplementation in schizophrenic patients' *Human Psychopharmacology* **11**: 39–46.

Melrose, S and Shapiro, B (1999) 'Students' perceptions of their psychiatric mental health clinical nursing experience: a personal construct theory exploration' *Journal of Advanced Nursing* **30**(6): 1451–1458.

Melville, MR, Packham, C and Brown, N *et al.* (1999) 'Cardiac rehabilitation: socially deprived patients are less likely to attend but patients ineligible for thrombolysis are less likely to be invited' *Heart* **82**(3): 373–377.

Men's Health Forum (2002) *Soldier It! Young Men and Suicide*. Available at: http://www.menshealthforum.org.uk/uploaded_files/mhfsuicideauditfinal.pdf

Mental Health Foundation (2002) *The Mental Health of Young Offenders. Bright Futures: Working with Vulnerable Young People*. London: The Mental Health Foundation.

Mental Health Foundation (2006) *Feeding Minds: The Impact of Food on Mental Health*. Available at: http://www.mentalhealth.org.uk/campaigns/food-and-mental-health

Mentality/NIMHE (2004) *Healthy Body and Mind: Promoting Health Living for People who Experience Mental Distress*. Available at: http://www.neyh.csip.org.uk/silo/files/hbhmprimarycare.pdf

Menzies, IEP (1959) 'The functioning of social systems as a defence against anxiety: a report on a study on the nursing service of a general hospital' *Human Relations* **13**: 95–121.

Mericle, BP (1999) 'Developing the therapeutic environment' in Keltner, NL, Schwecke, LH and Boston, CE (eds) *Psychiatric Nursing*, 3rd edn. London: Mosby.

Midgley, M (1989) *Wisdom, Information and Wonder: What Is Knowledge For?* London: Routledge.

Midgley, M (2003) *The Myths We Live By*. London: Routledge.

Milewa, T, Valentine, J and Calnan, M (1998) 'Managerialism and active citizenship in Britain's reformed health service: power and community in an era of decentralisation' *Social Science and Medicine* **47**(4): 507–517.

Miller, EJ and Gwynne, GV (1976) *A Life Apart*. London: Tavistock.

Miller, WB (1958) 'Lower class culture as a generating milieu of gang delinquency' *Journal of Social Issues* **14**(3): 5–19.

Miller, WR (1994) 'Motivational interviewing: Lll. On the ethics of motivational intervention' *Behavioural and Cognitive Psychotherapy* **22**: 111–123.

Miller, WR and Rollnick, S (2002) *Motivational Interviewing: Preparing People for Change*, 2nd edn. New York: Guildford Press.

Miller, WR, Zweben, A, Diclemente, CC and Rychtarik, RG (1992) *Motivational Enhancement Therapy Manual: A Clinical Research Guide for Therapists Treating Individuals with Alcohol Abuse and Dependence*. Rockville, MD: National Institute on Alcohol Abuse and Alcoholism.

MIND (2007) *Information: Lesbians, Gay Men and Bisexuals and Mental Health* [on-line]. Available at: http://www.mind.org.uk/Information/Factsheets/Diversity/Factsheetlgb.htm

Mishel, M (1988) 'Uncertainty in illness' *Image: Journal of Nursing Scholarship* 20: 225–232.

Mishra, R (1990) *The Welfare State in a Capitalist Society*. London: Harvester.

Mitchell, JT (1983) 'When disaster strikes: the critical incident debriefing process' *Journal of Emergency Medical Services* 8: 36–39.

Mitchell, L (2001) *Discovering and maintaining recovery for the consumer (A Consumers Perspective)* [on-line]. Available at: http://akmhcweb.org/recovery/RECOVERYMODEL.htm

Möller-Leimkühler, A (2003) 'The gender gap in suicide and premature death or why are men so vulnerable?' *European Archives of Psychiatry and Clinical Neuroscience* 253(1): 1–8.

Monahan, J (1988) 'Risk assessment of violence among the mentally disordered: generating useful knowledge' *International Journal of Law and Psychiatry* 11: 249–257.

Moore, M and Carr, A (2000) 'Depression and grief' in Carr, A (ed.) *What Works with Children and Adolescents? A Critical Review of Psychological Interventions with Children, Adolescents and their Families*. London: Routledge.

Moosajee, M (2003) 'A noxious cocktail of genes and the environment' *Journal of the Royal Society of Medicine* 96: 211–214.

Morgan, S (2004) 'The foundations of creative collaboration' in Ryan, P and Morgan, S (eds) *Assertive Outreach: A Strengths Approach to Policy and Practice*. London: Churchill Livingstone.

Morin, SM and Welsh, LA (1996) 'Adolescents' perceptions and experiences of death and grieving' *Adolescence* 31(123): 585–596.

Morrall, P (1998) *Mental Health Nursing and Social Control*. London: Whurr.

Morris, R, Cheek, B and Pell, K (with Thomson, G) (1996) *Advanced Ground Control and Restraint*. London: World Kobudo Federation.

Morrison, E (1990) 'The tradition of toughness: a study of nonprofessional nursing care in psychiatric settings' *Image: Journal of Nursing Scholarship* 22(1): 32–38.

Morrison, P (1991) 'The caring attitude in nursing practice: a repertory grid study of trained nurses' perceptions' *Nurse Education Today* 11: 3–12.

Morrison-Valfre, M (2005) *Foundations of Mental Health Care*. St. Louis, MO: Elsevier Mosby.

Mortimer, P (2006) 'Lucy in the sky with diamonds' *Openmind* **Jul/Aug**: 140.

Motluk, A (2005) 'How the food you eat could change your genes for life' *New Scientist* **188**: 12.

Mueser, K, Goodman, L, Trumbetta, S, Rosenberg, S, Osher, F, Vidaver, R, Auciello, P and Foy, D (1998b) 'Trauma and posttraumatic stress disorder in severe mental illness' *Journal of Consulting and Clinical Psychology* 66: 439–499.

Mueser, KT, Bond, GR, Drake, RE and Resnick, SG (1998a) 'Models of community care for severe mental illness: a review of research on case management' *Schizophrenia Bulletin* 24(19): 37–74.

Muir Gray, JA (2001) 'Using systematic reviews for evidence based policy making' in Egger, M, Smith, GD and Altman, I (eds) *Systematic Reviews in Health Care: Meta-analysis in Context*. London: BMJ Books.

Muir, WK Jr (1977) *Police: Streetcorner Politicians.* Chicago: University of Chicago Press.

Mukherjee, S, Schnur, DB and Reddy, R (1989) 'Family history of type 2 diabetes in schizophrenic patients' *Lancet* **1**(8636): 495.

Mullen, A and Murray, L (2002) 'Clinical placements in mental health: are clinicians doing enough for undergraduate nursing students?' *International Journal of Mental Health Nursing* **11**: 61–68.

Mulrow, CD (1987) 'The medical review article: state of the science' *Annals of Internal Medicine* **106**: 485–488.

Mulvey, E and Lidz, C (1984) 'Some considerations in the prediction of dangerousness in mental patients' *Clinical Psychology Review* **4**: 379–401.

Mulvey, E and Lidz, C (1995) 'Conditional prediction: a model for research on dangerousness to others in a new era' *International Journal of Law and Psychiatry* **18**(2): 129–143.

Murphy, K (2005) 'Psychosocial treatments for ADHD in teens and adults: a practice-friendly review' *Journal of Clinical Psychology* **61**(5): 607–619.

National Institute for Clinical Excellence (NICE) (2002a) *Guidance on the Use of Newer (Atypical) Antipsychotic Drugs for the Treatment of Schizophrenia. Technology Appraisal Guidance No. 43.* Available at: http://guidance.nice.org.uk/TA43/guidance/pdf/English

National Institute for Clinical Excellence (NICE) (2002b) *Schizophrenia: Core Interventions in the Treatment and Management of Schizophrenia in Primary and Secondary Care.* Available at: http://guidance.nice.org.uk/CG1/guidance/pdf/English

National Institute for Clinical Excellence (NICE) (2004) *Depression: Management of Depression in Primary and Secondary Care. National Clinical Practice Guideline No. 23.* Available at: http://guidance.nice.org.uk/page.aspx?o=236667

National Institute for Health and Clinical Excellence (NICE) (2005a) *Depression in Children and Young People: Identification and Management in Primary, Community and Secondary Care. Clinical Practice Guideline No. 28.* Available at: http://guidance.nice.org.uk/CG28/guidance/pdf/English

National Institute for Clinical Excellence (NICE) (2005b) *Violence: The Short-Term Management of Disturbed/Violent Behaviour in In-Patient Psychiatric Settings and Emergency Departments. National Clinical Guideline 25,* London, NICE. Available at: http://guidance.nice.org.uk/CG25/niceguidance/pdf/English/download.dspx

National Institute for Clinical Excellence (NICE) (2005c) *Post Traumatic Stress Disorder: The Management of PTSD in Adults and Children in Primary and Secondary Care. National Clinical Practice Guideline No. 23.* Available at: http://guidance.nice.org.uk/CG26/guidance/pdf/English/download.dspx

National Institute for Health and Clinical Excellence (NICE) (2006a) *Bipolar Disorder: The Management of Bipolar Disorder in Adults, Children and Adolescents, in Primary and Secondary Care.* Available at: http://guidance.nice.org.uk/cg38

National Institute for Health and Clinical Excellence (NICE) (2006b) *Violence: The Short-Term Management of Disturbed/Violent Behaviour in In-Patient Psychiatric Settings and Emergency Departments,* London, Royal College of Nursing. Available at: http://guidance.nice.org.uk/CG25/guidance/pdf/English/download.dspx

National Institute for Health and Clinical Excellence (NICE) (2007) *Depression (amended): Management of Depression in Primary and Secondary Care. NICE Clinical Guideline No. 23(amended).* Available at: http://guidance.nice.org.uk/CG23/guidance/pdf/English

National Institute for Mental Health in England (NIMHE) (2004a) *Cases for Change: User Involvement.* London: NIMHE.

National Institute for Mental Health in England (NIMHE) (2004b) *Mental Health Policy Implementation Guide: Developing Positive Practice to Support Safe and Therapeutic Management of Aggression and Violence in Mental Health In-patient Settings.* Leeds: NIMHE.

National Institute for Mental Health in England (NIMHE) (2005) *NIMHE Guiding Statement on Recovery*. Available at: http://www.psychminded.co.uk/news/news2005/feb05/nimherecovstatement.pdf

National Institute for Mental Health in England (NIMHE)/Care Services Improvement Partnership (CSIP) (2006) *Our Choices in Mental Health: A Framework for Improving Choice for People who Use Mental Health Services and their Carers*. Available at: http://www.csip-plus.org.uk/CPT/Our%20Choices%20Doc%20-%20Final.pdf

Naylor, DC (1997) 'Meta-analysis and the meta-epidemiology of clinical research' *British Medical Journal* **315**: 617–619.

Needham, I, Abderhalden, C and Halfens, RJG (2005) 'Non-somatic effects of patient aggression on nurses: a systematic review' *Journal of Advanced Nursing* **49**(3): 283–296.

Neimeyer, R (2001) 'Unfounded trust: a constructivist meditation' *American Journal of Psychotherapy* **55**(3): 364–371.

Neimeyer, RA (ed.) (2001) *Meaning Reconstruction and the Experience of Loss*. Washington, DC: American Psychological Association.

Neimeyer, RA and Hogan, NS (2001) 'Quantitative or qualitative? Measurement issues in the study of grief' in Stroebe, MS, Hansson, RO, Stroebe, W and Schut, H (eds) *Handbook of Bereavement Research, Consequences, Coping and Care*. Washington, DC: American Psychological Association.

Nelson-Jones, R (2003) *Basic Counselling Skills: A Helpers' Manual*. London: Sage.

Neville, K (2003) 'Uncertainty in illness: an integrative review' *Orthopaedic Nursing* **22**(3): 206–214.

Newburn, T and Stanko, EA (1994) 'Introduction: men, masculinity and crime' in Newburn, T and Stanko, EA (eds) *Just Boys Doing Business? Men, Masculinities and Crime*. London: Routledge.

Newman, J, Barnes, M, Sullivan, H and Knops, A (2004) 'Public participation and collaborative governance' *Journal of Social Policy* **33**(2): 203–223.

Newman, T and Blackburn, S (2002) *Transitions in the Lives of Children and Young People: Resilience Factors, Report for Scottish Executive Education and Young People Research Unit*. Available at: http://www.scotland.gov.uk/Resource/Doc/46997/0024005.pdf

NHS Executive (1996) *Patient Partnership: Building a Collaborative Strategy*. Leeds: NHSE.

NHS London (2006) *Report of the Independent Inquiry into the Care and Treatment of John Barrett*. Available at: http://www.london.nhs.uk/londonnhs-publications.aspx?id_Content=7300

NHS Service Delivery and Organisation (2006) *Achieving High Performance in Health Care Systems: The Impact and Influence of Organisational Arrangements*. London: National Co-ordinating Centre for NHS Service Delivery and Organisation Research and Development (NCCSDO).

Nicholas, D (2000) 'Men, masculinity and cancer: risk-factor behaviours, early detection and psychosocial adaptation' *Journal of American College Health* **49**(1): 27–33.

Nijman, H, Muris, P, Merckelbach, H, Palmstierna, T, Wistedt, B, Vis, A, van Rixtel, A and Allertz, W (1999) 'The staff observation aggression scale – revised (SOAS – R)' *Aggressive Behaviour* **25**: 197–209.

Nixon, S (1997) 'Exhibiting masculinity' in Hall, S (ed.) *Representation: Cultural Representations and Signifying Practices*. London: SAGE/Open University.

Noak, J (1995) 'Care of people with psychopathic disorder' *Nursing Standard* **9**(34): 30–32.

Noak, J (2001) 'Do we need another model for mental health care?' *Nursing Standard* **16**(8): 33–35.

Noblit, GW and Hare, RD (1988) *Meta-Ethnography: Synthesising Qualitative Studies*. London: Sage.

Nolan, P (1990) 'Psychiatric nursing – the first 100 years' *Senior Nurse* **10**(10): 20–23.

Nolan, P (1993) *A History of Mental Health Nursing*. London: Chapman and Hall.

Nolan, P, Haque, M, Badger, F, Dyke, R and Khan, I (2001) 'Mental health nurses' perceptions of nurse prescribing' *Journal of Advanced Nursing* **36**(4): 527–534.

Nolan, P, Haque, S and Doran, M (2007) 'A comparative cross-sectional questionnaire survey of the work of UK and US mental health nurses' *International Journal of Nursing Studies* **44**: 377–385.

Norman, R and Malla, A (2001) 'Duration of untreated psychosis: a critical examination of the concept and its importance' *Psychological Medicine* **31**: 381–400.

Nose, M, Barbui, C and Tansella, M (2003) 'How often do patients with psychosis fail to adhere to treatment programmes? A systematic review' *Psychological Medicine* **33**: 1149–1160.

Nursing and Midwifery Council (NMC) (2004a) *Standards of Proficiency for Pre-Registration Nursing Education* [on-line]. Available at: http://www.nmc-uk.org/aFrameDisplay. aspx?DocumentID=328

Nursing and Midwifery Council (NMC) (2004b) *The NMC Code of Professional Conduct: Standards for Conduct, Performance and Ethics*. Available at: http://www.nmc-uk.org/aFrameDisplay. aspx?DocumentID=201

Nursing and Midwifery Council (NMC) (2006a) *Circular 35/2006*. Available at: http://www. nmc-uk.org/aFrameDisplay.aspx?DocumentID=2286

Nursing and Midwifery Council (NMC) (2006b) *Nurse Prescribing and the Supply and Administration of Medication: Position Statement*. Available at: http://www.nmc-uk.org/aFrameDisplay. aspx?DocumentID=1219

O'Brien, L and Cole, R (2004) 'Mental health nursing practice in acute psychiatric close-observation areas' *International Journal of Mental Health Nursing* **13**: 89–99.

O'Sullivan, K (1984) 'Depression and its treatment in alcoholics: a review' *Canadian Journal of Psychiatry* **29**: 279–384.

Oades, L, Deane, F, Crowe, T, Gordon Lambert, W, Kavanagh, D and Lloyd, C (2005) 'Collaborative recovery: an integrated model for working with individuals who experience chronic and recurring mental illness' *Australasian Psychiatry* **13**: 279–284.

Ochocka, J, Nelson, G and Janzen, R (2005) 'Moving forward: negotiating self and external circumstances in recovery' *Psychiatric Rehabilitation Journal* **28**: 315–322.

Oehl, M, Hummar, M and Fleischhacker, WW (2000) 'Compliance with antipsychotic treatment' *Acta Psychiatrica Scandinavica* **102**(Suppl. 407): 83–86.

Office for National Statistics (ONS) (2007) *Suicides: Rate in UK men continues to fall* [on-line]. Available at: http://www.statistics.gov.uk/cci/nugget.asp?id=1092

Office of the Deputy Prime Minister (ODPM) (2005) *Transitions*. Available at: http://archive. cabinetoffice.gov.uk/seu/downloaddoccf3f.pdf?id=703

Oguisso, T (1995) 'Mental health nursing: a global perspective' *Journal of Psychiatric and Mental Health Nursing* **2**: 41–45.

Oliver, M (1992) *The Politics of Disablement*. Basingstoke: MacMillan.

Olofsson, B and Norberg, A (2001) 'Experiences of coercion in psychiatric care as narrated by patients, nurses and physicians' *Journal of Advanced Nursing* **33**(1): 89–97.

Olsen, DP (1997) 'When the patient causes the problem: the effect of patient responsibility on the nurse–patient relationship' *Journal of Advanced Nursing* **26**: 515–522.

Olsen, DP (2003) 'Influence and coercion: relational and rights-based ethical approaches to forced psychiatric treatment' *Journal of Psychiatric and Mental Health Nursing* **10**: 705–712.

Olstead, R (2002) 'Contesting the text: Canadian media depictions of the conflation of mental illness and criminality' *Sociology of Health and Illness* **24**(5): 621–643.

Onega, L (1991) 'A theoretical framework for psychiatric nursing practice' *Journal of Advanced Nursing* **16**: 68–73.

Onyett, S (2004) 'Functional teams and whole systems' in Ryrie, I and Norman, I (eds) *The Art and Science of Mental Health Nursing*. Maidenhead: Open University Press.

Orrell, M, Sahakian, B and Bergmann, K (1989) 'Self neglect and frontal lobe dysfunction' *British Journal of Psychiatry* **155**: 101–105.

Osborn, DPJ and Warner, J (1998) 'Assessing the physical health of psychiatric patients' *Psychiatric Bulletin* **22**: 695–697.

Palmstierna, T and Wistedt, B (1987) 'Staff observation aggression scale, SOAS: presentation and evaluation' *Acta Psychiatrica Scandinavica* **76**: 657–663.

Pannick, D (1992) *Advocates*. Oxford: Oxford University Press.

Papanicolaou, DA, Wilder, RL, Manolagas, SC and Chrousos, GP (1998) 'The pathophysiologic roles of Interleukin-6 in human disease' *Annals of Internal Medicine* **128**: 127–137.

Parenti, M (1978) *Power and the Powerless*. New York: St. Martin's Press.

Parish, C (2004) 'An exception to the rule' *Nursing Standard* **18**(20): 12–13.

Parkes, CM (1995) 'Guidelines for conducting ethical bereavement research' *Death Studies* **19**: 171–181.

Parkes, CM (2000) 'Counselling bereaved people – help or harm?' *Bereavement Care* **19**(2): 19–21.

Parkes, J (1996) 'Control and restraint training: a study of its effectiveness in a medium-secure psychiatric unit' *Journal of Forensic Psychiatry* **7**(3): 525–534.

Parliamentary Office of Science and Technology (POST) (2003) *Reform of Mental Health Legislation*. Available at: http://www.parliament.uk/post/pn204.pdf

Parsons, S (1998) 'What future for research in mental health nursing: share the objective statistics' *Journal of Psychiatric and Mental Health Nursing* **5**: 233–234.

Pashley, G (1992) 'Professional conceptions of mental illness and related illnesses' in Soothill, K, Henry, C and Kendrick, K (eds) *Themes and Perspectives in Nursing*. London: Chapman and Hall.

Paterson, B (2005) 'Thinking the unthinkable: a role for pain compliance and mechanical restraint in the management of violence?' *Mental Health Practice* **8**(7): 18–23.

Paterson, B and Tringham, C (1999) 'Legal and ethical issues in the management of aggression and violence' in Turnbull, J and Paterson, B (eds) *Aggression and Violence: Approaches to Effective Management*. Basingstoke: Macmillan.

Paterson, B, Bradley, P, Stark, C, Sadler, D, Leadbetter, D and Allen, D (2003a) 'Deaths associated with restraint use in health and social care in the UK: the results of a preliminary survey' *Journal of Psychiatric and Mental Health Nursing* **10**(1): 3–15.

Paterson, B, Bradley, P, Stark, C, Sadler, D, Leadbetter, D and Allen, D (2003b) 'Restraint-related deaths in Health and Social Care in the UK: learning the lessons' *Mental Health Practice* **6**(9): 10–17.

Paterson, B, Leadbetter, D and McComish, A (1998) 'Restraint and sudden death from asphyxia' *Nursing Times* **94**(44): 62–64.

Paterson, B, Leadbetter, D, Crichton, J and Miller, G (2007) 'Adopting a public health model to reduce violence and restraints in children's residential care facilities' in Nunno, M, Bullard, L and Day, DM (eds) *Examining the Safety of High Risk Interventions for Children and Young People*. Washington, DC: Child Welfare League of America.

Paton, C (1999) 'New Labour's health policy: the new healthcare state' in Powell, M (ed.) *New Labour, New Welfare State?* Bristol: Policy Press.

Pattison, S (2001) 'Are nursing codes of practice ethical?' *Nursing Ethics* **8**(1): 5–18.

Payne, S (2004) 'Gender influences on men's health' *The Journal of The Royal Society for the Promotion of Health* **124**: 206–207.

Pearson, A, Field, J and Jordan, Z (2006) *Evidence-Based Clinical Practice in Nursing and Healthcare.* Oxford: Blackwell Publications.

Pearson, A, Wiechula, R, Court, A and Lockwood, C (2005) 'The JBI model of evidence-based healthcare' *International Journal of Evidence Based Healthcare* **3**(8): 207–215.

Peck, E and Norman, I (1999) 'Working together in adult community mental health services: exploring the inter-professional role relations' *Journal of Mental Health* **8**(3): 231–242.

Peck, E and Parker, E (1998) 'Mental health policy in the NHS: policy and practice 1979–1998' *Journal of Mental Health* **7**(3): 241–259.

Peet, M (2004) 'Diet, diabetes and schizophrenia: review and hypothesis' *British Journal of Psychiatry* **184**(Suppl. 47): S102–S105.

Pendleton, D and King, J (2002) 'Values and leadership' *British Medical Journal* **325**: 1352–1355.

Penley, JA, Tomaka, J and Wiebe, J (2002) 'The association of coping to physical and psychological health outcomes: a meta-analytic review' *Journal of Behavioural Medicine* **25**(6): 551–603.

Penn, D and Wykes, T (2003) 'Stigma, discrimination and mental illness' *Journal of Mental Health* **12**(3): 203–208.

Penrod, J (2001) 'Refinement of the concept of uncertainty' *Journal of Advanced Nursing* **34**(2): 238–245.

Peplau, H (1952) *Interpersonal Relations in Nursing.* New York: Putman.

Peterkin, A (1993) 'Self help movement experiencing rapid growth in Canada' *Canadian Medical Association* **148**(5): 817–818.

Petersen, RC, Thomas, RG, Grundman, M, Bennett, D, Doody, R, Ferris, S, Galasko, D, Jin, S, Kaye, J, Levey, A, Pfeiffer, E, Sano, M, van Dyck, CH and Thal, LJ (2005) 'Vitamin E and donepezil for the treatment of mild cognitive impairment' *New England Journal of Medicine* **352**: 2379–2388.

Phelan, M, Stradins, L and Morrison, S (2001) 'Physical health of people with severe mental illness' *British Medical Journal* **322**: 443–444.

Phillips, D (2006) 'Masculinity, male development, gender and identity: modern and post-modern meanings' *Issues in Mental Health Nursing* **27**: 403–423.

Phillips, RJ (1934) 'Physical disorder in 164 consecutive admissions to a mental hospital: the incidence and significance' *British Medical Journal* **2**: 363–366.

Phillips, S (1996) 'Labouring the emotions: expanding the remit of nursing work?' *Journal of Advanced Nursing* **24**: 139–143.

Philo, G (1996) Media and Mental Distress. London: Longman.

Pickard, S (1998) 'Citizenship and consumerism in health care: a critique of citizens' juries' *Social Policy and Administration* **32**(3): 226–244.

Pilkington, E (2006) 'A child and his grief, one among thousands' *The Guardian*, 11 September, 18.

Pinker, S (1997) *How the Mind Works.* London: Penguin.

Platzer, H (2005) *Changing Families: Lesbian, Gay, and Bisexual Identity Work in Mental Health: an Evidence-Based Guide for People who Work with Families.* Available at: http://www.pace health.org.uk/NR/rdonlyres/AFCAD1FF-0F46-4C04-923A-B8062C62DE12/0/family_ service_good_practice_guidelines.pdf?knownurl=http%3a%2f%2fwww.pacehealth.org. uk%2fOneStopCMS%2fCore%2fCrawlerResourceServer.aspx%3fresource%3dAFCAD1FF-0F46-4C04-923A-B8062C62DE12%26mode%3dserve%26guid%3dffaaaf3138534364bcb260 eafd4fa43f

Playle, JF (1995) 'Humanism and positivism in nursing: contradictions and conflicts' *Journal of Advanced Nursing* **22**: 979–984.

Plunkett, WR, Attner, RF and Allen, GS (2005) *Management Meeting and Exceeding Customer Expectations.* Mason, OH: Thompson South Western.

Police Complaints Authority (2002) *Safer Restraint: Report of the Conference Held in April 2002 at Church House, Westminster.* London: PCA.

Polk, K (1994) 'Masculinity, honour and confrontational homicide' in Newburn, T and Stanko, EA (eds) *Just Boys Doing Business? Men, Masculinities and Crime.* London: Routledge.

Pollanen, MS, Chiasson, DA, Cairns, TJ and Yong, JG (1998) 'Unexpected death related to restraint for excited delirium: a retrospective study of deaths in police custody and in the community' *Canadian Medical Association Journal* **158**: 1603–1607.

Pollock, L (1988) 'The work of community psychiatric nursing' *Journal of Advanced Nursing* **13**: 537–545.

Pomeroy, EC, Kiam, K and Green, DL (2000) 'Reducing depression, anxiety and trauma of male inmates: an HIV/AIDS psychoeducational group intervention' *Social Work Research* **24**(3): 156–167.

Pope, LM, Adler, NE and Tschann, JM (2001) 'Postabortion psychological adjustment: are minors at increased risk?' *Journal of Adolescent Health* **29**: 2–11.

Pope, M and Denicolo, P (2001) *Transformative Education: Personal Construct Approaches to Practice and Research.* London: Whurr.

Porter, R (1987) *A Social History of Madness: Stories of the Insane.* London: Weidenfeld and Nicolson.

Porter, R (2004) 'Is mental illness inevitably stigmatising?' in Crisp, A (ed.) *Every Family in the Land.* London: Royal Society of Medicine Press Ltd.

Porter, S (1993) 'The determinants of psychiatric nursing practice: a comparison of sociological perspectives' *Journal of Advanced Nursing* **18**: 1559–1566.

Poster, EC and Ryan, J (1994) 'A multiregional study of nurses' beliefs and attitudes about work safety and patient assault' *Hospital and Community Psychiatry* **45**: 1104–1108.

Potts, MK, Burnam, MA and Wells, KB (1991) 'Gender differences in depression detection: a comparison of clinician diagnosis and standardised assessment' *Psychological Assessment* **3**: 609–615.

Powell, G, Caan, W and Crowe, M (1994) 'What events precede violent incidents in psychiatric hospitals?' *British Journal of Psychiatry* **165**: 107–112.

Primhe *et al.* (2005) *Running on Empty: Building Momentum to Improve Well-Being in Severe Mental Illness.* London: Sane. Available at: http://www.sane.org.uk/public_html/News/pdfs/RoE_Report_FINAL.pdf

Prins, H (Chair) (1993) *Report of the Committee of Inquiry into the Death in Broadmoor Hospital of Orville Blackwood and a Review of the Deaths of Two Other Afro-Caribbean Patients: 'Big Black and Dangerous?'* London: Special Hospitals Service Authority.

Prins, HA (1981) 'Dangerous people or dangerous situations? Some implications for assessment and management' *Medicine, Science and the Law* **21**: 125–133.

Prior, L (1993) *The Social Organization of Mental Illness.* London: Sage.

Punamaki, RL (1994) 'Self care and mastery among primary health care patients' *Social Science and Medicine* **39**(5): 733–741.

Rafferty, AM, Ball, J and Aitken, LH (2001) 'Are teamwork and professional autonomy compatible, and do they result in improved hospital care?' *Quality in Health Care* **10**(Suppl. 2): ii32–ii37.

Rasul, F, Stansfield, SA and Davey-Smith, G (2001) 'Sociodemographic factors, smoking and common mental disorder in the Renfrew and Paisley (MIDSPAN) study' *Journal of Health Psychology* **6**: 149–158.

Rawlinson, J (1995) 'Some reflections of the use of repertory grid technique in studies of nurses and social workers' *Journal of Advanced Nursing* **21**: 334–339.

Redelmeier, DA, Tan, SH and Booth, GL (1998) 'The treatment of unrelated disorders in patients with chronic medical diseases' *New England Journal of Medicine* **338**: 1516–1520.

Redman, BK (2005) 'The ethics of self-management preparation for chronic illness' *Nursing Ethics* **12**(4): 360–369.

Redman, BK and Fry, ST (2000) 'Nurses' ethical conflicts: what is really known about them?' *Nursing Ethics* **7**: 360–366.

Reed, P and Leonard, V (1989) 'An analysis of the concept of self neglect' *Advances in Nursing Science* **12**(1): 39–53.

Rees, J (2000) 'Food for thought: the canteen of a mental hospital' in Hinshelwood, RD and Skogstad, W (eds) *Observing Organisations: Anxiety, Defence and Culture in Health Care*. London: Routledge.

Reisner, AD (2005) 'The common factors, empirically validated treatments, and recovery models of therapeutic change' *The Psychological Record* **55**: 377–399.

Reith, M (1998) *Community Care Tragedies*. Birmingham: Venture Press.

Repper, J (2000a) 'Adjusting the focus of mental health nursing: incorporating service users' experiences of recovery' *Journal of Mental Health* **9**: 575–587.

Repper, J (2000b) 'Social inclusion' in Thompson, T and Mathias, P (eds) *Lyttle's Mental Health and Disorder*. London: Elsevier.

Repper, J (2006) 'Viewpoint' *Mental Health Today* **Feb**: 37.

Repper, J and Perkins, R (2003) *Social Inclusion and Recovery: A Model for Mental Health Practice*. London: Bailliere Tindall.

Rethink (2003) *Schizophrenia: The Experiences and Views of Self-Management of People with a Diagnosis of Schizophrenia* [on-line]. Available at: http://www.rethink.org/living_with_mental_illness/recovery_and_self_management/selfmanagement/index.html

Rethink (2005a) *A Report on the Work of the Recovery Learning Sites and Other Recovery-Orientated Activities and its Incorporation into the Rethink Plan 2004–08* [on-line]. Available at: http://www.rethink.org/living_with_mental_illness/recovery_and_self_management/recovery/index.html

Rethink (2005b) *Future Perfect*. Available at: http://www.rethink.org/how_we_can_help/news_and_media/press_releases/future_perfect.html

Rethink (2006) *You and Media*. Available at: http://www.rethink.org/how_we_can_help/news_and_media/press_releases/you_and_media.html

Rew, L (1988) 'Intuition in decision-making' *IMAGE: Journal of Nursing Scholarship* **20**(3): 150–154.

Rew, L and Barrow, E (1987) 'Intuition: a neglected hallmark of nursing knowledge' *Advances in Nursing Science* **10**(1): 49–62.

Rew, L and Barrow, EM (1987) 'Intuition: a neglected hallmark of nursing knowledge' *Advanced Nursing Science* **10**: 49–62.

Reyes-Ortiz, C (2001) 'Diogenes syndrome: the self-neglect elderly' *Comprehensive Therapy* **27**: 117–121.

Reynolds, W and Scott, B (2000) 'Do nurses and other professional helpers normally display much empathy?' *Journal of Advanced Nursing* **31**(1): 226–234.

Rhodes, LA (2004) *Total Confinement: Madness and Reason in the Maximum Security Prison*. Berkeley, CA: University of California Press.

Ribbens McCarthy, J (2006) *Young People's Experiences of Loss and Bereavement: Towards an Interdisciplinary Approach*. Maidenhead: Open University Press.

Ribbens McCarthy, J with Jessop, J (2005) *Young People, Bereavement and Loss, Disruptive Transitions*. York: Joseph Rowntree Foundation/National Children's Bureau.

Richards, D (2004) 'Self help: empowering service users or aiding cash strapped mental health services?' *Journal of Mental Health* **13**(2): 117–123.

Richter, D and Berger, K (2006) 'Post-traumatic stress disorder following patient assaults among staff members of mental health hospitals: a prospective longitudinal study' *BMC Psychiatry* **6**: 15.

Ricketts, T (1996) 'General satisfaction and satisfaction with nursing communication on an adult psychiatric ward' *Journal of Advanced Nursing* **24**(3): 479–487.

Rinaldi, M, McNeil, K, Firn, M, Koletsi, M, Perkins, R and Singh, SP (2004) 'What are the benefits of evidence-based supported employment for patients with first episode psychosis?' *Psychiatric Bulletin* **28**: 281–284.

Rinder, EC (2000) 'Combined group process–psychoeducation model for psychiatric clients and their families' *Journal of Psychosocial Nursing and Mental Health Services* **38**(9): 34–41.

Ritchie, JH (Chair), Dick, D and Lingham, R (1994) *The Report of the Inquiry into the Care and Treatment of Christopher Clunis*. London: HMSO.

Ritchie, S (1985) *Report to the Secretary of State for Social Services Concerning the Death of Mr Michael Martin*. London: SHSA.

Robbins, H and Finley, M (2000) *Why Teams Don't Work: What Went Wrong and How to Make it Right*. London: Texere.

Roberts, M (2005) 'The production of the psychiatric subject: power, knowledge and Michel Foucault' *Nursing Philosophy* **6**: 33–42.

Roberts, VZ (1994) 'The organisation of work: contributions from open systems theory' in Obholzer, A and Roberts, V (eds) *The Unconscious at Work: Individual and Organisational Stress in the Human Services*. London: Routledge.

Robertson, A (1998) 'The mental health experience of gay men: a research study exploring gay men's health needs' *Journal of Psychiatric and Mental Health Nursing* **5**: 33–40.

Robins, LN, Locke, BZ and Regier, DA (1991) *An Overview of Psychiatric Disorders in America*. New York: Free Press.

Robson, D and Gray, R (2005) 'Can we help people with schizophrenia stop smoking?' *Mental Health Practice* **9**(4): 14–18.

Robson, D and Gray, R (2007) 'Serious mental illness and physical health problems: a discussion paper' *International Journal of Nursing Studies* **44**: 457–466.

Robson, D, Wix, S and Gray, R (2005) 'Treatment planning, medication management and the forensic multidisciplinary team' in Wix, S and Humphries, M (2005) *Multidisciplinary Working in Forensic Mental Health Care*. London: Churchill Livingstone.

Roe, D, Chopra, M, Wagner, B, Katz, G and Rudnick, A (2004) 'The emerging self in conceptualizing and treating mental illness' *Journal of Psychosocial Nursing* **42**: 32–40.

Rogers, A and Pilgrim, D (2001) *Mental Health Policy in Britain*, 2nd edn. Basingstoke: Palgrave.

Rogers, A, Kennedy, A, Nelson, E and Robinson, A (2005) 'Uncovering the limits of patient-centeredness: implementing a self-management trial for chronic illness' *Qualitative Health Research* **15**(2): 224–239.

Rogers, C (1951) *Client-Centred Therapy: Its Current Practice, Implications and Theory*. Boston: Houghton Mifflin.

Rogers, P, Ghroum, P, Benson, R, Forward, L and Gournay, K (2006) 'Is breakaway training effective? An audit of one medium secure unit' *The Journal of Forensic Psychiatry and Psychology* **17**(4): 593–602.

Rolfe, G (1998) 'The marriage of heaven and hell: further remarks on the future of mental health nursing' *Journal of Psychiatric and Mental Health Nursing* **5**: 230–233.

Rolfe, G and Gardner, L (2006) 'Education, philosophy and academic practice: nursing studies in the posthistorical university' *Nurse Education in Practice* **6**(6): 326–331.

Rollnick, S, Mason, P and Butler, C (1999) *Health Behaviour Change: A Guide for Practitioners.* Edinburgh: Churchill Livingstone.

Rolls, L and Payne, S (2004) 'Child bereavement services: issues in UK service provision' *Mortality* **9**(4): 300–328.

Romanoff, BD (2001) 'Research as therapy: the power of narrative to effect change' in Neimeyer, RA (ed.) *Meaning Reconstruction and the Experience of Loss.* Washington, DC: American Psychological Association.

Rooney, C and Devis, T (1999) 'Recent trends in deaths from homicide in England and Wales' *Health Statistics Quarterly* **3**: 5–13. Available at: http://www.statistics.gov.uk/CCI/article.asp?ID=1216&Pos=2&ColRank=1&Rank224

Rose, D (2000) *User's Voices.* London: Sainsbury Centre for Mental Health.

Rose, D (2001) *Users' Voices: Perspectives of Mental Health Service Users on Community and Hospital Care.* London: Sainsbury Centre for Mental Health.

Rose, S, Bisson, J and Wessely, S (2004) 'Psychological debriefing for preventing post traumatic stress disorder (PTSD)' *The Cochrane Library, Issue 1.* Chichester: John Wiley & Sons.

Rosenstock, IM (1974) 'The health belief model and preventive health behaviour' *Health Education Monographs* **2**: 354–386.

Rosenthal, M, Stelian, J, Wagner, J and Berkman, P (1999) 'Diogenes syndrome and hoarding in the elderly: case reports' *The Israel Journal of Psychiatry and Related Sciences* **36**(1): 29–34.

Rowe, D (1996) 'The importance of personal construct psychology' in Walker, B, Costigan, J, Viney, L and Warren, B (eds) *Personal Construct Theory: A Psychology for the Future.* Melbourne: Australian Psychological Society.

Rowe, D (2006) 'What should mental health nurses do?' *Openmind* **Sept/Oct**: 141.

Rowe, R and Shepherd, M (2002) 'Public participation in the New NHS: no closer to citizen control?' *Social Policy and Administration* **36**(3): 270–290.

Rowley, J and Slack, F (2004) 'Conducting a literature review' *Management Research* **27**(6): 31–39.

Rowling, L (2003) *Grief in School Communities: Effective Support Strategies.* Buckingham: Open University Press.

Royal College of General Practitioners and Royal College of Nursing (2002) *Getting it Right for Teenagers in your Practice.* London: Department of Health.

Royal College of Nursing (RCN) (1999) *The Royal College of Nursing Mental Health Nursing Strategy.* London: RCN.

Royal College of Nursing (RCN) (2003) *Defining Nursing.* London: RCN.

Royal College of Paediatrics and Child Health (2003) *Bridging the Gaps: Health Care for Adolescents.* London: Royal College of Paediatrics and Child Health. Available at: http://www.rcpsych.ac.uk/files/pdfversion/cr114.pdf

Royal College of Psychiatrists (1993) *Consensus Statement on the Use of High Dose Antipsychotic Medication. Council Report CR 26.* London: Royal College of Psychiatrists.

Royal College of Psychiatrists (1995) *Strategies for the Management of Disturbed and Violent Patients in Psychiatric Units. Council Report CR 41.* London: Royal College of Psychiatrists.

Royal College of Psychiatrists (1997) *The Association between Antipsychotic Drugs and Sudden Death. Council Report CR 57.* London: Royal College of Psychiatrists.

Royal College of Psychiatrists (1998) *Management of Imminent Violence: Clinical Practice Guidelines to Support Mental Health Services.* London: Royal College of Psychiatrists.

Royal College of Psychiatrists (2000) *Anti-stigma Video.* GP Roadshow.

Royal Pharmaceutical Society of Great Britain (1997) *From Compliance to Concordance: Achieving Shared Goals in Medicine Taking.* London: Royal Pharmaceutical Society of Great Britain.

Royo, E and Món-Catalunya, M (2002) *International Forum on Gender, Humanitarian Action and Development Working Group: Gender and Masculinity.* Available at: http://www.europrofem. org/contri/2_04_en/en-masc/56en_mas.htm

Rozanski, A, Blumenthal, JA and Davidson, KW *et al.* (2005) 'The epidemiology, pathophysiology, and management of psychosocial risk factors in cardiac practice: the emerging field of behavioral cardiology' *Journal of the American College of Cardiology* **45**(5): 637–651.

Rozanski, A, Blumenthal, JA and Kaplan, J (1999) 'Impact of psychosocial factors on the pathogenesis of cardiovascular disease and implications for therapy' *Circulation* **99**: 2192–2217.

Rungapadiachy, D, Madill, A and Gough, B (2004) 'Mental health student nurses' perception of the role of the mental health nurse' *Journal of Psychiatric and Mental Health Nursing* **11**(6): 714–724.

Rusch, N and Corrigan, PW (2002) 'Motivational interviewing to improve insight and treatment adherence in schizophrenia' *Psychiatric Rehabilitation Journal* **26**(1): 23–32.

Ruschena, D, Mullen, PE, Burgess, P, Cordner, SM, Barry-Walsh, J and Drummer, OH (1998) 'Sudden death in psychiatric patients' *British Journal of Psychiatry* **172**: 331–336.

Ryan, MCM, Collins, P and Thakore, JH (2003) 'Impaired fasting glucose tolerance in first episode, drug naïve patients with schizophrenia' *American Journal of Psychiatry* **159**: 561–566.

Ryan, T (1998) 'Do you see what I see?' *OpenMind* **Nov/Dec**: 94.

Rydon, S (2005) 'The attitudes, knowledge and skills needed in mental health nurses: the perspective of users of mental health services' *International Journal of Mental Health Nursing* **14**: 78–87.

Ryrie, I, Agunbiade, D and Maris-Shaw, A (1998) 'A survey of psychiatric nursing practice in two inner city acute admission wards' *Journal of Advanced Nursing* **27**: 848–854.

Sabatini, MM (1998) 'Health care ethics: models of the provider–patient relationship' *Dermatology Nursing* **10**(3): 201–205.

Sabo, B (2006) 'Compassion fatigue and nursing work: can we accurately capture the consequences of caring work?' *International Journal of Nursing Practice* **12**(3): 136–142.

Sackett, DL, Rosenberg, WMC, Gray, JAM, Haynes, RB and Richardson, WS (1996) 'Evidence based medicine: what it is and what it isn't: it's about integrating individual clinical expertise and the best external evidence' *British Medical Journal* **312**: 71–72.

Sackett, DL, Straus, SE, Scott Richardson, W, Rosenberg, W and Haynes, RB (2000) *Evidence-Based Medicine: How to Practice and Teach EBM*, 2nd edn. Edinburgh: Churchill Livingstone.

Sadava, S (2001) 'Book review: Richard Sorrentino and Christopher Roney, The Uncertain Mind: Individual Differences in Facing the Unknown' *Canadian Psychology* **42**(4): 333–335.

Sainsbury Centre for Mental Health (SCMH) (1997) *Pulling Together: The Future Roles and Training of Mental Health Staff.* Available at: http://www.scmh.org.uk/80256FBD004F6342/ vWeb/pcPCHN6FTHWE

Sainsbury Centre for Mental Health (SCMH) (1998) *Acute Problems: A Survey of the Quality of Care in Acute Psychiatric Wards.* London: Sainsbury Centre for Mental Health.

Sainsbury Centre for Mental Health (SCMH) (2001a) *The Capable Practitioner.* London: SCMH.

Sainsbury Centre for Mental Health (SCMH) (2001b) *Mental Health Topics: Crisis Resolution.* Available at: http://www.scmh.org.uk/80256FBD004F3555/vWeb/flKHAL6RCJK2/$File/ Crisis_Resolution_MH_Topics.pdf

Sainsbury Centre for Mental Health (SCMH) (2002) *Breaking the Circles of Fear: A Review of the Relationship between Mental Health Services and African and Caribbean Communities.* London: SCMH.

Sainsbury Centre for Mental Health (SCMH) (2003) *Primary Solutions: An Independent Policy Review on the Development of Primary Care Mental Health Services* London: SCMH

Sainsbury Centre for Mental Health (SCMH) (2005) *Acute Care 2004: A National Survey of Adult Psychiatric Wards in England.* London: SCMH.

Salloum, A (2004) *Group Work with Adolescents after Violent Death: A Manual for Practitioners.* New York: Brunner-Routledge.

Sartorius, N (2002) 'Iatrogenic stigma of mental illness' *British Medical Journal* **324**: 1470–1471.

Savage, J (2007) *Teenage: The Creation of Youth 1875–1945.* London: Chatto and Windus.

Sayce, L (1995) 'Response to violence: a framework for fair treatment' in Crichton, J (ed.) *Psychiatric Patient Violence: Risk and Response.* London: Duckworth.

Sayce, L (2000) *From Psychiatric Patient to Citizen.* Basingstoke: Macmillan.

Sayce, L and Owen, J (2006) 'Bridging the gap: results of the DRC's formal investigation into physical health inequalities' *Mental Health Practice* **10**(2): 16–18.

Scherer, RW, Langenberg, P and von Elm, E (2005) 'Full publication of results initially presented in abstracts' *The Cochrane Database of Methodology Reviews* Issue 2, Art. No. MR000005. DOI:10.1002/14651858.MR000005.pub2.

Schön, D (1991) *The Reflective Practitioner: How Professionals Think in Action.* London: Ashgate Publishing.

Schwandt, TA (2001) *Dictionary of Qualitative Inquiry*, 2nd edn. Thousand Oaks: Sage.

Scott, P (2004) 'Commentary. The contribution of universities to the development of the nursing workforce and the quality of patient care' *Journal of Nursing Management* **12**: 393–396.

Scottish Association for Mental Health (SAMH) (2004) *'All you need to know?' Scottish Survey of People's Experience of Psychiatric Drugs.* Glasgow: Scottish Association for Mental Health.

Scourfield, J (2005) 'Suicidal masculinities' *Sociological Research Online* **10**(2). Available at: http://www.socresonline.org.uk/10/2/scourfield.html

Scraton, P and Chadwick, K (1987) ' "Speaking ill of the dead": institutionalized responses to deaths in custody' in Scraton, P (ed.) *Law, Order and the Authoritarian State.* Milton Keynes: Open University Press.

Scull, A (1981) *Madhouses, Mad-doctors and Madmen.* Athlone Press: London.

Scull, A (1993) *The Most Solitary of Afflictions: Madness and Society in Britain 1700–1900.* London: Yale University Press.

Scull, AT (1979) *Museums of Madness: The Social Organisation of Insanity in Nineteenth Century England.* London: Allen Lane.

Sequeira, H and Halstead, S (2002) 'Control and restraint in the UK: service user perspectives' *The British Journal of Forensic Practice* **4**(1): 9–18.

Sequeira, H and Halstead, S (2004) 'The psychological effects on nursing staff of administering physical restraint in a secure psychiatric hospital: "When I go home, it's then that I think about it" ' *British Journal of Forensic Practice* **6**(1): 3–15.

Sethi, D, Marais, S, Nurse, J and Burchart, A (2004) *Handbook of Interpersonal Violence Prevention Programmes.* Geneva: Department of Injuries and Violence Prevention, World Health Organisation.

Seymour, L (2003) *Not All in the Mind: The Physical Health of Mental Health Service Users.* Available at: http://www.scmh.org.uk/80256FBD004F3555/vWeb/flKHAL6PQLA9/$file/not+all+in+the+mind.pdf

Sharpe, S, Ribbens McCarthy, J and Jessop, J (2005) 'Young people's experiences of bereavement' in Ribbens McCarthy, J with Jessop, J (eds) *Young People, Bereavement and Loss: Disruptive Transitions.* York: Joseph Rowntree Foundation/National Children's Bureau.

Sharpe, S, Ribbens McCarthy, J and Jessop, J (2006) 'The perspectives of young people' in Ribbens McCarthy, J (ed.) *Young People's Experiences of Loss and Bereavement: Towards an Interdisciplinary Approach.* Maidenhead: Open University Press.

Shattell, M, McAllister, S, Hogan, B and Thomas, S (2006) '"She took the time to make sure she understood": Mental health patients' experiences of being understood' *Archives of Psychiatric Nursing* **20**(5): 234–241.

Shaw, C (1999) 'A framework for the study of coping, illness behaviour and outcomes' *Journal of Advanced Nursing* **29**(5): 1246–1255.

Sheild, H, Fairbrother, G and Obmann, H (2005) 'Sexual health knowledge and risk behaviour in young people with first episode psychosis' *International Journal of Mental Health Nursing* **14**: 149–154.

Sheppard, D (1996) *Learning the Lessons,* 2nd edn. London: The Zito Trust.

Sheridan, M, Henrion, R and Robinson, L *et al.* (1990) 'Precipitants of violence in a psychiatric in-patient setting' *Hospital and Community Psychiatry* **41**(7): 776–780.

Siddle, BK (1995) *Sharpening the Warrior's Edge: The Psychology & Science of Training.* Millstadt, IL: PPCT Research Publications.

SIGN (2001) *SIGN 50 A Guideline Developers Handbook.* Available at: http://www.sign.ac.uk/guidelines/fulltext/50/index.html

Sim, J (2004) 'The victimised state and the mystification of social harm' in Hillyard, P, Pantazis, C, Tombs, S and Gordon, D (eds) *Beyond Criminology: Taking Harm Seriously.* London: Pluto.

Simpson, EL and House, AO (2003) 'User and carer involvement in mental health services: from rhetoric to science' *British Journal of Psychiatry* **183**: 89–91.

Sirey, JA, Bruce, ML, Alexopoulos, GS, Perlick, DA, Friedman, SJ and Meyers, BS (2001) 'Perceived stigma and patient-rated severity of illness as predictors of antidepressant drug adherence' *Psychiatric Services* **52**: 1615–1620.

Skärsäter, I, Langius, A, Ågren, H, Häggström, L and Dencker, K (2005) 'Sense of coherence and social support in relation to recovery in first-episode patients with major depression: a one-year prospective study' *International Journal of Mental Health Nursing* **14**: 258–264.

Skills for Health (2005a) *MH30: Enable Individuals to Obtain and Maintain Household and Personal Goods* [on-line]. Available at: www.skillsforhealth.org.uk

Skills for Health (2005b) *MH32: Enable Individuals to Maintain their Personal Hygiene and Appearance* [on-line]. Available at: www.skillsforhealth.org.uk

Skolnick, JH and Fyfe, JJ (1993) *Above the Law: Police and the Excessive Use of Force.* New York: Free Press.

Slade, M, Thornicroft, G, Loftus, L, Phelan, M and Wykes, T (1999) *CAN: Camberwell Assessment of Need.* London: Gaskell.

Smith, G, Bartlett, A and King, M (2004) 'Treatments of homosexuality in Britain since the 1950's – an oral history: the experience of patients' *British Medical Journal* **328**: 427–429.

Smith, H and Brown, H (1992) 'Defending community care: can normalisation do the job?' *British Journal of Social Work* **22**(6): 685–693.

Snowden, LR and Wu, TW (1997) 'Ethnic differences in mental health services use among severely mentally ill' *Journal of Community Psychology* **25**: 235–247.

Social Exclusion Unit (2004a) *Mental Health and Social Exclusion.* London: Office of the Deputy Prime Minister.

Social Exclusion Unit (2004b) *Breaking the Cycle, Taking Stock of Progress and Priorities for the Future*. London: Social Exclusion Unit. Available at: http://archive.cabinetoffice.gov.uk/seu/docs/bc_takingstock.pdf

Social Services Inspectorate (2002) *Modernising Mental Health Services: Inspection of Mental Health Services*. London: Department of Health.

Sorrentino, R and Roney, C (2000) *The Uncertain Mind: Individual Differences in Facing the Unknown*. Hove: Psychology Press.

Soulliere, D (2005) 'Masculinity on display in the squared circle: constructing masculinity in professional wrestling' *Electronic Journal of Sociology*. Available at: http://www.sociology.org/content/2005/tier1/soulliere.html

Space, LG, Dingemans, P and Cromwell, RL (1983) 'Self-construing and alienation in depressives, schizophrenics and normals' in Adams-Webber, J and Mancuso, JC (eds) *Applications of Personal Construct Theory*. Ontario: Academic Press.

Sparks, R (1996) 'Masculinity and heroism in the Hollywood blockbuster' *British Journal of Criminology* **36**: 348–360.

Sperry, L (2003) *Handbook of Diagnosis and Treatment of DSM-IV Personality Disorders*, 2nd edn. New York: Brunner-Routledge.

Standing Nursing and Midwifery Committee (SNMAC) (1999) *Mental Health Nursing: 'Addressing Acute Concerns'* [on-line]. Available at: http://www.advisorybodies.doh.gov.uk/snmac/snmacmh.pdf

Stanton, AH and Schwartz, MS (1954) *The Mental Hospital: A Study of Institutional Participation in Psychiatric Illness and Treatment*. New York: Basic Books.

Stark, C, Paterson, B and Devlin, B (2004) 'Newspaper coverage of a violent assault by a mentally ill person' *Journal of Psychiatric and Mental Health Nursing* **11**: 635–643.

Steadman, H, Monahan, J, Robbins, P, Appelbaum, P, Grisso, T, Mulvey, E, Roth, P, Robbins, P and Klassen, D (1994) 'Designing a new generation of risk assessment research' in Monahan, J and Steadman, H (eds) *Violence and Mental Disorder: Developments in Risk Assessment*. Chicago: University of Chicago Press.

Stein, H, Allen, JG and Hill, J (2003) 'Roles and relationships: a psychoeducational approach to reviewing strengths and difficulties in adult functioning' *Bulletin of the Menninger Clinic* **67**(4): 281–313.

Steinberg, L (2002) *Adolescence*, 6th edn. Boston: McGraw-Hill.

Stephen, H (1998) 'Yellow card for violent patients' *Nursing Standard* **12**(52): 14.

Stevenson, C, Barker, P and Fletcher, E (2002) 'Judgement days: developing an evaluation for an innovative nursing model' *Journal of Psychiatric and Mental Health Nursing* **9**: 271–276.

Stokes, J and Crossley, D (1995) 'Camp Winston: a residential intervention for bereaved children' in Smith, SC and Pennells, M (eds) *Interventions with Bereaved Children*. London: Jessica Kingsley.

Stokes, J, Pennington, J, Monroe, B, Papadatou, D and Relf, M (1999) 'Developing services for bereaved children: a discussion of the theoretical and practical issues involved' *Mortality* **4**(3): 291–309.

Stokes, J, Wyer, S and Crossley, D (1997) 'The challenge of evaluating a child bereavement programme' *Palliative Medicine* **11**: 179–190.

Stonewall Scotland (2003) *Towards a Healthier LGBT Scotland*. Available at: http://www.lgbthealthscotland.org.uk/documents/Towards_Healthier_LGBT_Scot.pdf

Stover, E and Nightingale, EO (eds) (1985) *The Breaking of Bodies and Minds: Torture, Psychiatric Abuse and the Health Professions*. New York: WH Freeman and Co.

Stroebe, MS and Schut, H (2001) 'Meaning making in the dual process model of coping with bereavement' in Neimeyer, RA (ed.) *Meaning Reconstruction and the Experience of Loss*. Washington, DC: American Psychological Association.

Stroebe, MS, Hansson, RO, Stroebe, W and Schut, H (2001a) 'Introduction: concepts and issues in contemporary research on bereavement' in Stroebe, MS, Hansson, RO, Stroebe, W and Schut, H (eds) *Handbook of Bereavement Research, Consequences, Coping and Care.* Washington, DC: American Psychological Association.

Stroebe, MS, Hansson, RO, Stroebe, W and Schut, H (eds) (2001) *Handbook of Bereavement Research, Consequences, Coping and Care.* Washington, DC: American Psychological Association.

Stromwall, LK and Hurdle, D (2003) 'Psychiatric rehabilitation: an empowerment-based approach to mental health services' *Health and Social Work* **28**: 206–213.

Stroup, TS (2004) 'Antipsychotic drug treatment of schizophrenia: update on the CATIE trial' in *NCDEU Abstracts from the 44th Annual Meeting, June 1–4, Phoenix, AZ.* Bethesda, MD: Department of Health and Human Sciences, National Institutes of Health, National Institute of Mental Health.

Stuart, G (2001) 'Evidence-based psychiatric nursing: rhetoric or reality?' *Journal of the American Psychiatric Nurses Association* **7**(4): 103–114.

Stubbs, J and Gardner, L (2004) 'Survey of staff attitudes to smoking in a large psychiatric hospital' *Psychiatric Bulletin* **28**: 204–207.

Sullivan, P (1998) 'Therapeutic interaction and mental health nursing' *Nursing Standard* **12**: 39–42.

Swinton, J and Boyd, J (2000) 'Autonomy and parenthood: the forensic nurse as a moral agent' in Robinson, D and Kettles, A (eds) *Forensic Nursing and Multidisciplinary Care of the Mentally Disordered Offender.* London: Jessica Kingsley.

Symonds, B (1995) 'The origins of insane asylums in England during the 19th century: a brief sociological review' *Journal of Advanced Nursing* **22**: 94–100.

Tarbuck, P, Eaton, Y, McAuliffe, J, Ruane, M and Thorpe, B (1999) 'Care and responsibility training: survey of skills retention and diminution' in Tarbuck, P, Topping-Morris, B and Burnard, P (eds) *Forensic Mental Health Nursing: Strategy and Implementation.* London: Whurr.

Tardiff, K (1988) 'Management of violent patient in an emergency situation' *Psychiatric Clinics of North America* **11**: 539–549.

Taylor, CA and Sorenson, SB (2002) 'The nature of newspaper coverage of homicide' *Injury Prevention* **8**: 121–127.

Taylor, D (2002) 'Antipsychotic prescribing – time to review practice' Psychiatric Bulletin **26**: 401–402.

Taylor, D, Paton, C and Kerwin, R (2005) *The South London and Maudsley NHS Trust & Oxleas NHS Trust 2005–2006 Prescribing Guidelines*, 8th edn. Abingdon: Taylor & Francis.

Taylor, PJ and Gunn, J (1999) 'Homicides by people with mental illness: myth and reality' *British Journal of Psychiatry* **174**(1): 9–14.

Taylor-Piliae, R and Molassiotis, A (2001) 'An exploration of the relationship between uncertainty, psychological distress and type of coping strategy among Chinese men after cardiac catheterisation' *Journal of Advanced Nursing* **33**(1): 79–88.

Teagarden, JR (1989) 'Meta-analysis: whither narrative review?' *Pharmacotherapy* **9**: 274–284.

The United Kingdom Parliament (2004) *Lord Hansard Written Answers 16 January 2004.* Available at: http://www.publications.parliament.uk/pa/ld200304/ldhansrd/vo040116/text/40116w01.htm#40116w01_wqn5

Thomas, P (2006a) 'General medical practitioners need to be aware of the theories on which our work depends' *Annals of Family Medicine* **4**(5): 450–454.

Thomas, S (2006b) 'From the editor – Introduction to the guest editors of this special issue on men's mental health' *Issues in Mental Health Nursing* **27**: 331–332.

Thompson, C and Dowding, D (2001) 'Responding to uncertainty in nursing practice' *International Journal of Nursing Studies* **38**: 609–615.

Thompson, D and Watson, R (2001) 'Academic nursing: what is happening to it and where is it going?' *Journal of Advanced Nursing* **36**(1): 1–2.

Thompson, N (ed.) (2002) *Loss and Grief: A Guide for Human Services Practitioners*. Basingstoke: Palgrave.

Thompson, SG (1995) 'Why sources of heterogeneity in meta-analysis should be investigated' in Chalmers, I and Altman, DG (eds) *Systematic Reviews*. London: BMJ Publishing Group.

Thorne, S (2006) 'Patient–provider communication in chronic illness' *Family Community Health* **29**(1S): 4S–11S.

Thorne, S, Jenson, L, Kearney, MH, Noblit, G and Sandelowski, M (2004) 'Qualitative meta-synthesis: reflections on methodological orientation and ideological agenda' *Qualitative Health Research* **14**(10): 1342–1365.

Thornicroft, G (2006) 'Tackling discrimination' *Mental Health Today* **Jun**: 26–29.

Thornicroft, G, Rose, D, Huxley, P, Dale, G and Wykes, T (2002) 'What are the research priorities of mental health service users?' *Journal of Mental Health* **11**: 1–5.

Thornton, A and Lee, P (2000) 'Publication bias in meta-analysis: its causes and consequences' *Journal of Clinical Epidemiology* **53**: 207–216.

Thyer, G (2003) 'Dare to be different: transformational leadership may hold the key to reducing the nursing shortage' *Journal of Nursing Management* **11**: 73–79.

Tierney, M, Charles, J, Naglie, G, Jaglal, S, Kiss, A and Fisher, R (2004) 'Risk factors for harm in cognitively impaired seniors who live alone: a prospective study' *Journal of the American Geriatrics Society* **52**(9): 1435–1441.

Tolmunen, T, Voutilainen, S, Hintikka, J, Rissanen, T, Tanskanen, A, Viinamäki, H, Kaplan, GA and Salonen, JT (2003) 'Association of dietary folate and depressive symptoms are associated in middle-aged Finnish men' *Journal of Nutrition* **133**: 3233–3236.

Took, M (2002) 'Mental breakdown and recovery in the UK' *Journal of Psychiatric and Mental Health Nursing* **9**: 635–637.

Towell, D (1975) *Understanding Psychiatric Nursing: A Sociological Study of Modern Psychiatric Nursing Practice*. London: RCN.

Townsend, PN, Davidson, N and Whitehead, M (1988) *Inequalities in Health*. London: Penguin.

Toynbee, P (2006) 'Compassionate conservatism sounds uncannily familiar' *The Guardian*, 13 June, 29.

Trenoweth, S (2003) 'Perceiving risk in dangerous situations' *Journal of Advanced Nursing* **42**(3): 278–287.

Truax, C and Mitchell, K (1971) 'Research on certain therapist interpersonal skills in relation to process and outcome' in Garfield, SL and Bergin, A (eds) *Handbook of Psychotherapy and Behaviour Change*. Chichester: John Wiley & Sons.

Tuck, I (1997) 'The cultural context of mental health nursing' *Issues in Mental Health Nursing* **18**: 269–281.

Tusaie, K (2004) 'Resilience: a historical review of the construct' *Holistic Nursing Practice* **Jan/Feb**: 3–8.

Tversky, A and Kahneman, D (1974) 'Judgment under uncertainty: heuristics and biases' *Science* **185**: 1124–1131.

Ungvari, G and Hantz, P (1991) 'Social breakdown in the elderly: I. Care studies and management' *Comprehensive Psychiatry* **32**: 440–444.

UNICEF (2007) *HIV/AIDS and Children*. Available at: http://www.unicef.org/aids/index_orphans.html

United Kingdom Central Council for Nursing, Midwifery and Health Visiting (UKCC) (1998) *Guidelines for Mental Health and Learning Disabilities Nursing: A Guide to Working with Vulnerable Clients*. London: UKCC. Available at: http://www.nmc-uk.org/aFrameDisplay.aspx?DocumentID=521

United Kingdom Central Council for Nursing, Midwifery and Health Visiting (UKCC) (2002) *The Recognition, Prevention and Therapeutic Management of Violence in Mental Health Care* [online]. Available at: http://www.nmcuk.org/aFrameDisplay.aspx?DocumentID=663

United States Department of Health and Human Sciences (2007) *Pediatric Terrorism and Disaster Preparedness: A Resource for Pediatricians*. Available at: http://www.ahrq.gov/research/pedprep/resource.htm

University of Manchester (2006) *National Confidential Inquiry into Suicide and Homicide by People with Mental Illness: Avoidable Deaths*. Available at: http://www.medicine.manchester.ac.uk/suicideprevention/nci/Useful/avoidable_deaths.pdf

University of Melbourne (2005) *Conducting a Literature Review. University of Melbourne Getting Started Guides*. Available at: http://www.lib.unimelb.edu.au/postgrad/litreview/getting-started.html

Van Deusen, KM and Carr, JL (2004) 'Group work at the university: a psychoeducational sexual assault group for women' *Social Work with Groups* **27**(4): 51–63.

Vaughan, K and McConaghy, N (2004) 'Megavitamin and dietary treatment in schizophrenia: a randomised, controlled trial' *Australian and New Zealand Journal of Psychiatry* **33**: 84–86.

Vere-Jones, E (2007) 'What's happened to the mental health nursing review?' *Nursing Times* **103**(15): 14–16.

Vick, N, Birke, S and McKenzie, R (2002) 'Risk assessment and the Care Programme Approach: an independent sector initiative' *British Journal of Forensic Practice* **4**(2): 11–18.

Villegas, M, Feixas, G and Lopez, N (1986) 'Phenomenological analysis of autobiographical texts: a design based on personal construct psychology' *Phenomenological Inquiry* **10**: 43–59.

Vinestock, M (1996) 'Risk assessment: "a word to the wise?"' *Archives in Psychiatric Treatment* **2**: 3–10.

Viney, LL (1987) *Interpreting the Interpreters*. Malabar, FL: Krieger Publishing Co.

Viney, LL and Westbrook, MT (1976) 'Cognitive anxiety: a method of content analysis for verbal samples' *Journal of Personality Assessment* **40**(2): 140–150.

Vose, CP (2000) 'Drug abuse and mental illness: psychiatry's next challenge!' in Thompson, PL and Mathias, P (eds) *Lyttle's Mental Health and Disorder*. London: Elsevier.

Vostanis, P and Dean, C (1992) 'Self-neglect in adult life' *British Journal of Psychiatry* **161**: 265–267.

Waddington, JL, Youssef, HA and Kinsella, A (1998) 'Mortality in schizophrenia: antipsychotic polypharmacy and absence of adjunctive anti-cholinergics over the course of a 10-year prospective study' *British Journal of Psychiatry* **173**: 325–329.

Wahl, OF (1999) 'Mental health consumers' experience of stigma' *Schizophrenia Bulletin* **25**: 467–478.

Walker, BM (1996) 'A psychology for adventurers: an introduction to personal construct psychology from a social perspective' in Walker, BM and Kalekin-Fishman, D (eds) *The Construction of Group Realities: Culture, Society and Personal Construct Theory*. Malabar, FL: Krieger Publishing Co.

Walker, H and MacAulay, K (2005) 'Assessment of the side effects of antipsychotic medication' *Nursing Standard* **19**(40): 41–46.

Walker, L, Jackson, S and Barker, P (1998) 'Perceptions of the psychiatric nurse's role: a pilot study' *Nursing Standard* **12**(16): 35–38.

Walsh, D and Downe, S (2004) 'Meta-synthesis method for qualitative research: a literature review' *Journal of Advanced Nursing* **50**(2): 204–211.

Walsh, E, Moran, P, Scott, C, McKenzie, K, Burns, T, Creed, F, Tyre, P, Murray, R and Fahy, T (2003) 'Prevalence of violent victimisation in severe mental illness' *British Journal of Psychiatry* **183**: 233–238.

Walsh, M (1998) *Models and Critical Pathways in Clinical Nursing: Conceptual Frameworks for Care Planning.* London: Bailliere Tindall.

Walter, G and Rey, JM (1999) 'The relevance of herbal treatments for psychiatric practice' *Australian and New Zealand Journal of Psychiatry* **33**: 482–489.

Walter, T (1999) *On Bereavement: The Culture of Grief.* Buckingham: Open University Press.

Warner, R (1985) *Recovery from Schizophrenia: Psychiatry and Political Economy.* London: Routledge and Kegan Paul.

Watkins, M (2000) 'Competency for nursing practice' *Journal of Clinical Nursing* **9**(3): 338–346.

Watkins, P (2001) *Mental Health Nursing: The Art of Compassionate Care.* Edinburgh: Butterworth-Heinemann.

Watson, R (2006) 'Is there a role for higher education in preparing nurses?' *Nurse Education in Practice* **6**(6): 314–318.

Weaver, ICG, Cervoni, N, Champagne, FA, D'Alessio, AC, Sharma, S, Seckl, JR, Dymov, S, Szyf, M and Meaney, MJ (2004) 'Epigenetic programming by maternal behaviour' *Nature Neuroscience* **7**: 847–854.

Weaver, T, Madden, P, Charles, V, Stimson, G, Renton, A, Tyrer, P, Barnes, T, Bench, C, Middleton, H, Wright, N, Paterson, S, Shanahan, W, Seivewright, N and Ford, C (2003) 'Comorbidity of substance misuse and mental illness in community mental health and substance misuse services' *British Journal of Psychiatry* **183**: 304–313.

Weaver, T, Renton, A, Stimson, G and Tyrer, P (1999) 'Severe mental illness and substance misuse: research is needed to underpin policy and services for patients with comorbidity' *British Medical Journal* **318**: 137–138.

Weed, M (2005) 'Meta interpretation: a method for the interpretive synthesis of qualitative research' *Forum: Qualitative Social Research* **6**(1): Art. 37.

Weeks, J (1991) *Against Nature: Essays on Sexuality, History and Identity.* London: Rivers Oram.

Weidner, G and Cain, V (2006) 'The gender gap in heart disease: lessons from Eastern Europe' *American Journal of Public Health* **93**(5): 768–770.

Wenk, E, Robison, J and Smith, G (1972) 'Can violence be predicted?' *Crime and Delinquency* **12**: 393–402.

Werner, E (1989) 'High risk children in young adulthood: a longitudinal study from birth to 32 years' *American Journal of Orthopsychiatry* **59**: 72–81.

Wertheimer, A (2001) *A Special Scar: The Experiences of People Bereaved by Suicide*, 2nd edn. Hove: Brunner-Routledge.

West, A and West, R (2002) 'Clinical decision-making: coping with uncertainty' *Postgraduate Medical Journal* **78**: 319–321.

Westbrook, MT (1976) 'Positive affect: a method of content analysis for verbal samples' *Journal of Consulting and Clinical Psychology* **44**(5): 715–719.

Westmarland, L (2001) 'Blowing the whistle on police violence: gender, ethnography and ethics' *British Journal of Criminology* **41**: 523–535.

Wetli, CV and Fishbain, DA (1985) 'Cocaine-induced psychosis and sudden death in recreational cocaine users' *Journal of Forensic Sciences* **30**: 873–880.

White, C (2003) 'Doctors fail to grasp concept of concordance' *British Medical Journal* **327**(642): 20.

Whitehead, M (1987) *The Health Divide: Inequalities in Health in the 1980s.* London: Health Education Council.

Whittington, CJ, Kendall, T, Fonagy, P, Cottrell, D, Cotgrove, A and Boddington, E (2004) 'Selective serotonin reuptake inhibitors in childhood depression: systematic review of published versus unpublished data' *The Lancet* **363**(9418): 1341–1345.

Whittington, D and McLaughlin, C (2000) 'Finding time for patients: an exploration of nurses' time allocation in an acute psychiatric setting' *Journal of Psychiatric and Mental Health Nursing* **7**: 259–268.

Whittington, R and Balsamo, D (1998) 'Violence: fear and power' in Mason, T and Mercer, D (eds) *Critical Perspectives in Forensic Care: Inside Out.* Basingstoke: Macmillan.

Whittington, R and Wykes, T (1992) 'Staff strain and social support in a psychiatric hospital following assault by a patient' *Journal of Advanced Nursing* **17**: 480–486.

Whittington, R and Wykes, T (1994) 'Violence in psychiatric hospitals: are certain staff prone to being assaulted?' *Journal of Advanced Nursing* **19**(2): 219–225.

Whittington, R and Wykes, T (1996) 'Aversive stimulation by staff and violence by psychiatric patients' *British Journal of Clinical Psychology* **35**: 11–20.

Wilkinson, RG (1996) *Unhealthy Societies: The Affliction of Inequality.* London: Routledge.

Williams, GC, Freedman, ZR and Deci, EL (1998) 'Supporting autonomy to motivate patients with diabetes for glucose control' *Diabetes Care* **21**: 1644–1651.

Williams, J and Bean, D (1998) 'Coping with loss: the development and evaluation of a children's bereavement project' *Journal of Child Health Care* **2**(2): 58–65.

Williams, JW Jr, Mulrow, CD, Chiquette, E, Hitchcock, N, P'Aguilar, C and Cornell, J (2000) 'A systematic review of newer pharmacotherapies for depression in adults: evidence report summary: clinical guideline, part 2' *Annals of Internal Medicine* **132**: 743–756.

Williams, R (2005) 'Professional capability: evidence- and values-based frameworks for psychiatrists and mental health services' *Current Opinion in Psychiatry* **18**: 361–369.

Willis, B and Gillett, J (2003) *Maintaining Control: An Introduction to the Effective Management of Violence and Aggression.* London: Arnold.

Wilson, C, Nairn, R, Coverdale, J and Panapa, A (1999) 'Constructing mental illness as dangerous: a pilot study' *Australian and New Zealand Journal of Psychiatry* **33**: 240–247.

Wilson, R (2006) 'A place of safety?' *Openmind* **Jul/Aug**: 140.

Wilson, V and Pirrie, A (2000) *Multidisciplinary Teamworking: Beyond the Barriers? A Review of the Issues.* Edinburgh: Scottish Council for Research in Education.

Wilson-Barnett, J (2006) '30th Anniversary Invited Editorial Reflecting on Smith JP (1978) "Higher Education and Nursing"' *Journal of Advanced Nursing* **3**(3): 219–220.

Wimpenny, P (2006) *Literature Review on Bereavement and Bereavement Care, Aberdeen. The Joanna Briggs Collaborating Centre for Evidence-Based Multi-professional Education/Faculty of Health and Social Care Robert Gordon University.* Available at: http://www.rgu.ac.uk/files/Bereavement-Final.pdf

Wing, J and Brown, GW (1970) *Institutionalism and Schizophrenia: A Comparative Study of Three Mental Hospitals.* Cambridge: Cambridge University Press.

Winlow, S (2001) *Badfellas: Crime, Tradition and New Masculinities.* Oxford: Berg.

Winlow, S, Hobbs, D, Lister, S and Hadfield, P (2001) 'Get ready to duck: bouncers and the realities of ethnographic research on violent groups' *British Journal of Criminology* **41**: 536–548.

Winston's Wish (2006) *Family Assessment, Guidelines for Child Bereavement Practitioners.* Cheltenham: Winston's Wish.

Winter, DA (1992) *Personal Construct Psychology in Clinical Practice: Theory, Research and Applications*. London: Routledge.

Winter, R and Maisch, M (1996) *Professional Competence and Higher Education*. Lewes: Falmer Press.

Wolfensberger, W (1972) *The Principles of Normalisation in Human Services*. Toronto: National Institute of Mental Retardation.

Women and Equality Unit (2006) *Getting Equal: Proposals to Outlaw Sexual Orientation Discrimination in the Provision of Goods & Services*. Available at: http://www.womenandequalityunit.gov.uk/publications/sexo_consult_paper.pdf

Woodbridge, K and Fulford, B (2004) *Whose Values? A Workbook for Values-Based Practice in Mental Health Care*. London: Sainsbury Centre for Mental Health.

Woods, P, Reed, V and Robinson, D (1999) 'The behavioural status index: therapeutic risk, insight, communication and social skills' *Journal of Psychiatric and Mental Health Nursing* **6**: 79–90.

Woolf, Lord Justice H and Tumim, S (1991) *Prison Disturbances April, 1990*. London: HMSO Cm.1456.

Worden, WW (1996) *Children and Grief: When a Parent Dies*. New York: The Guilford Press.

Work Group on Palliative Care for Children of the International Work Group on Death, Dying and Bereavement (1999) 'Children, adolescents and death: myths, realities and challenges' *Death Studies* **23**: 443–463.

World Health Organization (1991) *World Health Organization Project on Human Rights*. Available at: http://www.who.int/mental_health/policy/legislation/mental_health_and%20_human_rights_factsheet_may_2006.pdf

World Health Organization (2002a) *Adolescent Friendly Health Services, An Agenda for Change, Geneva, WHO*. Available at: http://www.who.int/child-adolescent-health/publications/ADH/WHO_FCH_CAH_02.14.htm

World Health Organization (2002b) *Gender and Road Traffic Injuries*. Geneva: WHO, Department of Gender and Women's Health.

Wright, S (1999) 'Physical restraint in the management of violence and aggression in in-patient settings: a review of issues' *Journal of Mental Health* **8**(5): 459–472.

Wright, S, Gray, R, Parkes, J and Gournay, K (2002) *The Recognition, Prevention and Therapeutic Management of Violence in Acute In-Patient Psychiatry: A Literature Review and Evidence-Based Recommendations for Good Practice*. London: UKCC.

Young Minds (2006) *A Work in Progress: The Adolescent and Young Adult Brain*. A Briefing Paper. London: Young Minds.

Young, J (1994) *Cognitive Therapy for Personality Disorders: A Schema-focussed Approach*. Sarasota, FL: Professional Resource Exchange.

Young, J (1999) *The Exclusive Society: Social Exclusion, Crime and Difference in Late Modernity*. London: SAGE.

Young, J (2002) 'Crime and social exclusion' in Maguire, M, Morgan, R and Reiner, R (eds) *The Oxford Handbook of Criminology*, 3rd edn. Oxford: Oxford University Press.

Youth Justice Board (2005) *Persistent Young Offenders*. London: Youth Justice Board.

Zabin, LS, Hirsch, MB and Emerson, MR (1989) 'When urban adolescents choose abortion: effects on education, psychological status and subsequent pregnancy' *Family Planning Perspectives* **21**(6): 248–255.

Zeidner, M, Boekaerts, M and Pintrich, PR (2000) 'Self regulation, directions and challenges for future research' in Boekaerts, PR and Zeidner, M (eds) *Handbook of Self Regulation*. London: Academic Press.

Zohar, D and Marshal, I (1994) *The Many Faces of Truth in the Quantum Society.* New York: William Morrow and Co.

Zubin, J and Spring, B (1977) 'Vulnerability: a new view of schizophrenia' *Journal of Abnormal Psychology* **86**: 260–266.

Index

Contemporary Issues in Mental Health Nursing, Edited by J. E. Lynch and S. Trenoweth
© 2008 John Wiley & Sons, Ltd